ILLUSTRATED
DICTIONARY
OF
SPEECH-LANGUAGE
PATHOLOGY

ILLUSTRATED
DICTIONARY
OF
SPEECH-LANGUAGE PATHOLOGY

Sadanand Singh, Ph.D.
San Diego State University

Raymond D. Kent, Ph.D.
University of Wisconsin—Madison

With contributions from
Pam Rider

SINGULAR PUBLISHING GROUP
SAN DIEGO, CALIFORNIA

Singular Publishing Group, Inc.
401 West "A" Street, Suite 325
San Diego, California 92101-7904

Singular Publishing Group, Inc., publishes textbooks, clinical manuals, clinical reference books, journals, videos, and multimedia materials on speech-language pathology, audiology, otorhinolaryngology, special education, early childhood, aging, occupational therapy, physical therapy, rehabilitation, counseling, mental health, and voice. For your convenience, our entire catalog can be accessed on our website at *http://www.singpub.com*. Our mission to provide you with materials to meet the daily challenges of the ever-changing health care/educational environment will remain on course if we are in touch with you. In that spirit, we welcome your feedback on our products. Please telephone (**1-800-521-8545**), fax (**1-800-774-8398**), or e-mail (*singpub@singpub.com*) your comments and requests to us.

Typeset in 9/11 Palatino by So Cal Graphics
Printed in the United States of America by Courier Westford

Library of Congress Cataloging-in-Publication Data Available

ISBN 0-76930-068-5

Contents

Preface

The editors of this dictionary are humbled by the vast expanse of multifaceted disciplines that now constitute Communication Sciences and Disorders. The vast scope and depth with which each aspect of the overall discipline must be delineated in such a dictionary inherently present tough challenges and boundless promises.

Here is a glimpse of the diversity of scope of study in Communication Sciences and Disorders: physics for knowing the nature of sound; anatomy and physiology for knowing the source; neurology to discover the relationship of the central nervous system to normal and disordered speech and language; chemistry to understand the nature of drugs that may influence communication; psychology to relate cognitive, developmental, educational, and social concomitance; sociology to explore facets of community and culture as both cause and effect of communication; anthropology to study important connections across time and space; linguistics as the foundation for formulating the content and structure of communication; and special education for applying communication specialties to improving learning and lifestyle. Besides these inherent dependencies, a significant number of medical specialties, for example, otolaryngology, pulmonology, anesthesiology, and radiology, have formed an inseparable bond with speech-language pathologists who deal with vocal laryngeal pathologies, along with the recent professional expansion into deglutition and swallowing disorders. Interdependence among the medical practices and speech-language pathology has given birth to an exciting new profession of medical speech-language pathology.

Communication Sciences and Disorders draws from each study area and specialty, with every aspect serving as a wellspring or selective source as the field grows and expands to accommodate more medically related disorders. A growing number of specialized functions that reside in "gray" areas have fallen within the scope of clinical responsibility of speech-language pathology. These new growth opportunities bring new challenges for "full" preparedness in training and continuing education. A speech-language pathologist who works predominantly in a medical setting needs to know a large array of terms and definitions, plus their clinical ramifications in treating patients with medically pegged communication disorders within the neurogenic, swallowing, and genetic realms across the spectrum of age—pediatrics through geriatrics.

As measurement techniques and technologies are perfected, the demand to best utilize the tools of the trade also stiffens. Objective measurements are acceptable and desired as part of clinical practice and are clinically feasible. This means we must have definitions of "who we are," "what function we perform," "what we need to know," and "how well can we perform the desired functions." Hence Singular's dictionaries.

The terms that have become part of the Communication Sciences and Disorders curriculum, clinical practice, and research have migrated from the wide variety of powerful disciplines with which we interface, some of which have been enumerated earlier. Although their innate meaning remains constant, the terms must be first and foremost gathered and defined in the context of persons working in the field of communication disorders and also for use by persons in the originating medical and allied fields. Stated plainly, this new home for these terms assumes an interacting environment that generates ongoing evolving perception of the terms. This dictionary, therefore, is not only for the daily use of the practitioners and students in the field of Communication Sciences and Disorders, but also for consults for and with the professions from which terms have entered our fields.

The two Editors of this dictionary have a combined experience of being students, teachers, and researchers for more than 65 years. As the American Speech-Language-Hearing Association (ASHA) celebrates its 75th anniversary, we have been there when most of these terms knocked on our doors and found a new venue and fresh outlook. It is our feeling that an attempt needed to be made now to present "standardized" contemporary definitions to serve as anchored reference points for current understanding and future discussions.

It needs to be said that (1) all terms could not be included, (2) some that are included perhaps need not have been, and (3) the definitions are subject to scrutiny and scrutiny is welcome. Our own biases are part of the weakness. Detachment is a virtue reserved for hermits and poets.

Notes

In "Plan of a Dictionary of the English Language," 1747, the grandfather of modern dictionaries, Dr. Samuel Johnson, wrote, "The value of a work must be estimated by its use. it is not enough that a dictionary delights the critic, unless at the same time it instructs the learner," (from *Dictionaries: The Art and Craft of Lexicography*, by Sidney I. Landau (1984), p. 50. New York: Charles Scribner's Sons).

Singular's Illustrated Dictionary of Speech-Language Pathology is designed and developed with users in prime consideration.The following are pointers on putting this work to maximum and efficient use.

- Entries are placed in alphabetical order in a variety of ways. The traditional ordering by noun (followed by modifier) is common, but logical usage is also employed and many entries are provided in more than one place. There is an entry for **free morpheme** in **F** (**free morpheme**) and in **M** under **morpheme**. In a similar vein there are entries for both **amnesia, retrograde** and **retrograde amnesia**. The redundancy is intentional. We trust it helps users to locate entries quickly.

- As users from a variety of fields reference this work, variations in meaning of a given term are not numbered, but are separated by semicolons. We do not imply that one meaning is more correct than another, just that a term can have more than one application.

- Abbreviations follow spelled out main entries. The appendices include a listing of common abbreviations and their full forms.

We invite your input on this work. Please send us your suggestions for entries in future editions through our Website at

http://www.singpub.com

Acknowledgments

1. Angie S. Singh

   The authors are profoundly grateful to Angie Singh for her enthusiasm, which lifted this project from the normal arena of a book to an impressive ensemble of product line, consisting of handy pocket guide, elaborate tabletop, and CD-ROM. The CD-ROM was entirely her idea and it enhanced the value of these dictionaries manyfold.

2. Sandy Doyle

   Just as no book at Singular could see the bindery without the keen oversight of Sandy Doyle, the Singular dictionaries were no exceptions. Sandy monitored this highly complex project with a will to protect both Singh and Kent—the people for whom she would place no limits on herself. The authors express a deep sense of appreciation.

3. Linton M. Vandiver

   Van has checked and crosschecked the definitions, illustrations, and the content of this dictionary multiple times. He has proofed them, and made substantial comment about many aspects of the dictionary. He is a perfectionist and that was a great help, but he was also a great help because of his friendship with the authors.

4. In addition— Joan Bade of the University of Wisconsin did the spade work; Kristin Banach provided editorial support; and Brad Bielawski navigated this highly involved production to a successful completion. Our colleagues Jay Rosenbeck, Charles Speaks, Thomas Murry, and Marie Linvill added needed expertise.

5. With all of the help of these able people, the authors are certain that if there are flaws in this work, they belong to Singh and Kent.

Dedication

Dedicated to ASHA's commemoration of its 75th anniversary
and
the profound impact its members have made for the quality of life
of communicatively disordered individuals
around the world

A

Alveolus, Alveoli

Schematic representation of cluster of alveoli with capillary bed. Lower portion shows a cross section through alveoli and terminal bronchiole.

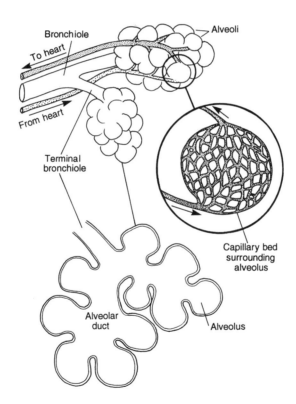

a- prefix: without; lack of, not

Aarskog syndrome x-linked recessive mutation of hypertelorism, hypodontia, brachydactyly, inguinal hernias, shawled scrotum, short stature, occasional cognitive impairment, with jaw and dental anomalies leading to articulation disorders; possible hypernasality and VPI from clefting

-ab prefix: away from

abbreviation expansion memory-resident utility software that provides keyboard assistance. A short string of letters and/or numbers is used to represent a larger, expanded set of keystrokes. When a given string is activated, the expanded stream of keystrokes replaces the short form. The expansion may be any type of data, such as words, phrases, salutations, or computer commands. For example, "MS" = My name is Mike Smith"

abdomen region of the body between the thorax and pelvis; the diaphragm separates the thoracic and abdominal cavities

abdominal cavity that part of the torso between the diaphragm and the pelvis, containing many important organs including the stomach, liver, intestines, spleen, and kidney

abdominal fixation process of impounding air within the lungs through inhalation and forceful vocal fold adduction that results in increased intra-abdominal pressure

abdominal viscera organs of the abdominal region; the cavity containing inferior portion of the esophagus, stomach, intestines, colon, rectum, liver, spleen, pancreas, kidneys, cecum, appendix, gallbladder, and bladder

abduct to move apart from the median plane of the body, to separate

abduction to draw a structure away from midline. The muscles that perform such a function generally are called abductors

abduction quotient the ratio of the glottal half-width at the vocal processes to the amplitude of vibration of the vocal fold

ablation removal (as by surgery)

aboral away from or opposite to the oral cavity or mouth

abscess cavity containing pus in midst of inflamed tissue, caused by an infection

absolute jitter a discrete measure of very short term (cycle-to-cycle) variation of vocal pitch periods expressed in microseconds. This parameter is dependent on the fundamental frequency of the voicing sample. Therefore, normative data differs significantly for men and women. Higher pitch results in lower values

absolute refractory period action potential period following depolarization of a cell membrane during which stimulation will not result in further depolarization

abstraction ability to perceive relationships among isolated aspects of objects, events, or persons

abulia inability to initiate or complete activities or make decisions because of decreased or absent initiative

acalculia an inability, often associated with aphasia, to make simple mathematical calculations

acceleration the rate of change of velocity with respect to time (measured in millimeters per square second: mm/s^2)

acceleration techniques communication aid and computer techniques used to speed up system use. Prestored messages, word prediction, and abbreviation expansion are methods of acceleration

access barriers obstacles to an individual's use of AAC caused by limitations in an individual's capabilities, attitudes, or resources. Cognitive, perceptual, motoric, and literacy deficits are examples of access barriers

access method (scanning, direct select, encoding): the method that an individual employs to access an alternative or augmentative communication device

- **acoustic access** access through the auditory channel, either unaided or aided, to acoustic information

- **adaptive computer access** hardware and/ or software that allows persons to use computers with or without standard input or output devices. For example, adaptive access can be accomplished via alternative keyboards, touch boards, Braille, screen enlargement, speech synthesis, voice recognition, with access through the game port or switches with scanning

- **direct selection** AAC access method that allows the user to indicate choices directly by pointing with a body part or technological aid to make a selection; the most rapid method of entering information into a computer

- **motor access** the ways in which an individual physically approaches and uses an AAC system

accessory features of stuttering distinctive audible and visible characteristics of stutter events that result from excessive effort and tensing

accommodation process of cognitive adaptation that modifies an existing scheme in response to new experiences. Also, making facilities and programs accessible to and usable by persons with disabilities through appropriate modifications, including policy modifications, task restructuring, modified schedules, equipment acquisition or modification, training or provision of qualified readers or interpreters, and other similar provisions

account type of narrative in which the speaker evaluates and interprets the significance of events

acculturation the process by which an individual adapts cognitively and emotionally to a new culture, as well as adapting to its communication system

acetylcholine (ACh) common central and peripheral cholinergic neurotransmitter released at synapses of some pre- and postganglionic parasympathetic neurons, preganglionic sympathetic neurons, somatic neurons, and some central neuron synapses. After relaying a nerve impulse, acetylcholine is rapidly broken down by the enzyme cholinesterase

achalasia, esophageal dysfunction of the esophagus, consisting of failure or incomplete relaxation of the lower esophageal (cardioesophageal junction) sphincter and absent peristalsis of the esophagus, often leading to dilation of the thoracic esophagus

acidosis a condition of either respiratory or metabolic origin in which there is a decrease of alkali in body fluids in relation to acid content. Respiratory acidosis results from respiratory retention of CO_2 due to hypoventilation or inadequate pulmonary ventilation

acid-perfusion test test whereby acid is dripped into the distal esophagus through a nasogastric tube and the patient's symptoms are recorded; used to help determine whether a patient has gastroesophageal reflux (GER)

acoustic of or relating to science of sound or to organs, nerves, or physical sense of hearing

acoustic access access through the auditory channel, either unaided or aided, to acoustic information

acoustic cue acoustic information in a segment of speech that contributes to phonetic recognition

acoustic feedback sound produced when the amplified sound from a receiver device is picked up again by the microphone and reamplified; a high-pitched squeal

acoustic nerve (or cranial nerve or vestibulocochlear nerve) CN VIII, the eighth cranial nerve, important for transmitting auditory and balance sensation from the inner ear to the brain

- **high spontaneous rate auditory nerve fibers** fibers that require a high level of stimulation to fire and respond to the higher level of human signal intensity auditory range and that have little or no background firing noise

- **low spontaneous rate auditory nerve fibers** fibers that respond to very low signal intensities and that display random firing

acoustic neuroma benign tumor of cranial nerve VIII arising from Schwann cells; often grows in the internal auditory canal. Signs and symptoms are produced in cerebellum, lower cranial nerves, and brainstem. Can cause tinnitus, progressive hearing loss, headache, dizziness, and unsteady gait, with later stage symptoms of paresis and speaking/swallowing difficulty. Also known as acoustic neurofibroma, bellopontine angle tumor, acoustic schwannoma

acoustic power the physical measure of the amount of sound energy produced and radiated into the air per second (measured in watts)

acoustic reflex a bilateral reflex of the stapedius muscle in the middle ear; it is activated by sounds of high intensity and reduces the transmission of energy into the inner ear, providing protection from loud noise

- **crossed acoustic reflex** stapedius muscle contraction recorded with sound stimulus to one ear and immittance recording probe in the other ear

acoustics the branch of physics that deals with the study of sound

- **classroom acoustics** the background noise and reverberation properties characteristic of a classroom, determined by the size and surfaces of the room, the sound sources inside and outside, furnishings, people, and other factors

acoustic zero decibels 0.0002 microbar

acquired immunodeficiency syndrome (AIDS) cell-mediated immunity defect, resulting in the inability to resist infection manifested by opportunistic infections, including candidiasis, pneumocystis, carinii pneumonia, oral hairy leukoplakia, herpes zoster, cervical dysplasia and carcinoma, Kaposi's sarcoma, toxoplasmosis, non-Hodgkin's lymphoma. Prognosis is poor. AIDS is highly contagious through transmission of the HIV-1 and HIV-2 viruses (mainly through blood and semen)

acquisition, simultaneous learning two languages at the same time

acquisition, successive learning a second language following establishment of a first language

acrolect dialect that approximates the accepted standard usage of a language (its common or major dialect)

acromegaly overproduction of growth hormone, causing bones of the face, jaw, and extremities to continue to grow after normal growth has been completed

actin one of two muscle proteins; actin forms thin fibrils as part of the contractile portion of muscle action

acting voice trainer a professional with extra training who may work with injured voices as part of a medical voice team in an effort to optimize speaking voice performance

action level noise exposure level at which a worker must be enrolled in an occupational hearing conservation program; OSHA defines this level as 85dBA for an average of 8 hours in 1 day

action potential (AP) sequential electrochemical polarization and depolarization associated with longitudinally propagated change of potential across a cell membrane, reflecting activation of excitable cells such as nerve or muscle

- **auditory evoked potential (AEP)** small electrical potential superimposed by auditory input on the steady-state electrical activity of the brain. Usually detectable only by signal averaging

- **differential recording** the electrophysiologic technique based on the recording of action potentials from a limited spatial region by use of bipolar electrodes connected to a differential amplifier

- **discharge** electrical signals defined and recorded as action potentials or spikes by electrical recording micropipettes placed within the cell or near and outside the cell.

Neurons and muscles have distinct membranes with channels that will transiently open to allow specific ions to move across the membrane into or out of the cell. The movement of ions creates a current that can be measured as a voltage, the action potential. Discharge is the number of action potentials that a neuron or muscle fiber will produce

- **electrophysiological recording** technique of using micropipettes or metal to record action potentials inside or outside of neurons and muscle cells. Micropipettes placed in these two types of cells can record action potentials in millivolts. Micropipettes and metal electrodes placed outside this tissue records extracellular signals that are much smaller—in the microvolt range

- **endocochlear potential** constant positive potential of the inner ear's scala media

- **hair cell intracellular resting potential** negative electrical potential difference between the ear's endolymph—the potential of the hair cells

- **membrane potential/resting potential/ standing potential** to some degree, each cell in one's body pumps ions across cell membranes to keep an electrical potential difference across the membrane; ions travel in and out of a cell through channels in the membrane; passive channels allow free movement; chemically gated channels are selective, for example, with sodium-selective channels pumping sodium (and some calcium) out of cells and allowing potassium in; voltage gated channels are only open for some potentials

active matrix screen a laptop computer monitor that uses one transistor for every pixel element refreshing of the screen. Screen graphics are sharp without ghosting of images

activity of daily living (ADL) common term used by rehabilitation specialists for primary aspects of daily life, such as personal hygiene, dressing, grooming, eating, drinking, walking, and sitting

acute abrupt initial symptoms and consequences of impairment, injury, or disease, usually subsiding after a fairly short duration

ad- prefix: toward (consonant assimilates to initial consonant of roots beginning with c, f, g, p, s, or t); combining form meaning toward

Adam's apple prominence of the thyroid cartilage seen as a bulge in the neck, primarily in males

adaptation the cognitive process of organizing new experiences to achieve equilibrium in one's understanding of the world

adaptive device a device that permits participation in an activity that otherwise would not be possible

A/D converter analog to digital converter; a device that converts an analog (A) signal to a digital (D) form. The conversion process involves both sampling and quantization operations. A/D converters for personal computers typically are expansion boards that fit into the computer

addiction habitual, compulsive physiological and/or psychological dependence on a substance (i.e., drug or chemical) or practice. The overpowering physical or emotional urge to do something repeatedly that an individual cannot control, accompanied by a tolerance for a substance and withdrawal symptoms if use is discontinued. Alcohol and/or drugs become the central focus of life

additive bilingualism the second language (L2) adds to and does not replace the first language (L1)

adduct to draw two structures closer together or to move toward midline

adduction A movement that draws a body part, such as an arm or a leg, toward the center or midline of the body. The muscles that perform such a function generally are called adductors

adenoid facies clinical presentation often secondary to hypertrophied nasopharyngeal tonsil (adenoid); characterized by a persistent open mouth, mouth breathing, and a generally dull expression; often in combination with pinched nose

adenoidectomy surgical removal of the adenoids

adenoids normal small masses of lymphoid tissue on nasopharynx posterior wall forming pharyngeal tonsils; in children, enlarged or hypertrophied pharyngeal tonsil

adenoma sebaceum facial rash associated with tuberous sclerosis

adiadochokinesis inability to make a sequence of rapid alternating movements

adipose connective tissue of fat cells arranged in lobules

aditus of mastoid antrum entryway to the tympanic antrum

adjective word that typically modifies a noun, specifying a quality of the thing, indicating amount or extent or distinguishing from another thing

- **comparative** adjective form that expresses the relative degree of an attribute in comparing two items (e.g., bigger is the comparative form for big)

admittance a technical term quantifying ease of energy flow through a vibratory system; unit of measure is the acoustic mho; electrical: reciprocal of impedance measured in siemens

adrenergic innervation characterized by synapses that release the neurotransmitter norepinephrine and are found particularly in the sympathetic division of the autonomic nervous system

adult respiratory distress syndrome (ARDS) severely impaired lung function with a number of etiologies, marked by alveolar and/or interstitial hemorrhage and edema; also called wet lung

adventitious sound an auditory event that may accompany typical breathing sounds, but not easily heard, such as wheezes, crackles, and gurgles

adverb word that modifies a verb, adjective, another adverb, preposition, a phrase, a clause, or a sentence to express a relationship of manner or quality, location, time, amount, cause

aer- or aero- prefix: pertaining to air or gas

aeration the process of introducing air (usually oxygen) to a space or cavity; oxygen replacement of CO_2 in lungs

aerobic an organism, such as bacteria, that requires molecular oxygen to live. It is the aerobic bacteria, such as those of the *Pseudomonas* species, which appear to bind to cells of the trachea

affect expressive monologues instances in which preschoolers talk to themselves as they reflect on their emotions

affect (flat) absence or near absence of any signs of expression (usually facial but also vocal) of feeling, emotion, or mood

affective control ability to control emotions

afferent carrying toward a central location; generally, sensory nerve impulses; inflowing

- **afferent fibers** sensory fibers that carry nerve impulses from stimulation of the sensory end organs to the central nervous system (CNS)

- **afferent roots** peripheral nerve bundles carrying sensory information to the ventral horns of the spinal cord

- **afferent tract** sensory pathway of the nervous system in the spinal cord that transmits impulses toward the brain, also ascending tract

- **general somatic afferent** sensory nerves that communicate sensory information from skin, muscles, and joints, including pain, temperature, mechanical simulation of skin, length and tension of muscle, along with movement and position of joints

- **general visceral afferent** nerves that transmit sensory information from receptors in visceral structures, such as the digestive tract

affricate a speech sound that involves the two phases of a stop (vocal tract obstruction) and a prolonged frication; consonant with a stop onset and fricative release

affricate consonants obstruent consonants produced with characteristics of both stop consonants and fricative consonants. Examples are the first and last sounds in the words church and judge

affrication phonological error pattern of stops or fricatives pronounced as affricates, such as "see" pronounced as [tsi]

aftercare in alcohol and other drug addiction rehabilitation, the package of services offered clients after completion of a short-term intensive (after residential) treatment program

agenda outline of steps toward goal, including the steps that proceed toward that goal

aggressive conversational style conversational style characteristic of some persons who have hearing loss, characterized by hostility, belligerence, and bad attitude

aging process of growing old, partly from body cells slowing or stopping replacement of dead or weak body cells, with special influence on cells incapable of mitotic division (i.e., neurons)

agitation a chronic restless inability to keep still. Agitation is most often psychomotor agitation, that is, having emotional and physical components. Agitation can be caused by anxiety, overstimulation, or withdrawal from depressants and stimulants

aglossia-adactylia syndrome concurrent congenital absence of the tongue and digits

agnosia impairment of sensory recognition of familiar items caused by damage to sensory association areas or association pathways of the brain; often named to denote the sensory system involved; for example, visual agnosia, auditory agnosia

agonist muscle contracted for purpose of a specific motor act, with the contraction opposed by another muscle (antagonist); also a substance such as a drug that promotes a receptor-mediated biologic response

agrammatism aphasia type noted by lack of use of proper function words, such as articles and prepositions, and lack of appropriate endings to words such as plurals, tenses, and possessives; may be seen in written and/or spoken language; inability to create sentences because of syntactic, morphological, and semantic deficits; can result from lesion in dominant temporal lobe

agranulocytosis a disorder of severe acute deficiency of certain blood cells (neutrophils) because of bone marrow damage from toxic drugs or chemicals; characterized by fever, with ulceration of the mouth and throat and possible rapid progression to prostration and death

agraphia loss of writing ability in the absence of abnormality of a limb and usually associated with damage to brain language centers. Characterized by spelling errors, reversals, impaired word order, and other manifestations of faulty written language use, such as alexia and aphasia. Sometimes called dysgraphia

aided communication communication modes that require equipment in addition to the communicator's body. Examples are pencil and paper, typewriters, headpointers, picture communication boards, eye gaze boards, dedicated augmentative communication devices, and computers with speech synthesis

aided language stimulation interactive, receptive, and expressive communication training that uses picture communication displays to model language skills

aided thresholds hearing thresholds obtained from a patient using hearing aids, indicated by an "A" on the audiogram

air-bone gap variance between the threshold for hearing acuity by bone conduction and by bone conduction

air conduction a general name for the test paradigm in which sound is presented to the listener through an earphone coupled to the ear; sound information travels through the air, enters the external auditory canal, and progresses through the middle ear, inner ear, and then to the brain; air conduction thresholds are represented by a "O" (right ear) and "X" (left ear) on the audiogram

air pressure force of air per unit area, measured in pascals

airflow the volume of air moved in a unit of time, for example, milliliters per second or liters per minute

air volume quantity of air contained in a vessel, usually measured in liters or milliliters in human physiology

airway tube for passage of air into and out of the lung, trachea, bronchi, and bronchioles

- **acute upper airway obstruction** occlusion of the route for passage of air into and out of the lungs, most commonly due to foreign bodies lodging in or around the larynx

- **anatomical airway** anatomical dead space; conducting airways that do not participate in gas exchange

- **artificial airway** a means of securing an airway to ensure patency (e.g., an endotracheal tube). Often used to connect with mechanical ventilation

- **conducting airway** air passage from the nose to a bronchiole

- **lower airway** air passage from the subglottis to the bronchiole level

- **respiratory airway** the location in the airway where there is an interchange of gasses and includes the respiratory bronchioles, alveolar ducts, sacs, and alveoli

- **upper airway** air passage from the nose or mouth to and including the larynx

akathisia restless overactivity, involuntary movements induced by antipsychotic drugs

akinesia diminished or absent motor activity

ala wing-like structure

Alagille syndrome may include speech-language delay secondary to mild cognitive impairment, evidenced by small stature, broad forehead, heart anomalies, vertebral anomalies, hepatic anomalies, occasional cognitive impairment, small genitals

albinism genetic absence of pigment of the eyes or of the eyes, hair, and skin that can include late-onset sensorineural hearing loss

albumen a protein found in mammals, often measured in a blood analysis to determine an individual's nutritional needs. Low levels of albumen can impede the weaning process by decreasing inspiratory muscle strength and affecting the ability to tolerate increases in the work of breathing

alcohol abuse pattern of excessive and/or inappropriate alcohol use distinguishable from addiction by the degree of free choice the individual has in when (or whether) to start or stop use

alcoholic dementia an organic brain syndrome associated with prolonged, heavy ingestion of alcohol, characterized by impairment of long- and short-term memory, abstract thinking and judgment, and other disturbances of higher brain function

alexia impairment in reading the printed word; may be acquired or developmental. Acquired alexia is a reading impairment that accompanies or is a part of aphasia. Frequently called dyslexia and also known as word or text blindness or visual aphasia

Alezzandrini syndrome appears first in adolescence and young adulthood and evidenced by unilateral degenerative retinitis, depigmentation of facial hair and scalp, along with facial blotching and often bilateral hearing loss

-algia suffix: pain

algorithm a step-by-step procedure or formula for solving a particular type of problem; must have unambiguous rules and a clear stopping point

aliasing artifacts or errors generated during sound digitization because sound energy in the analog signal exists at frequencies higher than one-half of the sampling frequency

alimentation feeding; nourishment

alkalosis a condition of either respiratory or metabolic origin in which there is an excessive alkaline content in the blood. Conversely, there is a reduction of the acid content of the blood; respiratory form caused by hyperventilation and subsequent CO_2 loss

allele one of two or more varying forms of a gene occupying corresponding locations on homologous chromosomes

allergic reaction (drug) adverse response of antibodies produced in reaction to drugs; may appear as skin rash, fever, joint pain, breathing difficulty; drug allergies can develop gradually or appear suddenly; some allergic reactions are life-threatening

allergy bodily (immune) hypersensitive response to foreign substances or organisms; anaphylactic shock is a severe form of allergy response, with symptoms including dizziness, loss of consciousness, labored breathing, swelling of the tongue and breathing tubes, blueness of skin, low blood pressure; possible death

allophone a variant of a phoneme. The phoneme is a family of speech sounds that occur in various phonetic environments or that can be selected by a speaker without disturbing phonemic identity. For example, vowels in English can either be nasalized or not. The nasal allophone of a vowel is a variant produced with velopharyngeal opening as in the difference of the /æ/ in dance (nasalized) and cat (not nasal). Most speakers produce nasalized vowels when they occur adjacent to nasal consonants. Similarly, many consonants can be produced with lip rounding when they occur adjacent to lip-rounded sounds

- **complementary distribution** allophones with distinctive phonetic environments; as in the aspirated /p/ in pie has a different sound than the unaspirated /p/ in spy; the aspirated form is generally in the initial positions and the unaspirated occurs after an initial /s/ sound; these /p/ pronunciations can never exchange positions and are in complementary distribution; also termed noncontrastive distribution

- **free variation** a relationship between allophones in which they can be freely exchanged for one another in different contexts

alphabet board a low-tech communication aid displaying letters of the alphabet that may also contain a few words or sentences. An AAC user points to letters to spell words to communicate a message

Alphabet, International Phonetic (IPA) an alphabet designed to provide universal symbols to represent all the known speech sounds used in human languages

alphabet, manual series of hand configurations that correspond to each letter in the alphabet; used to fingerspell words in manual communication

Alport syndrome dysphagia, apnea, nephritis, sensorineural hearing loss, myopia, stridor, apnea, with normal speech and language development

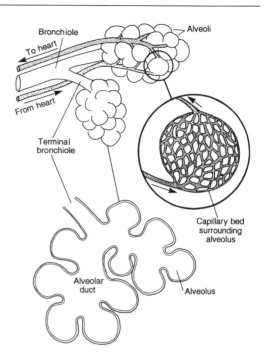

alveolus, alveoli (plural) small cavity; as in alveolus of lung, the air sac wherein gas exchange occurs

---

altered speech human speech that is recorded and then altered in some manner

alternation the variations in linguistic structure and speaking style in response to the roles and audience in a particular setting

alternative communication a method of communication other than oral; one that replaces oral-verbal communication

alve- prefix: channel, socket

alveolar consonant class of productions from constriction between articulators at the alveolar ridges (immediately behind upper front teeth). American English alveolar consonants are [t], [d], [s], [z], [n], [l], and [r]

alveolar pressure (P_A) air pressure measured at the level of the alveolus in the lung

alveolar process dental arch of the bony seat for teeth formed by a portion of the maxilla, or mandible (jaw)

alveolus, alveoli (plural) small cavity; as in alveolus of lung, the air sac wherein gas exchange occurs

Alzheimer disease a progressive and irreversible mental deterioration. Often begins with intermittent states of mental confusion, disorientation, and loss of recent memory. Sub-

Sign Language

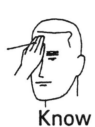 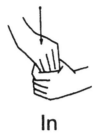 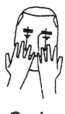

Know   In   Sad

American Sign Language (ASL) a manual system of communication used by members of the Deaf Culture in the United States; sometimes referred to with the term Ameslan. Having a distinct grammar and syntax, ASL is a separate language

---

sequently leads to severe impairment in all realms of thinking, memory, language, and communication

ambient noise noise in a particular listening environment: usually a mix of near and distant sounds

ambiguity material having more than one interpretation, direction, development, or meaning

ambisyllabic consonant description used by some who consider a given sound belong to two syllables. Some view the second [m] in "mama" to be ambisyllabic

amblyopia reduced vision with no apparent pathologic or structural etiology, sometimes linked with squinting; toxic amblyopia can be caused by tobacco, alcohol, or other drugs

ambulation walking

amenorrhea abnormal absence or suppression of menstruation; can be an adverse effect of certain drugs and is one symptom of depression

American Academy of Audiology (AAA) professional society for audiologists, founded in 1988

American National Standards Institute (ANSI) group that determines standards for measuring instruments, including audiometers. The American national standards body that represents the U.S. with the International Organization for Standardization (ISO) and the International Electrotechnical Commission (IEC). ANSI standards are voluntary. ASCII is an ANSI character set

American Sign Language (ASL) a manual system of communication used by members of the Deaf Culture in the United States; sometimes referred to with the term Ameslan. Having a distinct grammar and syntax, ASL is a separate language

American Speech-Language-Hearing Association (ASHA) [formerly American Speech and Hearing Association] professional organization of speech and hearing professionals, including speech-language pathologists, audiologists, and speech and hearing scientists

Americans with Disabilities Act (ADA) United States law enacted in 1990 (Public Law 101–336) to provide equal access to persons with disabilities

Amerind a type of sign language based on American Indian sign language in which gestures are used to facilitate or augment oral communication; used especially with patients who have word-finding difficulties

amino acid organic chemical composition of one or more basic amino groups, along with one or more acidic carboxyl groups. More than 100 amino acids occur in nature, with 20 of these being the building blocks of peptides that form proteins. The 8 amino acids that form complete proteins are termed essential

amnesia the partial or total loss of long-term memory; a phenomenon in which an area of experience becomes inaccessible to conscious recall

- **amnesia, aphasic** lack of capacity to remember spoken words or the words for labels for characteristics, circumstances, or objects

- **amnesia, apraxic** loss of ability to move in response to a request, because the request is quickly forgotten

- **anterograde amnesia** inability to learn and form new memories following trauma that led to problem

- **retrograde amnesia** loss of memory for events that occurred before the brain injury or the neurologic disorder

amniocentesis removal of fluid surrounding a fetus, which allows laboratory analysis for genetic and other studies.

amniotic fluid fluid surrounding fetus in the uterus

amphi-, amph-, ampho- prefix: on both sides, surrounding

amphiarthrodial bony articulation in which bones are connected by cartilage, allowing motion in more than one direction, as of the human lower jaw

amplification increasing the magnitude of a stimulus signal, such as increasing the loudness of an acoustic signal, to intensify its perception

- **linear hearing aid amplification** hearing aid amplification system in which there is a one-to-one correspondence between the input and output until the maximum output level is reached

- **nonlinear amplification** amplification system that does not provide a one-to-one correspondence between input and output at all input levels

amplifier a device that increases the amplitude of an input signal. Electronic amplifiers are used to increase signal gain for recording, playback, or analysis

- **differential amplifier** an amplifier that removes common mode components from two signals, for example, by inverting one input and then summing the two

amplitude the magnitude of displacement for a sound wave. The waveform of a sound is represented on a two-dimensional graph in which amplitude is plotted as a function of time. To a certain degree, amplitude of sound determines the perceived loudness of the sound. Also, maximum excursion of an undulating signal from the equilibrium; the amplitude of a sound wave is related to the perceived loudness; mostly it is expressed as a logarithmic, comparative level measure using the decibel (dB) unit

- **amplitude perturbation quotient** a relative evaluation of short term (cycle-to-cycle) variation of peak-to-peak amplitude expressed in percentage.

  smoothed amplitude perturbation quotient (sAPQ) a relative evaluation of long-term variation of the peak-to-peak amplitude within the analyzed voice sample, expressed in percentage

- **amplitude spectrum** a display of relative amplitude versus frequency of the sinusoidal components of a waveform

- **amplitude to length ratio** the ratio of vibrational amplitude at the center of the vocal fold to the length of the vocal fold

- **amplitude tremor** regular (periodic) long-term amplitude variation (an element of vibrato)

- **amplitude tremor frequency** this measure is expressed in hertz and shows the frequency of the most intensive low-frequency amplitude-modulating component in the specified amplitude-tremor analysis range

- **amplitude tremor intensity index** the average ratio of the amplitude of the most intensive low frequency amplitude modulating component (amplitude tremor) to the total amplitude of an analyzed sample. The algorithm for tremor analysis determines the strongest periodic amplitude modulation of the voice. This measure is expressed in percentage

- **coefficient of amplitude variation** this measure, expressed in percent, computes the relative standard deviation of the peak-to-peak amplitude.

ampulla rounded, flasklike structure or dilation of any tiny lymphatic or blood vessel, duct, or tube; a part of the vestibular mechanism

amygdaloid almond-shaped or resembling a tonsil

amyloidosis condition resulting from deposition of amyloid (starchlike carbohydrate-protein substance) in abnormal amounts in various tissues throughout the body; seen in such chronic conditions as amyloidosis, tuberculosis, rheumatoid arthritis, and Alzheimer disease

amyotrophic lateral sclerosis (ALS) neuromuscular disorder characterized by degeneration of both upper and lower motor neurons in the central nervous system; also known as Lou Gehrig's disease

amyotrophy progressive loss of muscle bulk associated with weakness of these muscles; a feature of chronic neuropathy; combined with spasticity characterizes motor neuron disease

an- prefix: not, without; lack of

ana- prefix: up, again

anabolic steroid derived from synthetic male hormones or testosterone to increase muscle mass and counteract effect of endogenous estrogen and may cause irreversible deepening or hoarseness of the voice

anaerobe a microorganism, such as bacteria, that cannot live in the presence of molecular oxygen. Anaerobic bacteria are usually cultured from saliva

anaerobic infection infection caused by anaerobic bacteria, that is, those that do not require (and in most cases cannot tolerate) the presence of oxygen and that usually are found in deep puncture wounds; examples include tetanus and gangrene

analgesia relief from pain; the state of insensibility to pain without loss of consciousness

analgesics pain-relieving drugs

analog signal a signal whose waveform has continuous variations in amplitude. The radiated sound-pressure waveform of speech is an analog signal, because its amplitude varies continuously in time

analogy similarity between items in a portion of otherwise unlike items and association based on such affinity

anaphoric reference the linguistic effect in which pronouns replace nouns or noun phrases and refer to their occurrence earlier in the context; relationship of grammatical elements to antecedents

anaphylaxis abnormal reaction to a particular antigen, in which histamine is released from body tissues; an allergic attack is an example of localized anaphylaxis; rare, but very serious, is anaphylactic shock, with widespread histamine release causing swelling, bronchiole constrictions, heart failure, and sometimes death

anarthria the inability to articulate because of neuromuscular involvement

anastomosis, anastomoses pathological or surgical linkage of two nerves, blood vessels or other tubular structures

- **neural anastomosis** surgical or pathological linkage of two tubes; surgery connecting a branch of an undamaged nerve to a damaged nerve; treatment for some dysarthric clients; a branch of the intact XIIth cranial nerve may be connected to the damaged VIIth cranial nerve to restore function and appearance

anatomic position erect body, with face, palms, arms, and hands facing forward hanging down and a bit out from the torso and feet slightly apart. considered as standard neutral stance for describing places or motions of various anatomical structures

anatomy the study, description, and classification of structure and organs of an organism

- **applied anatomy** the subdiscipline of anatomy concerned with diagnosis, treatment, and surgical intervention
- **comparative anatomy** study of homologous structures of different animals
- **developmental anatomy** study of anatomy of growth and development
- **gross anatomy** study of the body and its parts as visible without the aid of microscopy
- **microscopic anatomy** study of structure of the body by microscopy
- **pathological anatomy** branch exploring structural changes accompanying disease
- **surface anatomy** study of the body and its surface markings, as related to underlying structures
- **systematic anatomy** descriptive anatomy

Anderson syndrome articulation impairment secondary to malocclusion caused by abnormal jaw growth and position, evidenced by maxillary hypoplasia, mandibular prognathism, scoliosis, thin calvarium

androgen a steroid that increases male-specific features; the best known natural androgen is testosterone

anemia abnormally low number of red blood cells or hemoglobin; below the normal range of 4.2 million/mm³ to 6.1 million/mm³

- **aplastic anemia** disordered white blood production

anesthesia loss of sensation caused by nerve function depression created by a pharmacologic agent; may be topical, local, regional, or general; clinical speciality for administering anesthetic drugs (usually in surgery)

anesthetic a substance that causes partial or total loss of consciousness and insensibility to pain

- **topical anesthetic** anesthetics applied to a local region through injection or direct application by touch or spraying for pain relief

aneurysm abnormal dilation or ballooning of a blood vessel (typically an artery); often a potential site for a hemorrhage because of acquired or congenital vessel wall weakness; subarachnoid hemorrhage can result from a burst brain aneurysm

angina, Ludwig's cellulitis; painful, soft-tissue infection and swelling of the floor of the mouth capable of compromising (blocking) the airway

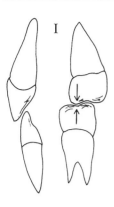
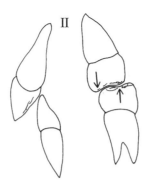
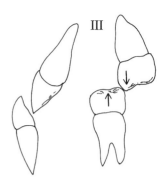

Angle's classification of malocclusion   identification of dental malocclusion, based on the mesiodistal association of the permanent molars and incisors. There are three classes, identified by Roman numerals

---

angio-, angei-, angi- prefixes: referring to a vessel, usually blood vessel; a covering; an enclosure

angiogram a radiographic test that permits visualization of the course and condition of a person's blood vessels after injection of a radiosensitive dye directly into the bloodstream

angiography X-ray study for viewing the flow of blood in the body canals

angiology science dealing with blood vessels and the lymphatic system

angioma tumor containing blood or lymphatic vessels, generally benign; can be congenital

Angle's classification of malocclusion identification of dental malocclusion, based on the mesiodistal association of the permanent molars. There are three classes, identified by Roman numerals; I = neutrocclusion, II = distocclusion, III = mesiocclusion

angular gyrus a folded convolution of the inferior parietal lobe of the cerebrum that is considered to be important in language processing; typically associated with Brodmann area 39

anhedonia inability to appreciate pleasure from typically pleasing activities; a symptom of depression

anion an ion carrying a negative charge

anisotropic property of a material that produces different strains when identical stresses are applied in different directions; an example is a transmission speed that is faster in one direction than in another; a structure whose appearance varies with the angle of observation

ankyloglossia complete or partial fusion of the tongue to the mouth floor; tongue movement limited and speech often impaired because of a short or absent lingual frenum

ankyglossia superior syndrome congenital malformation, with tongue attached to the hard palate

anlage the embryological foundation for subsequent development; in embryology, the earliest recognizable appearance of a developing part or organ (primordium); in psychoanalysis, the genetic propensity for personality characteristic or trait

anomaly a deviation from typical structure or pattern; abnormality (i.e., a cochlear anomaly); congenital malformation, such as extra finger or absent limb

anomia inability to retrieve common, well-known words from one's mental dictionary; a form of aphasia with substantive or meaningful words (such as persons and objects seen, heard, or felt) disproportionally omitted; generally from a lesion in the brain's language areas

anorexia loss of appetite; aversion to food

anorexia nervosa severe disorder manifested by extreme fear of obesity, usually by young women, in which aversion to food leads to emaciation, amenorrhea, hyperactivity, and distortion of body image; can be life-threatening

anosmia absence or impairment of the sense of smell (olfaction)

anosognosia the denial of illness or deficit caused by organic or biological factors; generally applies to neurological defect, particularly paralysis—generally by persons with nondominant parietal lobe lesions who deny their hemiparesis

anoxia lack of oxygen from inspired gases, arterial blood, or tissues (a reduction of oxygen is hypoxia)

ansa anatomical structure that forms a loop or arc

antagonist agent, such as a drug or a muscle, that opposes the action of another (the agonist) or competes for same site; antagonist drugs prevent an original drug from binding to receptors and exerting its effect

ante- prefix: before in time or in place; front

anterior in front of; before

anterior commissure of the vocal fold the junction of the vocal folds in the front of the larynx

antero- prefix: before, earlier

anthropology the study of humans, with the cultural branch dealing with behavior, including speech and language, thought systems, social constructs, and artifacts and the physical anthropology discipline dealing with anatomical aspects

anti-, ant- prefix: against

antibiotic drug used to combat infection (bodily invasion by a living organism such as a bacteria or virus). Most antibiotics have action specifically against bacteria and are soluble elements developed from bacteria or molds that discourage the growth of other microorganisms

antibody (Ab) an immunoglobulin secreted in response to viruses, bacteria, or other antigenic agents; each antigen is specific to its own antibody; experimentally used to identify the presence of a protein, as an antibody will bind with its antigen; antibodies can be protective or injurious; protective antibodies destroy harmful bacteria and neutralize toxins, while injurious antibodies combined with foreign substances cause allergic reactions

anticholinesterase agent drug that causes acetylcholine to accumulate at the junctions of cholinergic nerve fibers and their effector organs or sites, prompting stimulation of the fibers throughout the central and peripheral nervous systems; used for treatment of myasthenia gravis, among other conditions, as anticholinesterase agent drugs allow acetylcholine to transmit nerve impulses

anticoagulant substance preventing or slowing blood coagulation

anticonvulsant drug preventing or reducing seizure severity

antidepressant measure or substance to prevent or relieve depression

- **monoamine oxidase (MAO) inhibitors (antidepressants)** increase accumulation of epinephrine, norepinephrine, and serotonin in nervous system storage sites; adverse effects can be significant

- **tricyclic antidepressant agents** impede reuptake of amine neurotransmitters

antiformant in vocal tract acoustics, a transfer function property in which energy does not travel effectively; opposite in effect to a formant. Antiformants, or zeros, arise because of divided passages or constrictions in the vocal tract

antigen (Ag) any material that induces sensitivity and/or immune response and reacts in a recognizable manner with immune cells and/or antibodies of a sensitized subject; a substance that can be recognized as foreign by the immune system because it reacts with specific receptors on lymphocytes

antihistamine drug to combat response to histamine, which is activated in allergic, inflammatory reactions

antineoplastic about a substance or process that hampers malignancy; a chemotherapeutic agent controlling or killing cancer cells

antinode a peak in a standing wave pattern. A point, line, or surface in a standing wave where some characteristic of the wave field has maximum amplitude.

antiparkinsonian about a procedure or substance for treating parkinsonism. Medications are categorized as ones that compensate for dopamine loss in patients' corpus striatum and as anticholinergic agents

antipsychotics a group of drugs used to treat psychotic disorders; sometimes referred to as major tranquilizers or neuroleptics

antiresonance a resonance phenomenon in which energy transmission is impeded

antisocial personality disorder a pervasive pattern of disregard for and violation of the rights of others. The disorder is characterized in part by risk taking, criminality, and pathological lying

antitragus region posterior and inferior to the tragus, a small extension of the ear's auricular cartilage

antitrismus tonic muscular spasm forcing the opening of the mouth

antonyms two words whose meanings contrast due to opposite values in a single semantic feature, as in *hot* and *cold*

antrum an incompletely closed cavity, especially one with bony walls

- **mastoid antrum** cavity in the temporal bone petrous portion, linking with the mastoid cells and the epitympanic recess of the middle ear
- **maxillary antrum** maxillary sinus

anular ringlike; also spelled annular

anus ring of muscular tissue at terminal end of large bowel

anxiety disorders a group of disorders characterized by unrealistic fear, panic, or avoidance behavior. Manifestations range from mild, chronic tenseness to more intense states of irritability and apprehension. These disorders include (among others) panic attacks, phobias, obsessive-compulsive disorders, and generalized anxiety disorders

- **generalized anxiety disorder** a disorder characterized by at least 6 months of persistent and excessive anxiety and worry not caused by exposure to a drug or medication

anxiolytics minor tranquilizers with antianxiety and tension relief effects; example is benzodiazepine

aperiodic irregular behavior that has no definite period, is usually either chaotic or random; waveform without periodic vibrations; not oscillatory

Apert syndrome speech production often delayed secondary to cognitive impairment, chronic upper airway obstruction, and severe occlusal anomalies, with compensatory articulation from possible cleft palate; language often delayed and/or impaired and voice can be harsh and breathy from laryngeal calcification; condition marked by craniosynostosis, syndactyly, symphalagism, short upper arms, hydrocephalus, choanal stenosis/atresia, acne

apex peak; uppermost extremity (in anatomy, especially the peak of a conical or pyramidal structure)

- **apex of arytenoid cartilage** upper pointed end of cartilage that supports the corniculate cartilage and aryepiglottic fold

Apgar score a numeric value between 1 and 10, assigned to a newborn to describe physical status at birth; determined by the baby's color, heart rate, respiration, muscle tone, and responsiveness, with a rating of from 8 to 10 considered optimal

aphasia impairment in the comprehension and production of language symbol systems that results from fairly localized damage to the brain, especially in right-handed persons. Usually accompanies focal areas of damage to the left cerebral hemisphere. Affects reading, writing, speaking, understanding, gestures, and other symbol systems used in communication

- **Broca's aphasia** characterized by loss of fluency, agrammatism, and paucity of vocabulary, usually arising from lesion to Brodmann areas 44 and 45 of the dominant cerebral hemisphere (Broca's area)
- **conduction aphasia** aphasia characterized by intact auditory comprehension but poor repetition of verbal materials; sometimes associated with damage to the arcuate fasciculus
- **expressive aphasia** common descriptor for people with aphasia who struggle to talk yet understand most of what is said to them; Broca's aphasia
- **fluent aphasia** category of aphasias characterized by a near normal "flow" of spoken words, although such utterances may not be clear or understandable, with problems noted in comprehension, reading, writing, or naming because of posterior lesions centered on the auditory association area of the left temporal or parietal lobe or both; includes Wernicke's aphasia, anomia, conduction aphasia, and transcortical sensory aphasia
- **global aphasia** aphasia in which all areas of speech and communication have severe impairment
- **motor aphasia** there is loss of speech production and/or language output that can be accompanied by loss of writing or signing (Broca's)
- **nonfluent aphasia** a category of aphasias characterized by halting, broken, or absent speech, word retrieval deficits, and motor planning deficits caused by lesion(s) in the anterior language area and left premotor cortex (Broca's area); includes Broca aphasia, transcortical motor aphasia, and global aphasia
- **receptive aphasia** sensory aphasia
- **sensory aphasia** comprehension of written and spoken language impaired and linked to effortless communication of malformed and substituted words
- **Wernicke aphasia** a type of aphasia named after the German neurologist who first described its features; characterized by fluent flow of speech, but with little or no comprehension of the spoken word; a severe fluent aphasia; also called receptive aphasia, sensory aphasia

aphasiology the study of aphasia

aphemia obsolete term for aphasia

aphonia the absence of vocal fold vibration; this term commonly describes people who have "lost their voice" after vocal fold injury. In most cases, such patients have very poor vibration, rather than no vibration; and they typically have a harsh, nearly whispered voice

- **hysterical aphonia** nonorganic voice loss attributed to psychogenesis

- **paralytica aphonia** paralysis of vocal folds; disease of laryngeal nerves

aphrasia aphasia form in which there is a problem communicating in sentences or phrases, although functional use of individual words remains

apical pertaining to the apex of a structure

apnea a transitory cessation of spontaneous respiration. Apnea during the respiratory cycle usually results from lack of stimulation to the respiratory center, secondary to inadequate CO_2 levels in the blood

- **deglutition apnea** required interruption of respiration during swallowing; interval during swallowing that is the pause time, usually between inspiration and expiration, to allow the bolus to pass over the closed airway

- **sleep apnea** a periodic cessation of breathing during sleep, often related to airway collapse from weakness of pharyngeal muscles. Symptoms include irregular breathing and loud snoring during sleep and excessive daytime sleepiness

apo- prefix: away from; separated or derived from

aponeurosis strong, fibrous sheet-like connective tissue that attaches muscle to bone when serving as a tendon or as a fascia in binding together muscles

apoplexy a common older, but now obsolete, medical term for a vascular stroke, cerebral stroke, intracranial hemorrhage, or "brain attack"

appendicular skeleton the skeleton, including upper and lower extremities

appendix of the ventricle of Morgagni a cecal pouch of mucous membrane connected by a narrow opening with the anterior aspect of the ventricle. It sits between the ventricular fold in the inner surface of the thyroid cartilage. In some cases, it may extend as far as the cranial border of the thyroid cartilage, or higher. It contains the openings of 60–70 mucous glands, and it is enclosed in a fibrous capsule, which is continuous with the ventricular ligament; also, called pyramidal lobe of thyroid gland

apposition a fitting together, as in layering of tissue cells

approximants liquids (/r/ and /l/) and glides (/j/ and /w/), having less prominent formants than vowels

approximate (verb) to bring closer together

apraxia inability to voluntarily execute a learned sequence of motor actions. The function may remain intact on an involuntary basis

- **apraxia of speech (AOS)** one of the major types of neuromotor articulatory speech disorders caused by brain damage that results in faulty planning, programming, or sequencing of the sounds of speech

- **ideational apraxia** perceptual loss of how to use an object; impaired ability to perform a complex or hierarchical motor act

- **motor apraxia** loss of ability to use an object when task is correctly understood

- **oral apraxia, primary** deficit in planning the nonspeech act, resulting in difficulty with imitating or producing voluntary nonspeech oral gestures, but without muscular weakness or paralysis

- **swallowing apraxia** In the context of swallowing, patients seem to have forgotten how to feed or how to initiate swallowing. This occurs primarily with unilateral lesions of the cerebral cortex, such as hemispheric infarcts, or with dementias

- **verbal apraxia,** primary deficit in planning the speech act, resulting in inconsistent phonemic distortions and substitutions with oral groping behaviors for voluntary verbal motor acts, but without muscular weakness or paralysis

aprosody a reduction or inability to use or appreciate the affective features of language, such as variations in intonation, rhythm, pitch, and loudness

APUD cells (amine precursor uptake and decarboxylation cells) class of cells producing hormones (such as insulin, ACTH, glycogen, and thyroxin) and amines (such as dopamine, serotonin, and histamine)

arachnodactyly long and slender fingers and toes (arachno- means spiderlike)

arachnoid fibrous delicate membrane that is the middle of the three coverings (meninges) of the central nervous system. The most external surface is close to the internal surface of the dura mater, with subdural space intervening and the arachnoid is held against the dura by the pressure of cerebrospinal fluid (CSF) between it and the innermost pia mater

arbitrary a capricious connection between words and their meanings that is highly personal

arch-, archi- prefix: beginning, origin

arch archlike structure or vault (in anatomy)

- **alveolar arch of mandible** margin of the alveolar process of the mandible that is free

- **Corti's arch** cochlear structure formed by the joining of the heads of Corti's inner and outer pillar cells

- **palatoglossal arch** pairs of ridges, or folds, of mucous membrane traveling from the soft palate to the side of the tongue; the palatoglossus muscle is enclosed in the arch, which forms the anterior margin of the tonsillar fossa. The arch also delineates the oral cavity from the isthmus of fauces; also known as anterior palatine arch, anterior pillar of fauces, arcus glossopalatinus, glossopalatine arch, glossopalatine fold

- **palatopharyngeal arch** one of a pair of ridges, or folds, of mucous membrane passing downward from the posterior margin of the soft palate to the pharynx lateral wall. The palatopharyngeus muscle is enclosed by the arch, which marks the posterior margin of the tonsillar fossa and also separates the isthmus of fauces from the oropharynx; also known as pharyngopalatine arch, posterior palatine arch, posterior pillar of fauces

arcuate arched, bow-shaped

arcuate fasciculus a primary association fiber tract within each cerebral hemisphere; connects Wernicke's area in the temporal lobe with Broca's area in the frontal lobe of the language-dominant hemisphere

arena assessment An assessment in which all team members are present throughout the entire evaluation

areola small cavity or space inside (more or less centered) a tissue

aria song, especially in the context of an opera

arm the upper extremity, especially the region from the elbow to the shoulder, often used for entire limb to wrist

Arnold-Chiari malformation congenital brainstem and lower cerebellum herniation extending though the foramen magnum into the cervical vertebra canal; can be associated with spina bifida and meningocele

array a selection of letters, numbers, punctuation marks, or computer commands commonly following predetermined plan or system; with personal computers, associated with scanning input

arrestor consonant following a vowel in a syllable

arrhythmia rhythm disturbance, generally cardiac; variety of etiologies, including adverse effect of drugs; alteration in force or rhythm

- **phasic sinus arrhythmia** dysrhythmia associated with respiratory rhythm, with speeded inspiration and slowed expiration

- **respiratory arrhythmia** irregularity in breathing rhythm other than phasic sinus arrhythmia; sometimes synonymous with phasic sinus arrhythmia

arterial blood gas (ABG) The oxygen and carbon dioxide dissolved in the arterial blood, measured by various means to assess patency of ventilation and oxygenation, as well as acid–base status. Concentration of O_2 is normally 95%, with partial pressure generally 80 to 100 mm Hg and CO_2 pressure usually 38 to 45 mm Hg. The typical pH of arterial blood is 7.40, ranging from 7.35 to 7.45

arteriogram an X-ray film of a damaged artery to determine its status, that is, whether it is open, blocked, weakened, or hemorrhaging

arteriosclerosis a chronic disease characterized by abnormal thickening and hardening of the arterial walls, with resulting loss of elasticity and blood supply—especially to the cerebrum and lower extremities

arthralgia pain in a joint without swelling or arthritis

arthritis inflammation of joints accompanied by movement limitation, pain, swelling

arthro-, arthr- prefix: joint; articulation

arthrology the study of joints

articulation the point of loose union between two structures, allowing movement between the units; also, shaping of vocal tract by positioning of its mobile walls such as lips, lower jaw, tongue body and tip, velum, epiglottis, pharyngeal sidewalls, and larynx; also, the modification of the vocal tone and airstream into distinctive connected speech or enunciation through movements of oral structures

- **coarticulation** the phenomenon in speech in which the attributes of successive speech units overlap in articulatory or acoustic patterns. That is, one feature of a speech unit may be anticipated during production of an earlier unit in the string (anticipatory or forward coarticulation) or retained during production of a unit that comes later (retentive or backward coarticulation)

- **manner of articulation** a phonetic feature of speech sounds that specifies the overall manner in which a sound is produced; the manner feature specifies whether a sound is voiced or voiceless, nasal or nonnasal, and so on

- **place of articulation** a phonetic feature of speech sounds that specifies the location in the mouth where the point of major constriction occurred when the sound was produced; the place feature specifies whether a sound is produced with a bilabial closure, an alveolar closure, and so on

- **tongue advancement** relative position of the tongue in the anterior–posterior (front-back) dimension of the vocal tract. As applied to vowels, tongue advancement relates primarily to the relative frequency of F_2 (second formant), or to the frequency difference between F_1 (first formant) and F_2. Front vowels tend to have relatively high F_2 values and a relatively large value of the F_2–F_1 difference

articulation disorder disorder of speech sound production; developmental disorder in which speech sounds are produced incorrectly or inadequately compared to normative standards; sometimes called a phonological disorder

articulators in speech production, the moveable and immobile structures used to produce the sounds of speech (tongue, lips, jaw, palate)

articulatory model a model that accounts for the movements of speech

articulatory synthesis a type of speech synthesis (machine-generated speech) in which the organs of the vocal tract are simulated and controlled to produce speechlike patterns

articulatory system in speech science, the system of structures involved in shaping the oral cavity for production of the sounds of speech

artifact what is incidental or not an actual occurrence, as phantom information in a histologic specimen or a graphic record that is caused by the study technique

- **chemical shift artifact** in an MRI, a dark area caused by a biochemical variation in resonant frequency of adjacent regions and not caused by a true anatomic separation

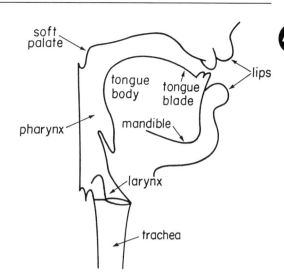

articulators in speech production, the moveable and immobile structures used to produce the sounds of speech (tongue, lips, jaw, palate)

aryepiglottic the arytenoid cartilage and the epiglottis; a fold of mucous membrane (aryepiglottic fold) and a muscle that is part of the fold (aryepiglottic muscle) that serve as a sphincter during swallowing

arytenoid cartilages paired, ladle-shaped cartilages to which the vocal folds are attached

arytenoid dislocation a condition frequently causing vocal fold immobility or hypomobility due to separation of the arytenoid cartilage from its joint and normal position atop the cricoid cartilage

ascending tract sensory pathway of the nervous system in the spinal cord that transmits impulses toward the brain, also afferent tract

Ascher syndrome articulation impaired by redundant and loose tissue of the upper lip; marked by drooping eyelids and benign thyroid enlargement

aspect character of the action of a verb as to its beginning, extent, fulfillment, or repetition and without reference to its position in time

asphyxia extreme hypoxia leading to consciousness loss and possibly death caused by such events as aspiration of vomit, foreign body in respiratory tract, drowning, electrical shock

aspirate speech sound characterized by breathiness ; in medicine, to remove by aspiration (by suction)

aspirate attack initiation of phonation preceded by air, producing /h/

aspiration the entry of foreign material into the airway past the level of the vocal folds. Also, in speech, the sound made by turbulent airflow preceding or following vocal fold vibration, as in /ha/; in medicine, breathing into the lungs substances that do not belong there, such as food, water, or stomach contents following reflux. Aspiration may lead to infections, such as pneumonia. Also, the penetration of secretions or ingesta below the level of the true vocal folds. This can interfere with effective air exchange (and lead to asphyxiation, for instance) or cause pulmonary inflammation and infection (so-called aspiration pneumonia). Aspiration may occur prior to the actual swallow through an unguarded larynx, during the pharyngeal stage of swallowing from overflow of residue contained in the pharyngeal recesses or from reflux of gastric contents

aspiration pneumonia infection of the lung following aspiration

aspiration pneumonitis inflammation (not necessarily due to infection) of the lung following aspiration

- **chronic aspiration** repeated or intractable episodes of aspiration

- **postprandial aspiration** aspiration in relationship to a meal

- **toxic aspiration** inhalation of substances such as strong acids, strong bases, or petrochemicals that lead to rapid, direct injury to the airspaces

assessment appraisal and/or evaluation; the process of conducting such appraisal, which includes interviewing, observing, and testing

- **arena assessment** assessment in which all team members are present throughout the evaluation

- **biopsychosocial** a holistic approach that takes into account a person's medical (biological), psychological, and social needs

- **criteria-based assessment** an assessment model that focuses on obtaining information in a decision tree format, as in determining which AAC system to implement

- **daily log** process for assessing conversational fluency and communication handicap, in which respondents self-monitor behaviors of interest and provide self-reports; usually completed more than once over a set period of time

- **dynamic assessment** approach to evaluation focused on the different ways by which an individual achieves a score rather than the score achieved; approach is characterized by guided learning to determine an individual's potential for change

- **feature matching** assessment process that matches the skills of the nonspeaking individual to the features of a given AAC system

- **informal assessment** assessment procedures that do not rely on formal or standardized tests; often designed by a clinical practitioner to accommodate the special abilities or limitations of an individual examined

- **maximal assessment** assessment model consisting of a thorough evaluation of an individual's abilities across cognitive, academic, perceptual, linguistic, and motor areas. Information is gathered across all domains

- **nonstandardized assessment** evaluation of abilities through informal procedures

- **objective assessment** demonstrable, reproducible, usually quantifiable evaluation, generally relying on instrumentation or other assessment techniques that do not involve primarily opinion, as opposed to subjective assessment

- **predictive assessment** assessment process consisting of a focused evaluation that evaluates those skills necessary for developing an AAC prescription by matching the skills of the nonspeaking individual to the features of a given AAC system. Predictive assessment is sometimes referred to as the "feature matching" process

- **standardized assessment** evaluation of abilities using formal test instruments

- **subjective assessment** evaluation that depends on perception and opinion, rather than independently reproducible quantifiable measures, as opposed to objective assessment

assimilation a process of cognitive adaptation in which new experiences are organized into existing schemes. Also, a process whereby an individual or group loses the heritage language and culture, which are replaced by the language and culture of the dominant group

assimilation processes a group of phonological processes in which the productions of dissimilar phonemes sound more alike; in phonological treatment, the objective is to eliminate such processes; major assimilation processes include:

- **devoicing** substitution of a voiceless sound for a voiced (e.g., /k/ for /g/ in final positions)

- **devoicing of final consonants** substitution of a voiceless final consonant for a voiced (e.g., /t/ for /d/ in syllable = final position)

- **labial assimilation** substitution of a labial sound for a nonlabial (e.g., /b/ for /d/)

- **nasal assimilation** substitution of a nasal consonant for a non-nasal (e.g., /n/ for /d/)

- **prevocalic voicing** substitution of a voiced sound for a voiceless sound preceding a vowel (e.g., /b/ for /p/ in prevocalic positions)

- **reduplication** repetition of a syllable, sometimes resulting in substitution of one syllable for another (e.g., wawa for water)

- **velar assimilation** substitution of a velar consonant for a nonvelar (e.g., /g/ for /d/)

assist-control mode (A/C) a mode of mechanical ventilatory support. The ventilator will respond to the patient's spontaneous breathing efforts by delivering air volume and a preset number of breaths if a patient fails to inspire within a set period; continuous mandatory ventilation is synonymous

assisted exercise an exercise requiring the assistance of another person or an adaptive device

assistive listening device (ALD) a system that improves communication with persons who are hearing-impaired by enhancing the signal-to-noise (S/N) ratio. The referees at NFL games switch on their FM systems when they want to be heard over the din of the crowd. Similarly, when a person with hearing impairment needs to get the clearest possible signal from the person talking, the best thing to do is to place the microphone for the ALD next to the mouth of the speaker and deliver the signal with as little distortion as possible to the ear of the listener. Some ALDs are FM radio systems functioning as miniature sending and receiving stations. Others use infrared (IR) modulation technology and still others are simply hand-held amplifiers attached to a set of earphones

assistive listening system a setup that delivers sound to individuals with peripheral or central auditory deficits to mitigate listening problems (e.g., frequency-modulated [FM] systems, personal amplifiers, infrared systems)

- **assistive technology** the use of aided tools to improve the skills, abilities, lifestyle, and independence of individuals with disabilities. Eyeglasses, hearing aids, Braille codes, bathroom and kitchen aids, wheelchairs, and AAC devices are examples

- **assistive technology device** commercially available, adapted, or custom designed equipment used to enhance the functional abilities of individuals with disabilities

assistive technology service defined by federal law as any service that directly assists an individual with a disability in the selection, acquisition, or use of an assistive technology device

associated features of stuttering effects of stuttered speech on the adjustment or behavior of an individual

associated monologue a mode of play behavior in which children playing together contribute individual monologues related to the same topic

association fibers neurons that transmit information between two regions of the same cerebral hemisphere

associative control ability to state issues relevant to a designated topic without using tangential remarks

astasia inability to stand or sit without help because of motor discoordination

astereognosis not capable of identifying shapes or forms by touch

asthenia debility, or weakness

asthma obstructive pulmonary (lung) disease most commonly associated with bronchospasm, and difficulty expiring air; marked by recurrence of wheezing with inspiration/expiration caused by bronchial constriction, along with paroxysmal dyspnea, coughing, and viscous mucoid bronchial secretions

astrocytes a form of large neuroglial cell having a star-like shape

astrocytoma brain tumor in which all grades of malignancy occur—from slow growth with fairly typical cells to rapid growth invasive tumors

asymmetrical tonic neck reflex (ATNR) a postural reflex often seen in children with cerebral palsy. When the head is rotated, the ATNR causes an extension in the arm and leg on the side to which the face is turned, while the opposite site increases in flexion; can be elicited by turning an infant's head laterally in a supine position. Visible evidence includes extension of the extremities on the chin side or flexion on the occiput side. The ATNR is commonly persistent in children with severe motor deficits. In typically developing infants, it disappears by about 6 months

asymmetry disproportion, imbalance, or inequality between two corresponding parts located on either side of a central axis

asymptomatic no obvious signs of a disease process

asynchronous a computer process in which one operation is completed before the following action is initiated

asynergy lack of coordination, often referring to the activation of agonist and antagonist muscles; decomposition of movement results when severe; found in disturbances of the cerebellum

ataxia deficit in motor coordination; also, total or partial inability to coordinate voluntary bodily movements, especially skilled muscular movements; often tied to injury to the cerebellum or posterior spinal cord columns; can involve the trunk, head, or limbs

ataxia-telangiectasia progressive cerebellar ataxia can lead to dysarthria, spasmodic dysphonia, and later (10 years of age) language problems from cognitive impairment; also marked by athetosis, relative small stature

ataxic dysarthria a type of motor speech disorder with a neuropathology of damage to the cerebellar system; characterized by slow, inaccurate movement and hypotonia; all aspects of speech may be involved, but articulatory and prosodic problems dominate; specific symptoms include imprecise consonants, excess and equal linguistic stress, and irregular articulatory breakdowns

atelectasis an area of collapsed lung (alveoli) that occurs when there is a failure of lung expansion or reabsorption of gas from the alveoli; may occur, for example, when there are excessive secretions in portions of the lungs

atherosclerosis an impairment of the blood vessels (especially arteries) due to a gradual accumulation of fatty deposits within their inner lining, if severe, normal blood flow may be permanently obstructed; characterized by fibrosis and calcification of afflicted vessels

atherosclerotic narrowing thickening and hardening of the medium- and large-sized coronary arteries, usually due to the formation of plaques (fat deposits)

athetosis constantly recurring series of writhing, slow, continuous, purposeless motions of the extremities (hands and feet), usually the result of a brain lesion (extrapyramidal) in the basal ganglia, tabes dorsalis, or conditions such as cerebral palsy

atlas the first cervical vertebra; articulating with the occipital bone and the axis

atmospheric pressure pressure of the atmosphere generated by its weight, at sea level, approximately 29.92 inches or 760 mm Hg (mercury), 1013.25 Mb (millibars) or 101,325 pa (pascals)

atonic normal tone is lacking, weak and without vigor, relaxed

atresia failure of development of a patent body opening

- **esophageal atresia** congenital breakdown of esophageal lumen development, often seen with tracheoesophageal fistula (TEF)

- **laryngeal atresia** may result in fusion or congenital webbing of the vocal folds or failure of development of the trachea, often near top or bottom of glottis

atrial septal defect (ASD) anomalous (usually congenital) opening between the two upper chambers of the heart

atrophy loss or wasting of tissue. Muscle atrophy occurs, for example, in an arm that is immobilized in a cast for many weeks (disuse atrophy) or in a limb that loses neural stimulation (denervation atrophy)

attachment the development of recognition and expectations for interaction between caregivers and infants; bonding

attention gateway to conscious experience; maintains primacy of certain information in ongoing information processing; mental concentration maintenance

alternating attention ability to shift attention between tasks that have different cognitive demands

- **divided attention skill** aspect of attention enabling a person to appropriately allocate focus and time between a series of activities

- **focused attention** attention required to recall information needed to complete an activity, usually under a timed constraint

- **joint attention** shared attention on a context by partners of visual and/or auditory attention

- **selective (focused) attention** ability to focus on relevant stimuli while ignoring simultaneously presented, but irrelevant stimuli (i.e., distractors)

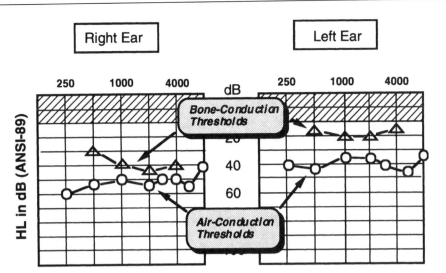

audiogram a graphic representation of hearing thresholds as a function of stimulus frequency. The two ears may be represented on separate graphs or on the same graph

- **sustained attention (vigilance)** ability to inhibit interference; requires sustained focus while waiting for a target stimulus to happen

attention deficit disorder (ADD) cognitive deficit that limits an individual's ability to pay attention and stay focused on a task; may involve restlessness, distractibility, and hyperactivity

attention deficit hyperactivity disorder (ADHD) persistent pattern of inattention and/or hyperactivity-impulsivity that is more frequent and severe than is typically observed in individuals at a comparable level of development; manifested in at least two settings; interferes with developmentally appropriate social, academic, or occupational functions; and has been present before age 7 years. Characterized by 3 types:

- **combined type** attention deficit characterized by hyperactivity-impulsivity and inattention

- **predominantly hyperactive-impulsive type** behavioral regulation disorder

- **predominantly inattentive type** presents with primary symptoms of inattention

attractor a geometric figure in state space to which all trajectories in its vicinity are drawn. The four types of attractors are point, limit cycle, toroidal, and strange. A point trajectory draws all trajectories to a single point. An example is a pendulum moving toward rest. A limit cycle is characteristic of periodic motion. A toroidal attractor represents quasiperiodic motion (often considered a subset of periodic

motion). A strange attractor is associated with chaotic motion

attribution relational words early relational words that refer to the attributes or characteristics of objects

attrition wearing away or loss

audible loud enough to be heard

audience persons whose presence may set the occasion for an address or naming response, influence whether an utterance occurs, or influence the form of the utterances that do occur

audile person who learns best by listening (audition) as opposed to looking

audiogram a graphic representation of hearing thresholds as a function of stimulus frequency. The two ears may be represented on separate graphs or on the same graph

- **corner audiogram** an audiogram that displays a profound hearing loss, with thresholds measurable only in the low frequencies

- **flat audiogram** audiogram configuration in which the thresholds across frequencies are similar

audio input, direct (DAI) hard-wired connection that leads directly from a sound source to a hearing aid or other listening device

audiologic rehabilitation term often used synonymously with aural rehabilitation or aural habilitation; sometimes may entail greater emphasis on the provision and follow up of listening devices and less emphasis on communication strategies training and speech perception training

audiologist specialist trained in the identification, assessment, and treatment/rehabilitation of hearing disorders who has academic accreditation in the practice of audiology

audiometer electronic instrument used for the measurement of hearing sensitivity

audiometric zone lowest sound pressure level that can just be detected by an average adult ear at any particular frequency; designated as 0 dB hearing level (HL) on an audiogram

audiometry specialized test for sensitivity of hearing

- **behavioral audiometry** test requiring a behavioral response from a patient

- **Békésy audiometry** an automatic process employing the Békésy audiometer that produces two readings for comparison of discrimination of interrupted tone and continuous tone, with results often informative for middle-ear, cochlear or CN VIII lesions; from Georg von Békésy (1899–1972)

- **impedance audiometry** battery of measures designed to assess middle ear functioning, including tympanometry and acoustic reflex threshold determination

- **industrial audiometry** assessment of hearing at regular intervals to assess the effects of noise exposure, as well as the measurement of industrial noise levels

- **play audiometry** behavioral method for testing the hearing thresholds of young children, in which correct identification of a stimulus presentation is rewarded by allowing the child to participate in a play-oriented activity

- **pure tone audiometry** checks an individual's capability of discriminating frequencies and includes comparison of air conduction and bone conduction tests

- **speech audiometry** measurement of speech listening skills, including speech awareness and speech recognition

- **visual reinforcement audiometry (VRA)** audiometric technique used with young children in which a correct response to a stimulus presentation is reinforced by a visual reward, such as the activation of a lighted toy

audiovisual combined or concurrent auditory and visual stimulation; learning aid employing visual and auditory aspects/symbols

audition hearing

auditory acuity sharpness and clarity with which sound is perceived

auditory-articulatory map knowledge a speaker of a language learns early in life that links specific movements of the person's articulators to the specific sounds caused by those movements

auditory association area cortical area surrounding the primary auditory cortex in the temporal lobe; responsible for interpreting the significance of sounds

auditory brainstem response (ABR) also called BAER (brainstem auditory evoked response); an electrophysiologic record of the synchronous discharge of auditory nerve fibers in response to a click or brief tone burst. It is the most commonly available procedure for assisting in the diagnosis of hearing impairment in infants and young children. It can also be used to uncover hidden damage to the auditory nervous system

auditory closure the ability to recognize a whole word despite the absence of certain elements

- **auditory closure, verbal** the ability to use spoken contextual information to facilitate speech recognition

auditory discrimination ability to differentiate specific sounds by their source or acoustical properties

auditory discrimination training treatment designed to teach clients to distinguish between correct and incorrect productions of speech sounds; often used on the assumption that auditory discrimination training is a precursor to speech sound production training; assumption questioned by some clinicians who believe that production training will induce discrimination as well; same as perceptual training

auditory evoked potential (AEP) small electrical potential superimposed by auditory input on the steady-state electrical activity of the brain. Usually detectable only by signal averaging

auditory meatus auditory canal

- **external auditory meatus** tubelike passage from the auricle to the tympanum of the middle ear

- **internal auditory meatus** short connection from the temporal bone to the fundus near the vestibule: contains CN VIII

auditory memory acquisition, storage, and retrieval of auditory sound patterns in both short-term and long-term form, frequently in a specified sequence

auditory nerve (or cranial nerve or vestibulocochlear nerve) CN VIII, the eighth cranial nerve, important for transmitting auditory and balance sensation from the inner ear to the brain

auditory perception identification, interpretation, or organization of sensory data received through the ear

- **natural auditory boundaries** enhanced abilities to discriminate between sounds; present at birth in the absence of experience and is not attributable to special language-acquisition devices, but instead to the natural operation of the auditory perceptual mechanism

auditory processing integrating what is heard with other knowledge, such as language understanding and usage

auditory scanning a scanning technique whereby an AAC user activates his or her switch when he or she hears the desired item spoken

auditory sequential memory ability to remember sounds, words, phrases, and sentences in a specified sequence

auditory targets, stored auditory memories of sounds contained in the native language that guide speakers' attempts to produce articulatory movements matching those sounds

auditory trainer, FM classroom assistive listening device in which the teacher wears a microphone and the signal is transmitted to the student(s) by means of frequency modulated (FM) radio waves

auditory training instruction designed to maximize an individual's use of residual hearing by means of both formal and informal listening practice

augmentative (assistive) and alternative communication (AAC) aided or unaided communication modes used as a supplement to or as an alternative to oral language, including gestures, sign language, picture symbols, the alphabet, and computers with synthetic speech

- **dedicated AAC systems** AAC equipment specifically designed to operate only as communication aids

- **nondedicated AAC systems** devices not specifically designed for communication that can be adapted to function as AAC devices (e.g., computers)

augmentative communication any system used to supplement or augment speech/voice or oral communication

aural habilitation sometimes used synonymously with aural rehabilitation; intervention for persons who have not developed listening, speech, and language skills; may include diagnosis of communication and hearing-related difficulties, speech perception training, speech and language therapy, manual communication, and educational management

aural/oral method an instructional method used to teach children with significant hearing loss using hearing, speechreading, and spoken language, but not manual communication

aural rehabilitation intervention aimed at minimizing or alleviating the communication difficulties associated with hearing loss; may include diagnosis of hearing loss and communication handicap, amplification, counseling, communication strategies training, speech perception training, family instruction, speech-language therapy, and educational management

auricle (also pinna) the outermost, visible, cartilaginous portion of the ear

auricular tubercle bulge on superior-posterior aspect of helix

auroscope instrument used for examining ears

auscultation a method of listening to body sounds, especially sounds in the lungs, for diagnosis. Cervical auscultation involves the placement of a stethoscope on the larynx to listen to the "sounds" of the swallow paired with inspiration and exhalation

autism developmental disorder affecting communication and social skills; characteristics may include delayed language, insistence on preservation of sameness and stereotypies

autoclave an appliance for heat sterilization that employs steam under high pressure

autoclitic a secondary verbal operant in which a conventional form (a tag, word, or order) comments on the relationships among the primary verbal operants; the behavioral equivalent to syntax and grammar

autoclitic frames B. F. Skinner's concept of certain orders in verbal responses that express relationships among stimuli

autocorrelation an analytic procedure in which a signal is correlated with a time-shifted version of itself (auto = self). If the signal is periodic, the autocorrelation function will have a peak at the time-shift value corresponding to a fundamental period. If the signal is aperiodic, the autocorrelation function will not have conspicuous peaks at any time-shift value. Autocorrelation is sometimes used to determine the fundamental frequency of a speech signal

autoimmune disease a disease characterized by alteration or sabotage of the body's immune system

automatic gain control (AGC) nonlinear hearing aid compression circuitry that changes gain as signal level changes and/or limits the output of a device (e.g., hearing aid) when the level reaches a specified value

automatic reinforcers sensory consequences of responses that reinforce those responses (e.g., the sensation a child with autism derives from banging his or her head)

automatic scanning a scanning technique in which the indicator moves automatically and continuously once the switch is hit, until the AAC user hits the switch again to interrupt the scanning at the selected communication item

automatic speech recognition (machine speech recognition) the recognition of speech by machine

autonomic independently functioning, acting independently of volition; relating to the autonomic nervous system

autonomic innervation part of the nervous system that innervates the visceral organs. It has two divisions, the sympathetic and parasympathetic

autonomic nervous system portion of nervous system controlling involuntary body functions such as the cardiac muscle, smooth muscle, and glands. It has two aspects, the parasympathetic and sympathetic

- **parasympathetic nervous system** autonomic nervous system craniosacral aspect, with effects including bronchiole and pupil constriction, alimentary canal smooth muscle contraction, heart rate moderation, and some glandular secretion

- **sympathetic nervous system** thoracolumbar autonomic nervous system portion, with effects including heart rate increase, bronchiole and pupil dilation, skin, viscera, and skeletal muscle vasodilation, peristalsis moderation, liver conversion of glycogen to glucose, and secretion of epinephrine and norephinephrine by the adrenal medulla. This system helps prepare the body to deal with stress

autosomal dominant inheritance a 50% risk of inheriting an abnormal trait because of the presence of an abnormal (mutant) dominant gene on one of the autosomes from one parent; dominant genes can be expressed in an offspring, even if only one parent codes for the trait

autosomal recessive inheritance a 25% risk of inheriting an abnormal trait because of the presence of an abnormal (mutant) recessive gene on one of the autosomes in both parents; both halves of a gene pair must be the same copy of the gene to be expressed. If only one gene copy is provided and the other pair member is not the mutant gene, the child is normal phenotypically, but is a carrier of the recessive trait, because he or she has one copy of the mutant allele

autosomes 22 pairs of human chromosomes are called autosomes and carry the majority of human genetic information, but do not play a role in sex determination

auxiliary respiratory muscles accessory muscles of breathing that assist in the expansion or compression of the rib cage by fixing, elevating, or depressing the ribs. They include muscles of the thoracic cavity, abdominal wall, and back. Contraction may allow for deep inhalation, forced exhalation, or performance of a Valsalva maneuver

auxiliary verb grammatical verbs that serve as helping verbs by conveying number and tense

avascular necrosis death of tissue due to lack of blood supply

A-weighted scale a filtering network used in a sound pressure level meter weighted to provide an equal loudness contour at 40 phones; sound level measurements made with this scale are designated with a dB(A)

axial in imaging, slices taken at 90° to the long axis of the body, the same axis as slices through a loaf of bread; orientation to long axis of the body

axial skeleton the bones of the axis of the skeleton, including the skull, veterbrae, ribs, sternum

axial tomograms radiographic slices taken at 90° to the long axis of the body

axis imaginary line through the center of the body

axoaxonic synapse synapse, with axon of one neuron actually touching axon of second neuron

axodendritic synapse synapse involving contact between the axon of one neuron and a dendrite of another

axodendrosomatic synapse synapse in which axon of one neuron touches dendrites and cell body of second neuron

axon the process of a neuron that conducts information away from the soma or body of the neuron. Axons tend to have few branches and can vary greatly in length; relays action potentials and self-propagating impulses

A

B

Bronchioles

small divisions of bronchial tree

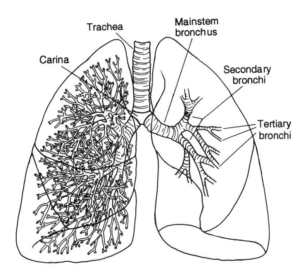

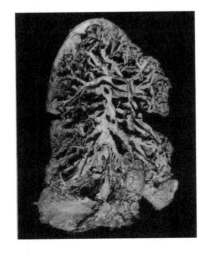

babbling nonmeaningful sequences of consonants and vowels produced by infants

- **fully resonant nuclei** infant tone productions (4 to 6 months) that closely approximate mature vowels

- **marginal babbling** infant sound productions with a variety of vowels and consonantlike productions that approximate CV syllables

- **nonreduplicated babbling (**also **variegated babbling)** final babbling state, which consists of strings of varied and multiple syllables, approximating true word form

- **reduplicated babbling** babbling in which a syllable is repeated in strings, as in *dadada*

Babinski reflex dorsiflexion of the great toe and spreading of other toes on stimulation of the ventral surface of the foot. This is normal in infants but is an indicator of a pyramidal tract lesion in children and adults

Babinski sign series of partial indicators of varying extent of upper motor neuron disease: no ankle jerk in sciatica; extensor plantar response with big toe extension and other toe adduction; more platysma on unaffected side during blowing or whistling; pronation of arm affected by paralysis that is placed in supination; and when patient attempts to sit from the supine position (with arms crossed over chest), thigh flexes and heel raises on affected side, with other leg continuing to be flat

Baby Jane Doe regulations U.S. Health and Human Services Department rules requiring state governments to check complaints about parental choices for treatment of infants with disability

baby talk characteristic speech patterns, including shorter phrases and exaggerated intonation, used when talking to infants

Bacillus genus of gram-positive aerobic, spore-producing bacteria in the Bacillaceae family

background noise extraneous noise that masks the acoustic signal of interest

backing phonological error pattern with alveolar consonants being replaced by velar consonants, such as "tee" being replaced by [ki]

backward chain series of sequenced behaviors, with the last steps of the sequence being taught first and teaching backward to the beginning of the chain; frequently used to teach self-help skills

bacterium, pl. **bacteria** tiny unicellular microorganism that generally reproduces by cell division; may be aerobic, anaerobic, parasitic or pathogenic

bagging, manual process of supplying breaths by a manual resuscitation bag, often used to oxygenate a patient before attempting intubation or when a patient is temporarily disconnected from mechanical ventilation

Baller-Gerold syndrome speech production onset and language may be delayed secondary to cognitive impairment and/or motor delay; marked by craniosynostosis, hypoplasia of the radius

Bamatter syndrome speech production may be delayed secondary to hypotonia, with articulation hampered by lax facial skin and muscle, as well as malocclusion from prognathism; face has an aged appearance

band-pass filter filter that allows frequencies only within a certain frequency range to pass

band-reject filter electrical device that attenuates signal frequencies within a specified frequency band between high and low extremes

bands range of adjacent parameter values; a frequency band is an ensemble of adjacent frequencies

bandwidth a measure of the frequency band of a sound, especially a resonance. Conventionally, bandwidth is determined at the half-power (3 dB down) points of the frequency response curve. That is, both the lower and higher frequencies that define the bandwidth are 3 dB less intense than the peak energy in the band

barbiturate a chemical derivative of barbituric acid that produces a calming effect; used to induce sleep and to control seizures; has potential for mental and/or physical dependence with prolonged frequent use

baritone the most common male vocal range; higher than bass and lower than tenor; singer's formant around 2600 Hz

barium swallow, modified (MBS) dynamic (moving) X-ray examination of oral and pharyngeal swallowing function, with a barium bolus studied through fluoroscopic observation

Bark scale a nonlinear transformation of frequency that is thought to correspond to the analysis accomplished by the ear, is closely related to the concept of critical band in auditory perception

baroreceptors pressure sensors; pressure-sensitive nerve endings in various cardiac walls that provide for physiologic adaptation to blood pressure changes; homeostasis depends on baroreception

barotrauma injury lung tissue secondary to a change in pressure. May occur when excessive lung volumes are used

Barrett's esophagus columnar metaplasia of the lower esophagus. The normal squamous epithelium is replaced by benign lesions caused by chronic reflux of acidic digestive juices, which severely damages the esophageal mucosa. Associated with chronic reflux esophagitis and considered a premalignant lesion that can lead to adenocarcinoma; symptoms include dysphagia, heartburn, and decreased lower esophageal sphincter pressure

barrier, access obstacle to an individual's use of AAC caused by limitations in an individual's capabilities, attitudes, or resources; cognitive, perceptual, motoric, and literacy deficits are examples of access barriers

barrier, opportunity barrier imposed by other persons or obstacles in the consumer's environment that impede an individual's ability to use AAC; outmoded policies, negative attitudes, limited knowledge, and lack of communication opportunities are examples of opportunity barriers

barrio Spanish for neighborhood. Used in the United States for areas where many Latinos live

basal ganglia (basal nuclei) nuclei deep within the cerebral hemispheres; currently synonymous with the caudate and lentiform nuclei (striate body), as well as the associated subthalamic nucleus and substantia nigra (see illustration, p. 30)

basal readers reading texts that use simplified vocabulary and syntax and are employed in class sets

base the lower, or supporting, portion of a structure

baselines recorded rates of responses for comparison with unknown aspects of planned intervention; baselines must reflect reliability or stability of repeated measurement; help establish clinician accountability; in treatment and research, baselines help rule out extraneous variables; preintervention measurement of a patient's skills

basement membrane delicate, noncellular structure immediately beneath the epithelium that secures the epithelium to the underlying tissue

base pair pairs of amino acids that connect two strands of intertwined sugar and phosphate molecules to form DNA

basic interpersonal communication skills (BICS) the language skills that are normally required by all members of a speech community as a first language and used for basic social interactions with other members of the speech community

basic unit of speech perception the question about whether the unit analyzed by listeners in speech perception is the phonetic feature, the phoneme, the syllable, or the word; research suggests that the unit of perception may vary with the task and that listeners analyze many different levels simultaneously during speech perception

basilar membrane a membrane forming the floor of the cochlear duct within the inner ear that supports the sensory end organ for hearing, the organ of Corti, along the length of the cochlea

bass baritone voice range between bass and baritone. Not as heavy as basso profundo, but typically with greater flexibility. Must be able to sing at least as high as F4. Also known as *basso contante* and *basso guisto*. Baritones with bass quality are also called *basse taille*

basso lowest male voice. Singers formant around 2300 Hz–2400 Hz

basso profundo deep bass; the lowest and heaviest of the bass voices. Can sing at least as low as D2 with full voice; singer's formant around 2200 Hz–2300 Hz

battered child syndrome child can exhibit bruises, scratches, burns, hematomas, or fractures of the long bones, ribs, or skull from abuse by an adult; there may be poor skin condition and malnutrition

battery a group of two or more voltaic cells that produce electricity; set of diagnostic tests

baud unit of measure of transmission speed; measure of the number of signal-state changes per second; for example, voltage or frequency changes; sometimes, but not always, the same as the number of bits per second; after J.M.E. Baudot (1845–1903); originally baud was used for telegraph transmissions and meant 1 Morse code dot per second

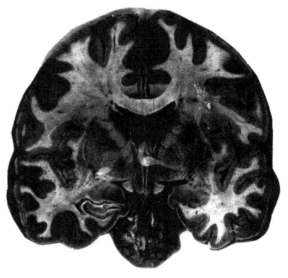

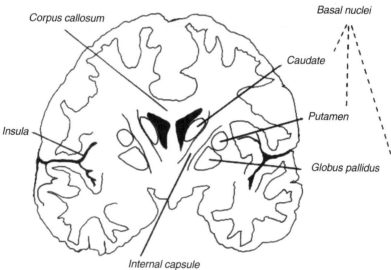

Corpus callosum

Basal nuclei

Caudate

Putamen

Insula

Globus pallidus

Internal capsule

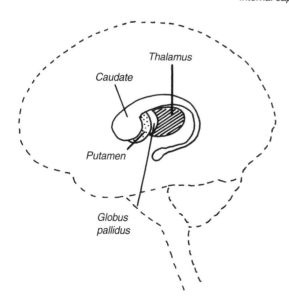

Thalamus

Caudate

Putamen

Globus pallidus

basal ganglia (basal nuclei) nuclei deep within the cerebral hemispheres; currently synonymous with the caudate and lentiform nuclei (striate body), as well as the associated subthalamic nucleus and substantia nigra

Beckwith-Wiedemann syndrome hypotonia and cognitive impairment can lead to speech-language delay, with articulation disorders secondary to large tongue and malocclusion (prognathism) common; marked by large birth size, ear lobe creases, and enlarged liver, spleen, and kidneys

behavior way of conducting oneself; response through action to stimulation

- **aberrant behavior** behavior that deviates from what is considered typical or desirable

- **chaotic behavior** distinct from random or periodic behavior. A chaotic system looks disorganized or random but is actually deterministic, although aperiodic. It has sensitive dependence on initial condition, has definite form, and is bounded to relatively narrow range (unable to go off into infinity)

- **conceptual behavior** responding to a variety of items that are related by some feature defining them as a class

- **incompatible behaviors** actions that cannot be produced simultaneously, such as sitting and walking; used to reduce certain undesirable behaviors

- **learned behavior** any behavior that primarily results from experience and interaction

- **noninteractive communication behaviors** characteristic of a passive conversational style; includes failure to contribute to the development of a conversational topic, minimal response to turn-taking signals, and a proclivity to bluff

- **operant behavior** behavior that is influenced by the consequences it produces

- **periodic behavior** action repeating over and over again over a finite time interval. Periodic behavior is governed by an underlying deterministic process

- **prechaotic behavior** predictable behavior preceding the onset of chaotic behavior. One example is period doubling

- **random behavior** action that never repeats itself and is inherently unpredictable

- **social behavior** any behavior that occurs in relation to others and influences their behavior

- **uncertainty behaviors (or verbal fragmentations)** excessive interjections and filler sometimes noted in utterances of aging individuals

behavioral audiometry tests of hearing that require a behavioral response from a patient

behaviorism a philosophical perspective on learning and behavior that emphasizes observable behaviors and their effects

Behçet's syndrome condition characterized by aphthous ulcers on various mucosal surfaces

behind-the-ear hearing aid (BTE) a hearing aid that is worn over the pinna and is coupled to the ear canal by means of an earmold

Békésy audiometry an automatic process employing the Békésy audiometer that produces two readings for comparison of discrimination of interrupted tone and continuous tone, with results often informative for middle-ear, cochlear, or CN VIII lesions (for George von Békésy, 1899–1972)

bel unit for sound intensity that is the logarithm (base 10) of the ratio of the power of a specific sound and the power for a reference sound, which is most commonly 10^{-16} per sq cm, the approximate threshold of hearing of the typical human ear at 1000 Hz

bel canto literally means "beautiful singing" and is a method and philosophical approach to singing voice production

Bell's palsy uncontrollable quivering or tremor of the facial nerve that is usually unilateral and can be permanent or transient

belly abdomen; the wide, fleshy portion of a muscle

benign tumors noncancerous tumors that are not able to metastasize or spread to distant sites

benzodiazepine a chemical class of psychoactive tranquilizer and hypnotic drugs that are used as sedatives, anxiety suppressants, and sleeping pills. This class includes diazepam (Valium), lorazepam (Ativan), chlordiazepoxide (Librium)

Bernoulli principle the effect dictating that given a constant volume flow of air or fluid at a point of constriction, there will be a decrease in air pressure perpendicular to the flow and an increase in velocity of the flow

Bernstein test a test whereby acid is dripped into the distal esophagus through a nasogastric tube and the patient's symptoms are recorded; used to help determine whether a patient has gastroesophageal reflux (GER)

beta blocker a medication that blocks action of the sympathetic or other adrenergic nerve fibers; often selective for cardiac receptors; generic drugs often end in "olol"

bi- prefix: two

bifurcate two-forked; to split into two parts or channels

bifurcation a sudden qualitative change in the behavior of a system. In chaos, for example, a small change in the initial parameters of a stable (predominantly linear) system may cause oscillation between two different states as the non-linear aspects of the system become manifest. This transition is a bifurcation

big books used frequently in whole language classrooms, they are teachers' books that are physically large enough for students to see and to be able to read along with the teacher

bilabial consonants formed using both lips. American English bilabial consonants are [p], [b], [m], [w]

bilateral on both sides

bilateral vocal fold paralysis loss of the ability to move both vocal folds caused by neurologic dysfunction

bilevel ventilation (BiPAP) a method of non-invasive mechanical ventilation which provides an inspiratory pressure as well as a lower expiratory pressure. It is a variation of CPAP

bilingual command of two languages

- **deficit model bilingual education** the child is perceived as having a language "deficit" that has to be compensated by remedial schooling. The problem is viewed as being in the child rather than in the school system or society or in the ideology of the perceiver. The opposite is an enrichment model

- **double immersion** schooling in which subject content is taught through a second and third language (e.g., Hebrew and French for first-language English speakers)

- **dual bilingual education (DBE)** two languages are used for approximately equal time in a curriculum

- **early exit/late exit bilingual education** early exit programs move children from bilingual classes in the first or second year of schooling. Late exit programs provide bilingual classes for three or more years of elementary schooling. Both programs exist in transitional bilingual education

- **enrichment bilingual education** develops bilingualism, thus enriching a person's life

- **immersion bilingual education** schooling in which some or most subject content is taught through a second, majority language

- **remedial bilingual education** also known as compensatory bilingual education. Uses the native tongue only to "correct" the students' presumed "deficiency" in the majority language

bilingualism the ability to speak two languages proficiently

- **additive bilingualism** the second language adds to and does not replace the first language

- **balanced bilingualism** approximately equal competence in two languages

- **exposure to language** simultaneous exposure to two different languages early in infancy or childhood

- **subtractive bilingualism** the second language replaces the first language

binaural for both ears

- **binaural advantage** the advantage of using both ears instead of one, such as better hearing thresholds and enhanced listening in the presence of background noise

- **binaural amplification** use of a hearing aid in each ear

- **binaural interaction** auditory processing involving the two ears and their neural connections

bio- prefix: living things

biofeedback a method used to reduce incorrect responses or shape and increase desirable responses in treatment; includes mechanical feedback given to the client on vocal pitch and intensity, respiration, galvanic skin response, and muscle action potential level; auditory and/or visual information on autonomic physiologic activities, with the individual learning, usually through trial-and-error, to self-control processes

biomechanics the study of the mechanics of human functioning, especially locomotion

biophysics the study of physical principles and methods in relation to living systems

biopsy removal of a small part of an organ tissue for diagnosis or treatment verification

biopsychosocial assessment a holistic approach to addiction assessment and treatment that accounts for a person's medical (biological), psychological, and social needs. This approach reflects the understanding that addiction affects the whole person and is influenced by a wide range of factors

biphasic a time-limited event or signal (including action potentials) possessing two distinct portions (e.g., one negative, another positive), as opposed to monophasic, triphasic, or polyphasic

bipolar disorder mood disorder in which there are episodes of either mania or depression; manic-depressive order is an older label

bipolar electrode electrode or electrode pair that measures electrical events (action potentials) at two distinct points; in electrophysiology, the resulting signals are usually supplied one to an inverting input, the other to a noninverting input of a differential amplifier; also pairs with one negative and one positive charge

bit a binary digit and the abbreviation for binary digit; the fundamental unit of information in a digital system. A bit has two possible values, conventionally expressed as 0 or 1; 16 bits equals one byte

bite occlusal relationship or chart of upper and lower jaws or teeth; gripping, holding cutting, or tearing with the teeth

- **persistent closed bite** the condition wherein supraversion of the anterior dental arch prohibits the posterior teeth from occlusion

- **persistent open bite** the condition wherein the incisors of upper and lower dental arches show a vertical gap from malocclusion of the posterior arch, which prohibits anterior contact

bite block a structure used experimentally or clinically to eliminate movement of the mandible during articulatory tasks; involves inserting a solid object into a person's mouth and requesting the individual to grip the item with his or her teeth

blackout a type of memory impairment that occurs when a person is conscious but cannot remember the blackout period. In general, blackouts consist of periods of amnesia or memory loss, typically caused by chronic, high-dose alcohol and/or drug abuse. Blackouts are most often caused by sedative-hypnotics such as alcohol and benzodiazepines; also temporary loss of consciousness from decreased cerebral blood supply

blade a wide, flat structure; a division of the tongue just posterior to the tip and anterior to the dorsum

-blast- combining form: elementary cell, such as embryonic germ cell; cell with ability to build tissue

blastocyst embryonic form in human development, a fluid-filled sphere containing embryonic cells formed about 8 days following fertilization, that implants in the uterine wall, also known as blastula (hollow ball of cells)

bleat fast vibrato, like the bleating of a sheep

blends consonant clusters

blended family nuclear family formed from two previously unrelated families; for example, a woman with her single biological child marries a man with his two biological children to form a blended family of two parents and three children

blepharitis eyelid inflammation from drugs or cosmetics put into the eye or on eyelid

Blissymbols a pictographic symbol system for communicatively impaired persons of all ages developed by Charles Bliss; composed of more than 2,000 graphic symbols; can be used on simple communication boards mounted on wheelchairs, on dedicated electronic devices with synthetic speech, and within computer software (see illustration, p. 34)

blocking Sudden obstruction or interruption in spontaneous flow of thought or speech

blood fluid pumped through body by the heart that transports nutrients and oxygen to the tissues and removes carbon dioxide and other waste byproducts for detoxification and/or excretion; basic plasma is a pale yellow/gray fluid, in which red and white blood cells are suspended

- **arterial blood gas (ABG)** The oxygen and carbon dioxide dissolved in the arterial blood, measured by various means to assess patency of ventilation and oxygenation, as well as acid–base status

- **blood gas determination** laboratory determination of blood pH and concentration/pressure of oxygen, carbon dioxide, and hydrogen ions

- **complete blood count** test determining count of red and white blood cells per cubic millimeter of blood

blood-brain barrier (BBB) a mechanism that prevents the transfer of most ions and large-molecular-weight compounds from the blood to brain tissue; the primary barrier is believed to be created by the modification of brain capillaries (as by reduction in fenestration and formation of tight cell-to-cell contacts) that prevents many substances from leaving the blood

Blissymbols

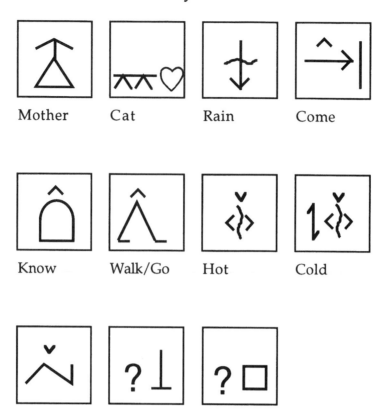

| Mother | Cat | Rain | Come |

| Know | Walk/Go | Hot | Cold |

| Sick | Who | What thing |

Blissymbols a pictographic symbol system for communicatively impaired persons of all ages developed by Charles Bliss; composed of more than 2,000 graphic symbols; can be used on simple communication boards mounted on wheelchairs, on dedicated electronic devices with synthetic speech, and within computer software.

and crossing the capillary walls into the brain tissues; similar capillaries are in the inner ear, retina, and iris; the BBB prevents or slows passage of some drugs, chemicals, radioactive ions, and such agents as viruses in the blood from entering the central nervous system

blood pressure (BP) the force or pressure of blood circulating through the arterial/vascular system

body hearing aid a hearing aid worn on the body; includes a box worn on the torso and a cord connecting to an ear-level receiver

bolus a ball or lump of masticated food ready to swallow; also, either a liquid or solid mass prepared for swallowing

bolus pressure (also luminal pressure) the pressure recorded within a liquid bolus within a free lumen. During pharyngeal and esophageal peristalsis, bolus pressure is typically much lower than squeeze pressure

bone hard, dense connective tissue of the body composing the skeleton; made of compact osseous materials that vary in porosity and flexibility

bone age skeletal age as estimated from the appearance of bones in X rays (also called anatomic age)

bone conduction transmission of sound through the bones in the body, particularly the skull

bone conductor vibrator or oscillator that is used to transmit sound to the bones of the skull through vibration

borderline personality disorder disorder beginning in early adulthood that features a pattern of unstable self-image, moods, and interpersonal relationships; marked by viewing persons or situations as either all good or all bad

bottom-up analyses analysis of an incoming message that proceeds by attempting to analyze the signal to determine which acoustic and phonetic features are contained in the message. The information that results from these analyses interacts with that derived by top-down analysis of speech

bottom-up model reading model that proposes reading proceeds from interpreting phonemes to words to phrases to sentences, and so forth

bottom-up processing information processing that is data driven; properties of the data are primary determinants of higher level representations and constructions

botulinum toxin (Botox) injection medical treatment procedure for neurogenic or idiopathic adductor spasmodic dysphonia and adductor spasmodic dysphonia that does not respond to behavioral treatment; botulinum toxin is injected into the thyroarytenoid muscle unilaterally or bilaterally; effects last about 3 months Also, a medical treatment for dystonias generally, as well as being used therapeutically to treat spasticity and for dermatological cosmetic procedures

botulism food poisoning from substances with the botulin toxin, which is destroyed by heat; toxin affects the central nervous system (CNS)

Boyle's law the law stating that, given a gas of constant temperature in a given container, the volume of a gas is inversely related to air pressure in the same conditions in the same container; the sum of pressure and volume of gas contained at a constant temperature remains constant; increase in gas volume will cause a decrease in air pressure and vice versa

brackets angled brackets ([ ]) enclosing sounds, indicating that the sound was produced without any claim that the sound is a phoneme of a language

brachy- short

brady- slow

bradycardia slowed heart rate

bradykinesia slowed physical movements; inability to make adjustments to posturing of the body; symptom of parkinsonism

brain attack a contemporary term for cerebral stroke; also used as a synonym for cardiovascular accident (CVA); term usage believed to help potential victims appreciate the urgency for rapid medical care with the onset of CVA symptoms, as is recognized for heart attack symptoms

brain imaging procedures used to map the structure and metabolic or electrophysiological properties of the brain; includes computed tomography (CT), magnetic resonance imaging (MRI), functional magnetic resonance imaging (fMRI), positron emission tomography (PET), regional cerebral blood flow, and brain electrical activity mapping

brain mapping procedure for identifying functional regions of the cerebral cortex by electrical stimulation during speech, reading, or other tasks

brainstem lower portion of the brain that connects the spinal cord to the midbrain and cerebral hemispheres; involved in the regulation of such motor, sensory, and reflex functions as breathing, blood pressure, and consciousness; composed of pons, medulla oblongata, and mesencephalon, mostly; the 12 cranial nerves (CN I–CN XII) arise from the brainstem

branchial pertaining to the anatomy of the throat and neck

• **branchial arches** the embryonic gill arches

bravura brilliant, elaborate, showy execution of musical or dramatic material

breath chewing a treatment technique involving the production of exaggerated chewing motions while vocalizing

breath group utterance produced on a single breath; sometimes used as a unit of prosody or intonation that can consist of several words or syllables

breathiness a voice quality that results when there is excessive air leakage during phonation because of inadequate approximation of the vocal folds; caused by various factors, this leads to air leakage (excessive airflow) during the quasiclosed phase, with this producing turbulence that is heard as noise mixed in the voice; treatment varies by cause

breathing exercises a treatment technique that focuses on achieving adequate respiratory support for speech

breathing, glossopharyngeal method of breathing than can possibly decrease an individual's dependence on mechanical ventilatory support; also called "frog breathing," it utilizes air injected into the lungs through the "gulping" action of the oral, pharyngeal, and pharyngeal muscles

breathing–swallowing coordination apnea that usually interrupts expiration in to protect the airway from food or liquid aspiration, with resumption of expiration after deglutition

brevis short; brief

Broca's aphasia aphasia characterized by loss of fluency and reduced paucity of vocabulary, usually arising from lesion in Brodmann areas 44 and 45 of the dominant cerebral hemisphere (Broca's area); characterized by good language comprehension, but poor speaking ability; patients often have anomia

Broca's area Brodmann areas 44 and 45 of the dominant cerebral hemisphere, responsible for motor planning for speech and components of expressive language; named after Pierre P. Broca (1824–1880)

Brodmann areas regions of the cerebral hemisphere identified by numeric characterization based on functional and anatomical organization; named for Korbinian Brodmann (1868–1918), scientific pioneer in studies of the mammalian cortex

bronch- prefix: windpipe

bronchi the two major branches from the trachea leading to right and left lungs

bronchial tree network of bronchi and bronchial tubes

bronchial tube divisions of the respiratory tree below the level of the mainstem bronchi

bronchiectasis lung condition following infection, often sustained in childhood. Also, chronic dilatation of the bronchi characterized by excessive sputum production and generally due to previous inflammation or infection of the airways

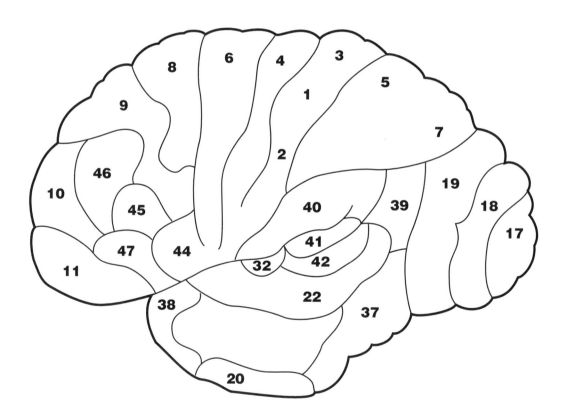

Brodmann Areas

Brodmann areas regions of the cerebral hemisphere identified by numeric characterization based on functional and anatomical organization; named for Korbinian Brodmann (1868– 1918), scientific pioneer in studies of the mammalian cortex

bronchioles small divisions of bronchial tree

bronchitis inflammation of the bronchial tubes in the lungs

- **chronic bronchitis** clinical syndrome of sputum production for at least 3 months in each of 2 successive years in a patient in whom other causes of chronic cough have been excluded

bronchoscope endoscope for inspecting the interior of tracheobronchial tree for diagnosis (including biopsy or culture retrieval) or to remove foreign objects or aspirate secretions from the respiratory tract; either standard tubular rigid metal instrument or flexible narrower fiberoptic bronchoscope

bronchospasm reflex constriction of the airways in response to a variety of stimuli, often associated with cough, wheezing, and mucus production

bronchus the primary division of the trachea, leading to the lungs on either side

bruit noise, especially an abnormal swishing or blowing sound heard during auscultation (as with a stethoscope)

bruxism grinding of the teeth

bucca- prefix: pertaining to the cheek

buccal cavity cavity lateral to the teeth, bounded by the cheek

buccal speech produced from air trapped inside cheeks that can be called "Donald Duck speech." Can be used to produce words and short phrases following tracheostomy

buffer a reserved area of memory (hardware device or a software routine) that temporarily holds a digital signal

bulbar pertaining to medulla oblongata (most caudal portion of brainstem)

bulbar palsy characterized by dysphagia, dysphonia, and/or dysarthria resulting from disease of the motor unit (i.e., including lower motor neurons [brainstem nuclei], cranial nerves, neuromuscular junctions, or muscles). Findings often include muscle atrophy and decreased reflexes of the face, tongue, and throat

bulimia serious eating disorder seen primarily in females, that is characterized by compulsive binge eating usually followed by self-induced vomiting or laxative or diuretic abuse; often accompanied by guilt and depression

burst noise created during the release of a stop consonant

bus a connecting system for the components of a microcomputer system. The type of bus determines the compatibility of add-in boards for a system

butterfly effect refers to the notion that in chaotic (nonlinear dynamics) systems a minuscule change in initial condition may have profound effects on the behavior of the system. For example, a butterfly flapping its wings in Hong Kong may change the weather in New York

buzzing a treatment technique involving the simultaneous reading aloud of rhyming sentences by a group

byte a unit of storage capable of holding a single character. A byte is equal to 8 bits on nearly all modern PCs. Large amounts of memory are indicated in terms of kilobytes (1,024 bytes), megabytes (1,048,576 bytes), and gigabytes (1,073,741,824 bytes)

C

Cleft

a fissure; divided: especially fissure that begins in an embryo, as the branchial cleft (facial cleft); clefts defined as craniofacial abnormalities can lead to serious problems in feeding and speech, which can be treated through surgery followed by therapeutic intervention

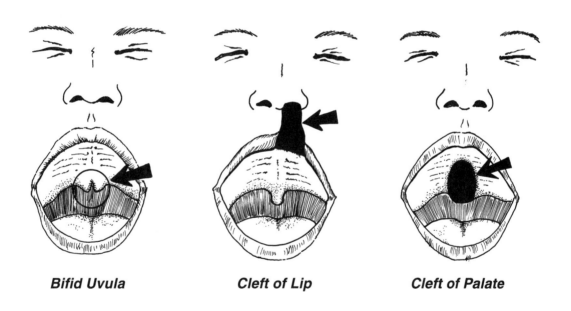

Bifid Uvula   **Cleft of Lip**   **Cleft of Palate**

cachexia profound weight loss, along with wasting, associated with emotional distress or chronic disease

café coronary collapse of a person while eating; characterized by choking, facial cyanosis, and eventual collapse caused by acute upper airway obstruction; generally caused by a bolus of meat

calcify to harden through the deposit of calcium salts

calcitonin gene-related peptide (CGRP) a neuropeptide that can serve as a transmitter within the CNS and is also present in the gastrointestinal tract

calendar age chronological age

CALP (cognitive academic language proficiency) level of language required to understand academically demanding subject matter in a classroom. Such usage is often abstract, lacking contextual supports such as gestures and viewing objects

canal a passageway or duct

cancer an abnormality in which cells no longer respond to the signals that control replication and growth. This results in uncontrolled growth and formation of various kinds of malignant neoplasms and may result in spread of tumor to distant locations (metastasis)

cancer staging process of defining scope and size of metastasis of a malignancy for developing treatment plan and predicting outcome

candida yeastlike fungus genus

Candida albicans microscopic fungal organism usually in the mouth mucous membranes, as well as intestinal tract and vagina. In some circumstances can cause superficial infections. Persons with HIV may have _C. albicans_ esophageal infection

cannula tracheostomy tube, a flexible tube for insertion into any body vessel, duct, or cavity to deliver medication or nutrition or to drain fluid

- **inner cannula** the internal portion of a tracheostomy tube that fits within the main or external structure of the tube; may be disposable or nondisposable

- **nasal cannula** delivers oxygen through the nose

- **outer cannula** the portion of the tracheostomy tube that forms the actual body of the tube (i.e., the external structure of the tube into which the inner cannula fits)

capacitance the ratio between the electrical charge given a conductive body and the potential difference between it and another adjacent charged body (unit: farad is the unit of capacitance equal to the capacitance of a capacitor between whose plates there appears a potential of 1 volt when it is charged by 1 coulomb of electricity); the property of a nonconductor of electricity allowing storage of energy from separation of the charge that occurs when opposite surfaces of the nonconductor are maintained at a difference of potential; also the measure of this property equal to the ratio of the charge on either surface to the potential difference between the surfaces

capillary microscopic blood vessel; the interface between the arterial and venous circulatory systems (joining arterioles and venules)

capillary hemangioma congenital vascular lesion, usually flat but may have elevated portions

capnography ongoing recording of the carbon dioxide level in expired air of patients who are mechanically ventilated; methods include infrared absorption and mass spectrometry

capsular referring to a capsule, which is a well-delineated anatomic entity enclosing an organ or other body part

caput the head

carcinogen a cancer-causing chemical or agent

carcinoma any of several forms of malignancy forming from epithelial tissue in more than one site

cardiac about the heart

cardinal vowel system set of vowel reference points introduced by the linguist Daniel Jones. It uses 8 primary vowels in a front-back arrangement, with variations in vertical tongue position for both front and back vowels

Front	*Back*
i	u
e	o
ɛ	ɔ
a	â

cardio- prefix: pertaining to the heart

cardiofaciocutaneous syndrome (CFC) delayed speech and language secondary to cognitive impairment and hypotonia; marked by large-appearing forehead with bitemporal depressions, sparse scalp hair, depressed nasal root, short neck, ptosis

cardiomegaly enlarged heart

cardiomyopathy group of diseases of the myocardium (middle layer of the heart walls, composed of cardiac muscle) characterized by the inability of the heart muscle cells to contract normally; World Health Organization limits to: "Primary disease process of heart muscle in absence of a known underlying etiology" in reference to idiopathic cardiomyopathy; synonym is myocardiopathy

cardiopulmonary pertaining to heart (cardio-) and lungs (pulmonary)

cardiovascular referring to the heart and its outgoing (arteries) and incoming (veins) blood vessels

cardiovascular disease disease of the heart or blood vessels composing several disorders, including coronary artery disease, cardiomyopathy, hypertension, hemorrhagic stroke syndrome, and heart rhythm disturbances

caretaker speech a simplified language used by parents with children to ensure understanding

Carhart's notch feature of an audiogram in which a dip occurs for bone conduction testing at about 2000 Hz; associated with otosclerosis

caries decay of teeth

carotid artery one of two main conduits of blood to the brain

carotid bruit an abnormal sound or murmur heard from the carotid artery during auscultation

carpal pertaining to the wrist

Carpenter syndrome delayed speech-language production onset secondary to cognitive impairment and articulatory impairment secondary to constricted maxilla; marked by craniosynostosis, polydactyly

carrier in physics, a waveform (typically a sinusoid) whose frequency or amplitude is modulated by a signal; in medicine, a person or other animal who is a carrier of an infectious agent but who has no symptoms or clinical evidence of disease. Nevertheless, that carrier is a potential source of infection for others; in genetics, an individual with a specified gene and capable of transmitting it to offspring, but not of demonstrating its typical expression, especially a trait that is heterozygous for a recessive factor

carrier phrase in speech audiometry or speech production tests, a phrase that precedes the target word, such as, "Say the word _____."

cartilage nonvascular connective tissue that is very firm and capable of withstanding signifi-

cant compressive and tensile forces; the three kinds of cartilage are hyaline cartilage, fibrocartilage, and elastic cartilage

- **arytenoid cartilage** one of two small pyramidal laryngeal cartilages articulating with the cricoid cartilage lamina; it provides attachment for the vocal process, vocal ligament, and other muscles

- **corniculate cartilage** small laryngeal cartilage flexibly attached near the apex of the arytenoid, in the region of the opening of the esophagus

- **cricoid cartilage** lowest of laryngeal cartilages, located below and behind the thyroid cartilage

- **cuneiform cartilage** nonarticulating cartilage attached in the mobile portion of each aryepiglottic fold

- **elastic cartilage** flexible, nonvascular connective tissue that is found primarily in the external ear, eustachian tube, and some laryngeal cartilages

- **epiglottis** elastic mucous membrane-covered cartilage at the foot of the tongue that is a diverter valve over the laryngeal opening during swallowing; it is erect during liquid swallows and is passively bent over the opening during solid food swallows

- **thyroid cartilage** largest of the laryngeal cartilages formed of two plates joined anteriorly to form the laryngeal prominence (Adam's apple)

- **tracheal cartilages** incomplete hyaline cartilage rings (16 to 20) making up the tracheal skeleton

cartilaginous constructed of cartilage

cartilaginous joint joint with cartilage connecting two bones

case frames concept of the early consistent word orders used by children to express semantic relationships from stages of language development of Roger Brown (1925–1997)

case grammar a generative grammar that emphasizes the cases or semantic roles assumed by nouns in relationship to the verb of a sentence

case identification assignment of a diagnosis to a set of signs and symptoms

castrato male singer castrated at around age 7 or 8 years old, so as to retain alto or soprano vocal range

cataphoric reference word (often pronoun) or phrase replacing nouns or noun phrases that occur later in the context (example: *her* is the cataphoric reference in "after her, Ann was followed by others")

cataract clouding of the lens of the eye

catecholamine a group of substances including dopamine, norepinephrine, and epinephrine that function as neurotransmitters, hormones, or both

categorical perception the observation that listeners hear classes of similar sounds within a continuous range of sounds

categorization the ability to group or sort items into categories based on common dimensions or features; requires more than simply the discrimination of two items from different classes; based on perceived similarity among discriminable items in a particular category

category voice type classified according to pitch range and voice quality; the most frequently used categories are bass, baritone, tenor, alto, mezzosoprano, and soprano, but many other subdivisions exist

category goodness the degree to which an item is judged to be representative of the category as a whole

cat eye syndrome speech and language usually delayed secondary to cognitive impairment, with possible compensatory articulation secondary to cleft palate; marked by coloboma of iris, choroid, and retina, as well as hypertelorism and kidney anomalies

catheter a small tube inserted into body passageways, canals, vessels, or cavities; for fluid withdrawal or injection or to assist in visualization

caudal toward the tail or coccyx

caudate nucleus a major deep brain cell body of gray matter that is part of the basal ganglia; the caudate and putamen form the striatum

causality understanding of cause-and-effect relationships

causation, multiple the concept that many variables are capable of simultaneously influencing a speaker's behavior

cause-effect pattern syntactic devices in text grammar that signal a cause-effect relationship is being proposed

-cele suffix: tumor, swelling, hernia

cell body the part of a neuron that contains the nucleus and its genetic material

cellulitis widespread inflammation of connective tissue

cementum thin layer of bone joining tooth and alveolus

centile charts standardized growth charts (height, weight, and head circumference) for children

central near the center of a structure

central auditory disorder (CAD) functional auditory disorder centered in the brainstem or cortex and not the peripheral hearing system (outer, middle, or inner ear)

central auditory nervous system (CANS) the auditory brainstem, subcortical pathways, auditory cortex, and corpus collosum

central auditory processes auditory system mechanisms and processes responsible for sound localization and lateralization; auditory discrimination; auditory pattern recognition; temporal aspects of audition including temporal resolution, temporal masking, temporal integration, and temporal ordering; auditory performance with competing acoustic signals; and auditory performance with degraded acoustic signals. These auditory system mechanisms and processes generate electrical brain waves or auditory evoked potentials (i.e., auditory brainstem response, auditory middle-latency response, auditory late-latency response, and auditory event-related response) in response to acoustic stimuli

central auditory processing processing of raw sensations into meaningful percepts. Creation of auditory space; auditory skill set, including discrimination, analysis, attention, and memory that integrate what is heard with language at the cortical level

central auditory processing disorder (CAPD) heterogeneous disorder involving an observed deficit in one or more of the central auditory processes responsible for generating the auditory evoked potentials (i.e., electrocochleography, auditory brainstem response, auditory middle-latency response, auditory late-latency response, and auditory event-related response) and such behavioral phenomena as sound localization and lateralization, auditory discrimination, auditory pattern recognition, temporal aspects of audition (including temporal resolution, temporal masking, temporal integration, and temporal ordering), auditory performance with competing acoustic signals, and auditory performance with degraded acoustic signals

central nervous system (CNS) the part of the nervous system contained within the bony cavities of the skull and spinal column; it consists of the brain and spinal cord components, to which sensory impulses are transmitted and from which motor impulses pass out, and that coordinates and supervises activity of the entire nervous system

central processing unit (CPU) controls the operation of a computer, performing arithmetical operations, along with decoding and executing instructions

cephalo- prefix: head or toward the head end

cephalocaudal moving in a head to tail direction, as in the typical developmental emergence of voluntary motor control

cepstrum a Fourier transform of the power spectrum of a signal used in speech analysis and machine speech recognition. The transform is described in terms of *quefrency* (note the transliteration from frequency), which has time-like properties. The cepstrum is used to determine the fundamental frequency of a speech signal. Voiced speech tends to have a strong cepstral peak, at the first *rahmonic* (note transliteration from harmonic)

cerebellum the lower, hindmost portion of the brain, primarily responsible for coordination and balance

cerebral asymmetry the idea that the two cerebral hemispheres are not equal in size or function

cerebral blood flow (CBF) flow of blood through the brain

cerebral cortex the "bark" of the cerebral hemispheres consisting of six layers of neurons forming a rind of gray matter around the cerebrum

cerebral dominance the concept that certain higher level brain functions, such as language, music, art, or logical thought are more localized in one hemisphere of the brain than the other. For speech, the left cerebral hemisphere is typically dominant

cerebral hemispheres the halves of the cerebrum, which are divided by the deep longitudinal fissure, with the corpus callosum connecting the hemispheres at the bottom of the fissure. Each hemisphere has four major lobes. The hemispheres have an outermost gray layer and internal white material surrounding gray matter islands called nuclei

cerebral palsy static encephalopathy related to perinatal brain injury, outwardly manifested by speech problems and dyscoordination

cerebrospinal fluid (CSF) serumlike fluid secreted from blood into brain ventricles, providing uniform pressure and cushioning of brain structures

cerebrovascular accident (CVA) any sudden disruption to the flow of blood to the brain that results in permanent injury or dysfunction; characterized by an occlusion or hemorrhage; known as stroke and the new term *brain attack*

- **embolic stroke** stroke resulting from a clot (thrombosis) traveling from the location of formation (such as heart, carotid artery, or aorta) to a brain artery (typically middle cerebral artery)

- **intracerebral stroke** CVA characterized by bleeding within the brain tissue

- **ischemic stroke** impaired flow of blood to the brain resulting from obstruction of a blood vessel, due either to narrowing of the vessel or to an embolism; blockage of cerebral blood vessels, leading to an area of reduced oxygen supply

cerebrovascular system vascular system and blood supply serving the brain

cerebrum the larger, most visible portion of the brain, consisting of two hemispheres overlying the rest of the brain and considered to be the home of conscious mental processes

cerumen the waxy secretion within the ear's external auditory meatus

cervical pertaining to the neck

cervical osteophyte bony outgrowth of the cervical vertebrae

chained association phenomenon in conceptual development in which a word occurs in successive contexts that are linked by one feature from the preceding situation

chaining a behavioral process in which responses are learned as fixed sequences in which each response leads to a subsequent response

- **forward chain** series of sequenced behaviors with first steps taught first and in order to the end; frequently used to teach academic skills

chains, focused narratives that organize a sequence of events around a character, but omit motivations for the character's actions

chains, unfocused narratives based on elements linked together

channel proteins specialized proteins in the cell membrane that allow specific ions to pass through the membrane

chanting a treatment technique involving vocalizations of repetitive tones

chant-talk a voice therapy technique characterized by speech that resembles chanting; consists of soft glottal attacks, raised pitch, prolonged syllables, even stress, and smooth blending of words; considered appropriate for hyperfunctional voice problems; helps reduce excessive muscular effort and tension associated with voice production

chaos a qualitative description of a dynamic system that seems unpredictable, but actually has a "hidden" order. Also a mathematic theory that involves fractal geometry and nonlinear dynamics

chaotic behavior distinct from random or periodic behavior. A chaotic system looks disorganized or random but is actually deterministic, although aperiodic. It has sensitive dependence on initial condition, has definite form, and is bounded to relatively narrow range (unable to go off into infinity)

checking action the use of muscles of inspiration to impede the outward flow of air during respiration for speech

chemical dependency involves loss of control, compulsion to use, continued use against one's own best interests, and, in spite of risk and adverse consequences, a belief in the efficacy of drugs and denial of a problem and the need to abstain from all mood-changing, addicting drugs for permanent recovery

chemical pneumonitis lung inflammation due to aspiration of irritating chemicals

chemical shift artifact an artifact in magnetic resonance scanning caused by a change in the resonant frequency of protons in different environments. For example, protons in fat may have different elements surrounding them than those in fluid or soft tissue. This produces slightly different spin frequencies when the two tissues are exposed to the same magnetic field. Because of this, there may be spatial misregistration between these two types of tissues

chemoreceptors sensory organs that are sensitive to properties of specific chemicals; also, specialized cells (i.e., neural receptors) in the central nervous system that respond to gas levels in the blood, especially levels of CO_2, for activating the muscles of inspiration

chemosensitive sensory fibers sensory fibers with receptors on the membranes of their terminals that respond to specific chemicals such as ammonium chloride

chemotherapy use of drugs to control/cure cancer

chereme minimal unit that signifies differences in meaning between specific manual signs. Examples include hand shape, location, and movement

chest voice heavy registration with excessive resonance in the lower formants

Chicano an ethnic identity marker for Mexican Americans who view themselves as different from first generation Mexican immigrants to the USA

child development specialists professionals specializing in evaluating child development and counseling parents

child-directed speech (CDS) characteristic speech directed to toddlers and preschoolers by caregivers

chin stick a device worn on an individual's head with a pointer that extends at the level of the chin, allowing the user to use head motion to point toward a symbol or object

choana a funnellike opening or channel

choanal atresia failure of the oronasal membrane to rupture (at about 6 weeks gestation), preventing the separation of nasal cavity from oral cavity. Thus, perinatal breathing is through the mouth, not the nose. Bilateral choanal atresia makes it impossible for an infant to suck, swallow, and breathe with coordination, thus oral feeding is usually impossible

cholecystokinin a peptide hormone secreted by the duodenum that regulates gastric motility and secretion, gall bladder contraction, and pancreatic enzyme secretion. It is also thought to be a neurotransmitter

cholesterol the most abundant of the naturally occurring steroid molecules (a subclass of lipid, or fat, molecules having a common structure); a constituent of many body components, such as hormones and vitamin D, and often associated with the lipoproteins in compounds such as high-density lipoproteins (HDL) and low-density lipoproteins (LDL)

cholinergic associated with nerve cells or fibers that use acetylcholine as the neurotransmitter

- **cholinergic innervation** neurons that secrete acetylcholine (ACh) at their terminals; includes neurons in the central nervous system, all of the alpha motor neurons that innervate skeletal muscle fibers, neurons in autonomic nervous system between pre- and postganglionic nerve fibers, and the postganglionic neurons that innervate cardiac and smooth muscle. Although ACh is the same transmitter released at all cholinergic synapses, the receptor on the postsynaptic membrane will differ for the type of synapse (i.e., muscarinic and nicotinic)

- **cholinergic neurons** neurons that secrete acetylcholine (ACh) at their terminals; includes neurons within the central nervous system, including all of the alpha motor neurons that innervate skeletal muscle fibers, neurons within autonomic nervous system between pre- and postganglionic nerve fibers, and some postganglionic neurons that innervate cardiac and smooth muscle. Although ACh is released at all cholinergic synapses, the receptor on the postsynaptic membrane will differ for the type of synapse (i.e., muscarinic and nicotinic)

chondral pertaining to cartilage

choral/unison reading a treatment technique involving two (unison) or more (choral) speakers simultaneously reading selected passages aloud

choral/unison speech a treatment technique that consists of the client speaking simultaneously with one (unison) or more (choral) speakers

chorea involuntary, nonstereotyped muscular movements, usually quick jerking movements

chorionic villi sampling antenatal test performed on minute parts of placental tissue

chromosomal disorder anomaly based on structure and/or number of chromosomes

chromosomes long strands of DNA (deoxyribonucleic acid) and protein that carry the genetic material (genes) that guides the formation of offspring. In a double strand of DNA, humans have 46 chromosomes or 23 pairs, 22 pairs are homologous pairs of autosomes and there is 1 pair of sex chromosomes; with reproductive fertilization, one member of each chromosome pair is contributed by each of two parents

chronic the symptoms or consequences of impairment, injury, or disease that persist for a long period of time

chronic obstructive pulmonary disease (COPD) a diagnosis that includes generalized airway obstruction; a combination of emphysema and bronchitis, sometimes with components of asthma. Emphysema is chronic alveolar distension caused by destruction of the lung tissue. Bronchitis is usually defined as the presence of a productive cough 3 months out of the year for a period of 2 years (consecutively) and excessive mucus production. Asthma is a narrowing of the bronchi. These conditions may be partly reversible with treatment, but severe COPD is usually considered irreversible

chronological age age from date of birth

cicatrix a scar

cilia hairlike projections from certain epithelial cells; usually serve a filtering and protective function; capable of a rhythmic beating motion

- **immotile cilia syndrome** a clinical syndrome of recurrent sinusitis and respiratory malfunctioning of the cilia and consequent diminished filtering action

ciliary defects dysfunction of the hairlike processes on airway cells that are normally responsible for propulsion of airway secretions, owing either to deficiency in the number or function of cilia

cingulum association fiber tract within the brain's cingulate gyrus that connects the callosal and hippocampal convolutions of the brain; also, a girdle or zone

circum- prefix: around

circumlocution a lack of precision with expressive language whereby the individual is unable to get to the point or "talks around" a topic or word

clarification requests one communicative partner signals to the other that there has been a communicative breakdown

clause a group of words that includes a subject and a predicate, but is not necessarily grammatically complete

- **nonrestrictive clause** the information in the clause merely elaborates on the topic, as in "which is comfortable" in "the weather, which is comfortable, is just what you wanted"

- **object noun complement** clause introduced by *that*, which serves an object phrases and completes a sentence (e.g., I see *that* he is here.)

- **restrictive clause** descriptive clause that is integral to the concrete meaning of the word it qualifies, as in "that you wanted" in "the weather that you wanted is not in the cards"

- **subordinate clause** an embedded clause that supplements the main clause in a complex sentence

-cle suffix: implies something very small

cleft a fissure; divided: especially fissure that begins in an embryo, as the branchial cleft (facial cleft); clefts defined as craniofacial abnormali-

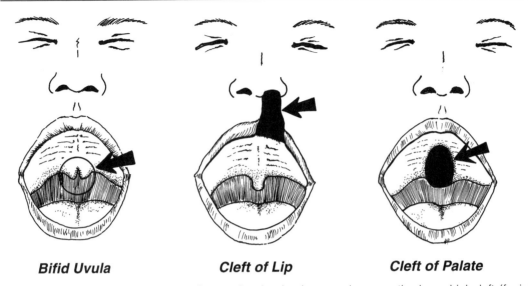

Bifid Uvula   **Cleft of Lip**   **Cleft of Palate**

cleft   a fissure; divided: especially fissure that begins in an embryo, as the branchial cleft (facial cleft); clefts defined as craniofacial abnormalities can lead to serious problems in feeding and speech, which can be treated through surgery followed by therapeutic intervention

ties can lead to serious problems in feeding and speech, which can be treated through surgery followed by therapeutic intervention

- **cleft jaw** embryonic development failure of the right and left mandibles to fuse, resulting in an abnormal jaw

- **cleft lip** a congenital defect resulting from failure of the premaxilla to fuse with the alveolus, resulting in one or more clefts in the upper lip

- **cleft palate** a congenital defect resulting from incomplete fusion of the horizontal palatal segments; fissure may be complete (extending into the nasal cavities from open hard and soft palates) or cleft may be incomplete, or partial; often accompanies cleft lip; seen about once in every 2,500 live births, affecting more females than males

- **cleft tongue** longitudinal fissure

- **cleft uvula** congenital failure of palatine folds to unite, causing uvula to be split in half

- **laryngeal cleft** a cleft in the larynx that may present with cough during feeding; stridor may be present at rest or increased with feeds; an anatomic abnormality resulting from incomplete closure of the tracheoesophageal septum or cricoid cartilage or both in the 6th to 7th week of fetal life

- **occult submucous cleft palate** a separation of the muscle fibers in the soft palate with an intact skin covering, but without a cleft uvula; on oral examination, the palate appears normal

- **submucous cleft palate** a separation of the muscle fibers in the soft palate and on occasion a separation of the palatal bone with an intact skin covering. The uvula is cleft (split); called a bifid uvula

- **synaptic cleft** the region between two communicating neurons into which a neurotransmitter is released

clonus a movement characterized by a rapid succession of contractions and relaxations in a muscle

closed captioning text or dialog that corresponds to the auditory speech signal from a television program or movie that is printed on the screen simultaneously with the speech signal

closed-head injury (CHI) nonpenetrating brain injury in which the skull (cranium) may be either intact or fractured, but the meninges are intact

closure the ability to subjectively complete and make whole an incomplete form. Listeners use language knowledge and inductive and deductive reasoning, as well as auditory and grammatical closure, to derive the meaning of words and messages

cloze reading comprehension probe in which a student supplies words that have been systematically deleted from a text

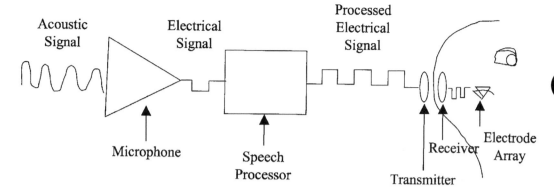

cochlear implant   device implanted in the skull that permits deaf persons to receive stimulation of the auditory mechanism; typically composed of a microphone, a speech processor, and an electrode array that is inserted into the cochlea; directly stimulates the auditory nerve by means of electrical current; most totally deaf patients with an implant can detect medium to loud sounds, including speech at comfortable listening levels; for many, cochlear implants aid in communication by improving lipreading ability, with persons able to use clues from the sounds and rhythms of speech and combine these with visual information; smaller amount of implant patients can discriminate words or sentences without lipreading.

cluster reduction phonological error pattern of deletion of one or more elements in a consonant cluster, as in [pid] or [sid] for "speed"

cluttering a speech-language disorder characterized by rapid speech rate, irregular speech rate, or both; a fluency disorder related to, but different from, stuttering; may coexist with stuttering. Also defined as a fluency disorder with rapid rate, indistinct articulation, and impaired language formulation, possibly suggesting poor organization of thought with reduced or absent awareness or concern about the problems. Certain elements of treatment are common to stuttering and cluttering

co- prefix: together

coaching a treatment technique in which a client is reminded about repeating previously practiced behaviors

coalescence melding of two or more sounds

coarctation narrowing, stricture, stenosis, constriction, usually of the aorta

coarticulation the phenomenon in speech in which the attributes of successive speech units overlap in articulatory or acoustic patterns. That is, one feature of a speech unit may be anticipated during production of an earlier unit in the string (anticipatory or forward coarticulation) or retained during production of a unit that comes later (retentive or backward coarticulation)

coccyx the most inferior portion of the vertebral column

cochlea the coiled shell-like cavity in the petrous portion of the temporal bone forming one of the labyrinth (internal ear) divisions; the cochlea contains the organ of Corti and other auditory structures that change sound to neural energy. Composed of three parallel canals: the scala vestibuli, scala media (cochlear partition), and the scala tympani. It is structured so that high-frequency sounds entering the cochlea are analyzed at the stiff, basal turn of the cochlea, with low frequency tones analyzed mostly at the apex at low intensities; the analysis of all signals seems to spread toward the stiff basal end as the intensity of the signals increases

cochlear aqueduct small opening between the scala vestibuli and the subarachnoid space of the cranial cavity

cochlear duct the membranous cochlear labyrinth, housing the sensory organs of the inner ear; also called the cochlear partition and scala media; middle space of the cochlea created by the membranous labyrinth and containing the organ of Corti, bordered at the top by Reissner's membrane and at the bottom by the basilar membrane. The major space in the scala media is filled with a fluid called endolymph, but the cells in the organ of Corti are protected from that fluid by a tight network called the reticular lamina. The cells of the organ of Corti are probably surrounded by perilymphatic fluid from the scala tympani

cochlear implant device implanted in the skull that permits deaf persons to receive stimulation of the auditory mechanism; typically composed of a microphone, a speech processor, and an electrode array that is inserted into the cochlea; directly stimulates the auditory nerve by means of electrical current; most totally deaf patients with an implant can detect medium to loud sounds, including speech at comfortable listening levels; for many, cochlear implants aid in communication by improving lipreading ability, with persons able to use clues from the sounds and rhythms of speech and combine these with visual information; smaller amount of implant patients can discriminate words or sentences without lipreading

cochlear microphonic stimulus-related auditory potential, being a direct electrical analog to the stimulus

cochlear nerve vestibulocochlear nerve; eighth cranial nerve (CN VIII), which emerges from the brain behind the facial nerve between the pons and medulla oblongata

cochlear nucleus initial brainstem nucleus of the auditory neural pathway found within the pons and subdivided into anteroventral, posteroventral, and dorsal cochlear nuclei; primary origin of source of the lateral lemniscus, or central auditory pathway

cochlear partition one of three canals, or scalae, within the cochlea; bounded by Reissner's membrane, basilar membrane, and spiral ligament

Cockayne syndrome after toddler years, progressive speech and language deterioration, with dysarthric component, secondary to progressive cognitive functioning deterioration; short stature, deficient subcutaneous fat, progressive peripheral neuropathy; central hearing impairment

cocktail party effect perception of conversation that is marked by speech sounds that often share the same intensity and spectral energy

coda in linguistics or phonology, the term for the consonant(s) that appear after the nucleus (vowel or diphthong) in a syllable; assumes a syllable structure of the type: onset + nucleus + coda.

code the systematic, orderly nature of language that allows speakers and listeners to express and comprehend meanings

- **paralinguistic codes** speech production aspects such as prosody, intonation, rate, rhythm, and stress that accompany a spoken message to express attitude or emotion

code switching a phenomenon in bilingualism in which speakers unknowingly include elements of one language in the other; dialects can also be code-switched

coefficient of amplitude variation this measure, expressed in percentage, computes the relative standard deviation of the peak-to-peak amplitude. It increases regardless of the type of amplitude variation

coefficient of fundamental frequency variation this measure, expressed in percentage, computes the relative standard deviation of the fundamental frequency. It is the ratio of the standard deviation of the period-to-period variation to the average fundamental frequency

coevolution influence of independent systems and/or individuals on and with one another, effecting mutual change or evolution, over time. Therapists have applied the concept to the changing relationship between family and therapist in which each affects the other

cognition process or act of knowing, including both judgment and awareness; also, a product of the process of thinking, including coordinating information from perception, memory, discrimination, and judgment

cognitive academic language proficiency (CALP) skill with the language taught in schools, which in the United States is usually English. CALP is the foundation of academic, analytical conversation and of independent acquisition of factual information. CALP is employed to use acquired information to find relationships, make inferences, and draw conclusions

cognitive approach, Vygotsky cognitive psychological approach that bases cognition and personality development on social interaction, dealing with macro- and microsocial influences during development; from Lev Semyonovich Vygotskii (1896–1934), variant contemporary English spelling of traditional Russian is Vygotsky

cognitive determinism a philosophy that emphasizes the primary role played by cognition in determining the acquisition of language

cognitive development, Piaget's stages developmental psychological processes as identified by Jean Piaget (1896–1980), an early theorist of the constructivist theory of instruction and learning

- **concrete operational stage (elementary and early adolescence)** operational thinking (capability to reverse mental actions) develops, with intelligence seen in systematic and logical symbol manipulation of concrete concepts; egocentrism diminishes

- **formal operational stage (adolescence and adulthood)** intelligence becomes linked to logical use of abstract concept symbols

- **preoperational stage (toddler and early childhood)** intelligence seen in symbol use, growing language maturity, and development of memory and imagination; egocentrism dominates

- **sensorimotor stage (infancy)** intelligence evidenced through motor activity without symbol use until very end of stage

cognitive reframing a relapse prevention skill training strategy that helps a patient who has been drug dependent find new responses to high-risk factors

cognitive style an individual's approach to processing information, problem solving, and cognitive tasks (e.g., bottom-up/top-down, impulsive/reflective, field dependent/field independent)

- **field-dependent cognitive style** organizing the world by focusing on the interrelatedness of constituent parts; meaning is contextually based

- **field-independent cognitive style** organizing the world by focusing on its constituent parts separately, with meaning derived from analysis of topics

Cohen syndrome delayed speech and language from cognitive impairment, with hypotonia influencing speech problems, along with misarticulations from open bite and maxillary constriction; also marked by obesity, short stature, delayed puberty, scoliosis, hypertensible joints, microcephaly

cohesion the relatedness of successive utterances in discourse

cohesive device units of identical or related intonation patterns that extend across utterance boundaries and that result in a sense of interconnectiveness among utterances

cohort in speech perception, a set of words that share a word-initial acoustic sequence. Also, a peer group or group of individuals having a statistical (e.g., age) factor in common

cold spots receptive fields of sensory nerve fibers that discharge in response to temperatures in a specific way. Stimulating this receptive field with a warm probe will elicit the perception of cold

collaborative team model an approach that views communication within the user's natural environments, considers the individual and fam-

ily as central to the process, and integrates natural supports, including friends and community members

collagen the primary protein (composing more than half in mammals) of the connective tissue white fibers of tissue, cartilage, and bone

collagen injection a medical treatment procedure for clients with paralyzed vocal folds; injected into the middle third of the folds, collagen increases the bulk and the chances of abduction

collection patterns language development syntactic devices associated with text grammar that indicate a listing of items

collective monologue a phenomenon in which children playing in proximity to each other talk simultaneously, but not necessarily to each other

colliculus a small elevation; hillock (anatomical)

- **colliculus of arytenoid cartilage** elevation on anterolateral side of arytenoid cartilage

- **inferior colliculus** paired ovoid eminence of the brainstem's mesencephalic tectum laminae: crucial way station in the central auditory pathway

coloboma any flaw—pathologic or congenital —especially of the eye

- **coloboma iridis** congenital cleft of iris

- **coloboma lobuli** congenital fissure of the ear lobule

- **macular coloboma** central retinal flaw resulting from arrested development or intrauterine retinal infection

coloratura in common usage, refers to the highest of the female voices, with range well above C^6. May use more whistle tone than other female voices. Coloratura actually refers to a style of florid, agile, complex singing that may apply to any voice classification. For example, the bass runs in Handel's *Messiah* require coloratura technique

com- combining form: with or together with

coma abnormal state of depressed responsiveness, with lack of response to tactile, thermal, proprioceptive, visual, auditory, olfactory, or verbal stimuli

command-driven a computer program that requires the user to type in explicit commands (cf. menu-driven, icon-based)

commissure angle, point, corner, or line of union or junction between two anatomical parts (as the lips at their angles, corner of eye, or adjacent heart valves); also connecting band of nerve tissue in the brain or spinal cord

common mode rejection ratio (CMRR) the ratio (often in dB) between the amplitude of the output of a differential amplifier, when a signal is fed to only one input, with the other input shorted to ground, and the amplifier output when the same signal is supplied to both inputs of a differential amplifier

common mode signal a signal or signal component presented to both inputs in a bipolar EMG electrode array, or to both inputs of a differential amplifier

common underlying proficiency (CUP) theory that basic language proficiency is based on acquisition of first and second languages

communication the process of sharing ideas between a sender who encodes a message and a receiver who decodes the message; may entail the use of a common system of symbols, speech, sign, writing, or hand gestures

- **aided communication** communication modes that require equipment in addition to the communicator's body. Examples are pencil and paper, typewriters, headpointers, picture communication boards, eye gaze boards, dedicated augmentative communication devices, and computers with speech synthesis

- **alternative communication** a method of communication other than oral—one that replaces oral-verbal communication

- **augmentative (assistive) and alternative communication (AAC)** aided or unaided communication modes used as a supplement to or as an alternative to oral language, including gestures, sign language, picture symbols, the alphabet, and computers with synthetic speech

- **basic interpersonal communication skills (BICS)** the language skills that are normally required by all members of a speech community as a first language and used for basic social interactions with other members of the speech community

- **manual communication** communication modes that entail the use of fingerspelling, signs, and gestures

- **nonverbal communication** conveying attitudes or ideas through gesture and facial expression, without the use of words, whether spoken, written, or gestured

- **simultaneous communication** educational approach used with individuals with severe and profound hearing loss that integrates aural/oral communication and manual communication; total communication

- **total communication** the simultaneous use of multiple modes of expression to enhance communication

- **total communication approach** educational philosophy for deaf children that emphasizes language development without regard to sensory system

- **unaided communication** communication aspects that use only the communicator's body; vocalizations, gestures, facial expressions, manual sign language, and head nods are examples

Communication Bill of Rights a set of guidelines developed by the National Joint Committee for the Communication Needs of Persons with Severe Disabilities, setting out individuals' basic rights to communication

communication board a communication aid that combines the use of the alphabet, whole words, and/or pictures. It allows expressive communication by pointing or gazing at a printed word, symbol, or picture. Communication boards are generally no-tech systems without spoken or written output

communication breakdown conversational point when one participant does not recognize the message presented by another

communication competence the knowledge required of a speaker to communicate appropriately within a given speech community, as well as the skills required to make use of that knowledge

communication disorder impairment in one's ability to communicate

communication displays general term for sets of organized picture communication symbols, including printed words. Communication displays appear in no-tech, low-tech, and high-tech devices

communication handicap psychosocial disadvantages resulting from such conditions as specific language impairment (SLI) and hearing loss, including the limitations that occur in performing the activities of everyday life

communication partner person with whom one engages in conversation

communication strategy a course of action taken to enhance communication

communication strategy training instruction provided to a person with communication disability or the person's frequent communication partner that pertains to communication strategies and the management of communication difficulties

communication system any single or combination of aided or unaided communication systems

communicative competence the ability of speakers to adjust their messages to effectively influence their listeners. Also, proficient use of a language in everyday conversations. This term accentuates being understood rather than being "correct" in using language rules

communicative functions intentions exhibited by infants and toddlers as classified by M. A. K. Halliday (1925–)

communicative intention a speaker's goal or objective in formulating a linguistic message; a speech act

compact one of the distinctive features originally proposed by Roman Jakobson and Morris Halle for classifying open vowels (+COMPACT) versus non-open vowels (!COMPACT). Also has been applied to consonants produced in the middle of the oral cavity, for example, the velar stops /k g/ are (+COMPACT) whereas labial and glottal consonants are (!COMPACT)

comparative adjective form that expresses the relative degree of an attribute in comparing two items (e.g., *big* vs. *bigger)*

comparison patterns language development syntactic devices associated with text grammar signaling that similarities or differences are being noted

compensation counteracting a defect or problem with a changed process or behavior

- **articulatory compensation** using an alternative or adapted articulation in place of the typical or expected pattern

- **swallowing compensation** lessening of a swallowing problem by learned behavior, increased use of alternative mechanisms, or the inherent plasticity of the nervous system and of swallowing functions. Compensation may occur through use of postures that change pharyngeal dimensions and redirect bolus flow; through adaptations in bolus volume, delivery, or consistency; or through the use of sensory reinforcements or prostheses

compensatory strategies a treatment technique employing atypical patterns to achieve the target behavior

competence versus performance in linguistics, a distinction between knowledge of grammatical rules (competence) and the ability to use the rules in language expression (performance)

complement part of a sentence or clause that acts to complete the action of a verb; also elements serving to complete a structure involving the verb "to be" (or similar verbs), for example, "She is sad."

complementary distribution allophones with distinctive phonetic environments; that is, the aspirated /p/ in pie has a different sound than the unaspirated /p/ in spy; the aspirated form is generally in the initial positions and the unaspirated occurs after an initial /s/ sound; these /p/ pronunciations can never exchange positions and are in complementary distribution; also termed noncontrastive distribution; contrasts with free variation

comprehensible input language delivered at a level understood by a learner

comprehension a sophisticated level of auditory-visual skill development, characterized by an ability to easily understand connected speech

- **compounding strategy** language development comprehension strategy in which all actions in a sentence are attributed to the first noun mentioned in the sentence

- **minimal distance principle** language development comprehension strategy in which the noun closest to the verb is assumed to be the agent

- **noun-verb-noun strategy** language development comprehension strategy that relies strictly on word order

- **order of mention strategy** language development comprehension strategy that assumes the first event mentioned occurred earlier than events in the remainder of the sentence

- **plausible event strategy** language development comprehension strategy that relies on determining the most probable state of affairs

compressed speech process employed in a challenge test of hearing in older adults in which speech segments are removed and the sample compressed in such a way that the frequency composition remains intact; comprehension is typically degraded for older adults with such compression, analysis of degradation allows for assessment and research

compression squeezing of a body or substance that decreases its size and/or volume, usually with an increase in density. Also (in hearing aid circuitry), nonlinear amplifier gain used to determine and limit output gain as a function of input gain

- **hearing aid compression** nonlinear amplifier gain used to determine and limit output gain as a function of input gain; compression ratio is the ratio in decibels between the acoustic input to a hearing-aid amplifier and its auditory output
- **medial compression** the degree of force that may be applied by the vocal folds at their point of contact

compression ratio the ratio in decibels between the acoustic input to a hearing-aid amplifier and its auditory output

compressive strength the ability to withstand crushing forces

computed tomography (CT) specialized X-ray scan that produces thin (usually 10-mm thick) cross-sectional reconstructions of the body using computer back-projection techniques; also called computerized axial tomography (CAT), an obsolete usage

- **dynamic computed tomography (CT)** employed to enhance vascular views through rapid injection of contrast medium
- **single-photon emission computed tomography (SPECT)** metabolic and physiological tissue function imaged by computer synthesis of single-energy photons emitted by radionuclides administered to the patient
- **spiral CT** scans produced by moving a patient at a constant rate through the bore of a CT scanner while the scanning tube is rotated around the patient. This produces a true volumetric dataset and allows standard transverse views, as well as images in any plane desired
- **trispiral tomography** allows a very thin and uniform focal plane, especially for inner ear visualization
- **ultrafast computed tomography** technique of CT scanning in which the X ray rapidly scans the patient in several planes quickly enough to freeze rapid motions such as occur in the oropharynx during swallowing

con- combining form: with or together with

conceptual behavior responding to a variety of items that are related by some feature defining them as a class

conceptualization formation of a concept and/or the conceptual interpretation

concert pitch also known as international concert pitch. The standard of tuning is A4. Reference pitch has changed substantially over the last 200–300 years

concha entrance to the ear canal; shell-like structure

- **cavum concha** deep portion of the concha

condensation an increase in density

conditioning modifying, molding, or adapting to conform; also to change so that a response or act once related to a given stimulus becomes linked to another

- **avoidance** teaching to learn to avoid punishing or unpleasant stimuli
- **classical (or respondent) conditioning** neutral stimulus (e.g., a bell) associated with an unconditioned stimulus (e.g., food) subsequently elicits conditioned responses similar to the unconditioned response (e.g., salivation)
- **head-turn conditioning** a technique used to test infants' discrimination of speech sounds between the ages of 6 and 12 months of age
- **operant (or instrumental) conditioning** desired behavior is reinforced when the behavior or a progressively closer approximation of the desired action is followed by a rewarding stimulus
- **reinforcers** stimuli that take on reinforcing properties through association with a know reinforcer

conduction aphasia aphasia often attributed to lesion of the arcuate fasciculus; characterized by intact auditory comprehension, but poor repetition of verbal materials

conduction velocity rate of conduction of impulse through a neuron

conductive hearing loss a hearing loss caused by obstruction to the normal sound-conducting mechanism of the outer and/or middle ears. Usually treatable by medicine or surgery. Relatively easy to manage with hearing aids, as direct amplification usually suffices

condyle rounded prominence at an extreme end of a bone; the process of the mandible that inserts into the temporomandibular joint (mandibular arch/process)

confabulation the filling in of memory gaps by inventing tales

confrontation naming naming a stimulus when asked to do so; a correct response to such questions as, "What is this?"

congenital conditions present at birth, which can be mental or physical traits, anomalies, diseases, malformations, and so on; may result from genetics or an influence during gestation; not necessarily negative

congestive heart failure a chronic failure of the heart to pump adequate amounts of blood throughout the body; congestion and fluid accumulation in various organs in the body (such as the lungs) result

conjoining linking two independent clauses into a single sentence

conjunction uninflected linguistic form that links sentences, clauses, phrases, or words

- **coordinating conjunction** in language development, a connecting word that links two structures into one sentence

- **subordinating conjunction** a conjunction that introduces a clause serving as an adverb to describe time, location, cause, or conditions related to the main clause

conjunctiva mucous membrane that coats the inner aspect of the eyelids and the outer surface of the eye

conjunctivitis inflammation of the conjunctiva

connective tissue tissue that bundles and links other body parts and tissue; types include cartilage, bone, and fibrous and loose tissue

consanguinity blood relationship; common parent or ancestry

consonant speech sound characterized by constriction or closure at one or more points in the breath channel. Consonants in American English are classified by voicing and manner of articulation. The broad classes of consonants are stop-plosives, nasals, fricatives, affricates, liquids, and glides (semivowels)

- **affricate consonants** obstruent consonants produced with characteristics of both stop consonants and fricative consonants. Examples are the first and last sounds in the words *church* and *judge*

- **continuant** a consonant produced without complete closure of the vocal tract

- **deletion of final consonant** an error pattern in which a child omits the consonant at the end of the word

- **devoicing of final consonant assimilation process** substitution of a voiceless final consonant for a voiced (e.g., /t/ for /d/)

- **glide** a consonant sound that has a gradual (gliding) change in articulation reflected by a

relatively long interval of formant-frequency shift

- **intervocalic** a consonant that occupies a position between two vowels; e.g., the second [p] in the word *paper* is intervocalic

- **labial** bilabial and labiodental consonants, with American English labial consonants being [p], [b], [m], [w], [f], [v]

- **nasal** class of consonants made with a lowered velum. American English nasal consonants are [m], [n], and [ŋ]

- **plosive consonant** produced by creating complete blockage of airflow, followed by the buildup of air pressure, which is then suddenly released, producing a consonant sound

- **sonorant consonant** a consonant produced with a narrowing of the vocal tract, but with no pressure buildup behind the narrowing

- **stop consonant** a consonant sound produced as a result of a complete closure formed by an articulator in the vocal tract

consonant-vowel-consonant (CVC) monosyllabic word structure; CVCs often are used as stimuli in isolated-word speech-recognition tests

consonant-vowel (CV) nonsense syllable composed of a consonant followed by a vowel (e.g., *ba*, *da*, *ga*). Also, any speech-sound sequence consisting of consonant and vowel

constituent equivalence the status given to pronouns in relation to the nouns or noun phrases they refer to (replace)

constituent structures the morphemes, words, and phrases that contribute to an overall sentence structure

constructive interference the interference of two or more waves such that enhancement occurs

content matter and/or topics in written work; part, element, or complex of parts; material dealt with in an area of study

context the overall collection of discourse stimuli that illuminate meaning; the interconnected circumstances within which something exists or happens

contextual information linguistic support available for identifying a target word, phrase, or sentence

contextualized language utterances that relate to the context in which they occur

context variability when a phonetic unit is produced in different contexts, for example, when the phonetic unit /d/ occurs in the syllable /di/ as opposed to /du/, its physical characteristics vary a great deal, even though we hear each /d/ as the same

contingent a conditional or interdependent relationship between stimuli

contingent queries a conversational device used to prompt for specific information that maintains the conversational flow

continuant a consonant produced without complete closure of the vocal tract

continuing care self-help groups, counseling, follow up, and individualized support for patients following discharge from treatment

continuity the ability to maintain an uninterrupted flow of speech

continuity hypothesis the phonological theory that the developmental sounds of babbling evolve into the sounds of speech

continuous discourse tracking (CDT) aural rehabilitation technique in which the receiver (listener) attempts to repeat text verbatim that is presented by a sender (speaker); performance is summarized as the number of words repeated per minute

continuous positive airway pressure (CPAP) a mode of noninvasive mechanical ventilation support that is noncycled; the ventilator provides a continuous flow of air to maintain a fairly constant pressure in the airway and at the alveolar level. CPAP is for patients capable of self-initiating respirations, but need help to maintain adequate arterial oxygen levels. CPAP can be administered through a ventilator and endotracheal tube, a nasal cannula, or into a hood enveloping the patient's head

contour, terminal the final pitch direction at the end of an utterance

contra- prefix: opposite, against

contrecoup injury brain injury evidenced on the side opposite the trauma to the skull, produced by the brain bouncing from the point of impact to the opposite side of the cranium

contraction a decrease in size, particularly of muscle; atypical shrinkage

- **off-contraction** a contraction that occurs with a latency period following the end of a stimulus. The off-contraction of esophageal smooth muscle, for example, is associated with depolarization of the muscle cells and the generation of spike potentials

- **tertiary contraction** simultaneous, nonpropulsive contraction that occurs at any level of the esophagus

contracture the shortening or tightening of tissue around a joint; a common consequence following a "brain attack" and often requiring active "range of motion" exercises to counteract

contraindication any factor negating a particular treatment

contralateral acting or occurring in concert with a part on the body's opposite side, as in the cerebral cortex controlling contralateral muscles (left brain side to right body side); opposite side of the body

contralto lowest of the female voices. Able to sing F_3 below middle C, as well as the entire treble staff; singer's formant at around 2800–2900 Hz

contrastive analysis phonological analysis that compares and contrasts two or more phonological systems; used especially for individuals who are learning a new language or languages to determine the relationship between the different phonological systems

contrastive sets/minimal pairs a treatment technique with a person being exposed to two (minimal pairs) or more (contrastive sets) sets of stimuli that differ in only one dimension. Usually, the individual is expected to discriminate between the sets of stimuli

contrastive stress drills a treatment method used to promote both articulatory proficiency and natural prosody, especially the stress and rhythm aspects of spoken language; used in treating apraxia of speech in adults; varying phrases and sentences are used to teach placing stress on different words; stressed words or terms may be used to promote articulatory proficiency or simply to vary prosodic features of speech

control to preserve influence over a situation or exercise restraint. In statistics: a case-control study control is a person not having the disease or outcome of interest; cohort study controls are persons not exposed to the studied independent variable; randomized controlled trial controls are a group getting a placebo or ordinary treatment and not the examined intervention

controlled mode ventilation (CMV) a mode of medical ventilation support that cycles to provide inspiratory breaths independent of the breathing efforts of a patient

controlled oral word association test (COWAT) a measure of word fluency or production in which the subject is asked to produce as many words as possible beginning with a given letter in a limited period of time; the Boston Naming Test is one example of a COWAT

control site an individual's point of contact with an AAC input device. Control sites can include body surfaces or the end of a head pointer

contusion (brain) a bruising, usually on the surface of the brain, from trauma to the head that causes minute bleeding, but with no skin broken or other structural abnormality

conus elasticus fibroelastic membrane extending inferiorly from the vocal folds to the anterior superior border of the cricoid cartilage. Also called the cricovocal ligament. Composed primarily of yellow elastic tissue. Anteriorly, it attaches to the minor aspect of the thyroid cartilage. Posteriorly, it attaches to the vocal process of the arytenoids

conventional the notion that language must be based on shared, customary, or implicitly agreed on patterns of behavior and meaning

convergence uniting toward a common point; coordination of eye movement allowing single-point imaging on retina

conversational acts functions of words and phrases within discourse classified by Dore: a combination of grammatical form (the utterance), propositional context (its meaning), and an illocutionary function (the intended effect)

conversational repairs devices used by individuals to clarify messages within a conversation

conversational rules implicit rules that guide the conduct of participants engaged in conversation

conversational style, aggressive conversational style characteristic of some persons who have hearing loss, characterized by hostility, belligerence, and negative attitude

conversational style, noninteractive characteristic of a passive conversational style; includes failure to contribute to the development of a conversational topic, minimal response to turn-taking signals, and a proclivity to bluff

conversational style, passive conversational style of some persons who have hearing loss, characterized by withdrawal from conversation, frequent bluffing, and avoidance of social interactions

conversational turn during the course of a conversation, the period during which a participant delivers a contribution to the conversation

conversational turn taking a pragmatic language skill and treatment target; often deficient

in clients with language disorders; involves appropriate exchange of speaker and listener roles during conversation

conversation linked adjacency pairs two remarks that often are linked in conversation, as when one communication partner asks, "How are you?" and another responds, "Fine, thank you."

convolutions turns; infoldings; also irregular furrows on the brain's surface, especially of the cerebrum

convulsion intense spasm or series of jerkings of the extremities, face, or trunk; synonymous with seizure, which is a sudden episode of uncontrolled electrical activity in the brain

cooing infant sound productions in the first few months that are vowel-like and associated with comfortable states

cooperative play play behavior in which children interact for common advantage

coping imagery a therapeutic technique in which the therapist leads a patient through an alternating series of images, one set pleasant and the other anxiety-provoking, to reduce anxiety by associating each anxiety-provoking situation with a pleasant image

copula verb that links its subject to a noun phrase, adjective, or prepositional phrase, especially sentence subject complement

copy synthesis a type of speech synthesis (machine-generated speech) in which stored copies of speech segments (such as syllables or words) are retrieved and assembled to form an utterance

cor- combining form: heart

cordectomy surgical removal of a vocal fold

core features of stuttering part-word or sound repetitions and prolongations that mark the occurrence of stutter events; may exist without accessory features

core subject a subject that is of prime importance in the curriculum. In the U.S., the three core subjects are mathematics, English, and science

core vocabulary highly functional, high-frequency words and phrases, typically related to basic needs

cornea transparent covering of the anterior part of the eye; primary refractory structure of the eye

Cornelia de Lange syndrome leads to neurogenically based articulation disorders, along with severely delayed speech production onset; cognitive impairment, microcephaly, seizures, hypertonia, cleft palate, with possible Robin sequence

corner vowels /a/, /i/, and /u/; vowels at the corners of a vowel triangle; they necessitate extreme placements of the tongue. Also, the vowels /a/, /æ/, /i/, and /u/ that define the points of the vowel quadrilateral

cornua horn

corona crown

coronal section a cross section dividing, by actually cutting or through imaging methods, the body or any body part in a vertical plane perpendicular to the median plane

coronary artery disease disease (such as myocardial infarction or heart attack) resulting from restriction or interruption of the blood supply to the heart muscle via the coronary arteries, commonly marked by the symptom of angina pectoris (pain)

corpor- prefix: body

cor pulmonale heart disease that occurs following lung disease, in which the right ventricle is enlarged

corpus body

corpus callosum a major bundle of commissural fibers in the brain forming an arched body beneath the longitudinal fissure and connecting the cerebral hemispheres

cortex outer layer of a body organ or structure

- **anterolateral cerebral cortex** a region of the cortex in front of the primary motor and premotor cortex regions

- **association cortex** cerebral cortex regions dealing with sensory information processing, integration of senses, or sensorimotor impulses

- **auditory cortex** region of cerebral cortex (more or less corresponding to Brodmann's areas 41 and 42) activated by auditory radiation from medial geniculate body, which receives input from the cochlear nuclei in the rhombencephalon

- **cerebellar cortex** thin gray surface layer of the cerebellum

- **cerebral cortex** dense, thin gray covering of the surface of the mammalian cerebral hemisphere. Layers classified by Brodmann are divided into three categories; molecular, or plexiform, layer; outer granular layer; pyramidal cell layer; inner granular layer; inner pyramidal (ganglionic) layer; and multiform cell layer. Brodmann designated 47 cerebral

cortex areas, which can be divided into three broad designations: motor cortex, sensory (auditory, visual, and somatic), and association area

- **frontal cortex** covering of the frontal lobe of the cerebral hemisphere (e.g., Brodmann areas 4 and 6)

- **motor cortex** the area of the cerebral cortex that most directly influences movement of face, neck, trunk, arm, and leg (Brodmann areas 4 and 6)

correlation coefficient a number or function implying the amount of agreement between two sets of data or between two arbitrary variables and that is equal to their covariance divided by the product of their standard deviations

corticosteroid potent substances produced by the adrenal cortex (excluding sex hormones of adrenal origin) in response to the release of adrenocorticoticotropic hormone (ACTH) from the pituitary gland, or related substances. Glucocorticoids influence carbohydrate, fat, and protein metabolism. Mineralocorticoids help regular electrolyte and water balance. Some corticosteroids have both effects to varying degrees. Corticosteroids may also be given as medications to alleviate various conditions, including inflammation, malignancy, suppressed immune system, and suppressed ACTH (adrenocorticotropic hormone) secretion, as well as for hormone replacement therapy

costa a rib

cost-benefit analysis (CBA) an economic evaluation of medical care costs that compares monetary benefit between a variety of health interventions

cost-effectiveness analysis (CEA) economic analysis for determining the best use of funds available for medical care. Often conducted on the basis of cost per unit achieved

cough forceful evacuation of the respiratory passageway, initiating with a deep inhalation through widely abducted vocal folds, tensing and tight adduction of the vocal folds, and elevation of the larynx, followed by forceful expiration; generally excited by mechanical or chemical irritation of bronchi or trachea or by pressure from adjoining structures

counseling a process of educating and supporting persons being treated and their families through verbal discussion, exchange of information, and offering of emotional support

countertenor male singing voice that is primarily falsetto, in the contralto range. Most countertenors are also able to sing in the baritone or tenor range. Countertenors are also known as contraltino or contratenor

count noun nouns that represent items that can be counted as individual units (e.g., pennies, forks); compare mass noun

coup injury brain injury at the point of impact from a blow to the head that results in the brain slamming against the point of impact

coupling act of pairing, joining, or linking together; in genetics, situation with nonalleles of two or more mutant genes near enough on same chromosome for likelihood of both being inherited

cover of vocal fold, the epithelium and superficial layer of lamina propria; in music, an alteration in technique that changes the resonance characteristics of a sung sound, generally darkening the sound; in commercial recording, a release of a song previously recorded, ordinarily by another artist

Cowden syndrome speech development may be impaired by lesions on lips, tongue, and gingiva, with hoarseness and breathiness secondary to laryngeal polyps

cranial relating to the head

cranial nerve nuclei groups of nerve cells associated with cranial nerves as sensory nuclei or motor nuclei

cranial nerves (CN) 12 nerve pairs originating at the base of the brain that carry messages for such functions as hearing, vision, swallowing, phonation, tongue movement, smell, eye movement, pupil contraction, equilibrium, mastication, facial expression, glandular secretion, taste, head movement, and shoulder movement. Starting with the most anterior, cranial nerves (CN) are enumerated by Roman numerals: (CN I) olfactory, (CN II) optic, (CN III) oculomotor, (CN IV) trochlear, (CN V) trigeminal, (CN VI) abducens, (CN VII) facial, (CN VIII) acoustic (vestibulocochlear), (CN IX) glossopharyngeal, (CN X) vagal, (CN XI) accessory, (CN XII) hypoglossal. Several cranial nerves, especially CN V, CN VII, and CN VIII, include two or more separate functions, which are considered as independent nerves by some scientists. That classification would separate the masticatory nerve from the trigeminal (CN V), the glossopalatine from the facial (CN VII), and the equilibrium from the acoustic (CN VIII), making 15 pairs (see illustration, p. 58)

craniostosis premature ossification of cranial sutures

craniotomy surgical removal of a portion of the skull to expose the cortex and meninges for inspection or biopsy; can be performed to relieve excessive intracranial pressure, as from subdural hematoma

cranium the bony portion of the skull containing the brain that is composed of the frontal, occipital, sphenoid, ethmoid and paired temporal and parietal bones; the bony brain case

creole a speech community's native language that has evolved from a pidgin, as in a mixture of English, Spanish, French, and African languages combining into grammatical forms seen in various portions of the Americas; the form for the language is not capitalized, but usage for the people of the speech communities is capitalized (Many older Creoles continue to primarily speak in creole)

crescendo to get gradually louder

crest ridge, bony prominence

CREST syndrome abbreviation for *c*alcinosis, *R*aynaud phenomenon, *e*sophageal dysfunction, *s*clerodactyly, and *t*elangiectasis

Creutzfeldt-Jakob disease progressive dementia, dysarthria, muscle wasting, and such involuntary movements as myoclonis and athetosis in a rare fatal encephalopathy

cricoarytenoid joint synovial joint in larynx, running from the base of each arytenoid cartilage and the top border of the cricoid cartilage lamina

cricoarytenoid muscle, lateral intrinsic laryngeal muscle that adducts the vocal folds through forward rocking and rotation of the arytenoids (paired)

cricoarytenoid muscle, posterior an intrinsic laryngeal muscle that is the primary abductor of the vocal folds (paired)

cricoid cartilage a solid ring of cartilage located below and behind the thyroid cartilage

cricopharyngeal bar posterior impingement of the pharyngoesophageal junction lumen as seen during radiographic studies. Symptomatic primarily in context of Zenker's (pharyngoesophageal) diverticulum and pharyngeal paralysis

cricopharyngeal incoordination normal swallowing reflex defect in which airway protection during food swallowing is compromised, which can lead to choking, air swallowing, nasal regurgitation, or pain in swallowing food

cricothyrodotomy procedure performed as an emergency airway management technique; the

Cranial Nerves, listed by Roman Numeral, Type (S = sensory, M = motor) and Innervated Region, and Function.

Nerve	Type / Innervated Region	Function
CN I	S / olfactory epithelium	Sense of smell
CN II	S / ganglion cells of retina	Sense of sight
CN III	M / eye muscles	Eye movement
CN IV	M / eye muscles	Eye movement
CN V	S / skin and head, dura mater	Facial sensation
	S / muscle spindles and mechanoreceptors in jaw muscles	Proprioception
	M / jaw muscles, tensor tympani	Chewing, ear drum
CN VI	M / eye muscles	Eye movement
CN VII	S / outer ear	Sensation
	S / taste buds in anterior tongue	Taste
	S / portion of nasopharynx	Taste
	M / salivary glands, lacrimal gland	Secretion
	muscles of facial expression and stapedius	Facial expression, stapedial reflex
CN VIII	S / Organ of Corti and vestibular apparatus	Hearing and balance
CN IX	S / outer ear	Sensation
	S / taste of posterior tongue	Taste
CN X	S / carotid body and sinus mucosa	Sensation
	M / parotid gland	Secretion
	M / pharynx (stylopharyngeus)	Pharyngeal action in speech and swallowing
	S / outer ear	Sensation
CN XI	M / shoulder and neck muscles	Head and shoulder movements
CN XII	M / tongue muscles	Tongue movements

cranial nerves (CN) 12 nerve pairs originating at the base of the brain that carry messages for such functions as hearing, vision, swallowing, phonation, tongue movement, smell, eye movement, pupil contraction, equilibrium, mastication, facial expression, glandular secretion, taste, head movement, and shoulder movement. Starting with the most anterior, cranial nerves (CN) are enumerated by Roman numerals: (CN I) olfactory, (CN II) optic, (CN III) oculomotor, (CN IV) trochlear, (CN V) trigeminal, (CN VI) abducens, (CN VII) facial, (CN VIII) acoustic (vestibulocochlear), (CN IX) glossopharyngeal, (CN X) vagal, (CN XI) accessory, (CN XII) hypoglossal. Several cranial nerves, especially CN V, CN VII, and CN VIII, include two or more separate functions, which are considered as independent nerves by some scientists. That classification would separate the masticatory nerve from the trigeminal (CN V), the glossopalatine from the facial (CN VII), and the equilibrium from the acoustic (CN VIII), making 15 pairs

creation of an incision between the cricoid and thyroid cartilages

cricothyroid muscle an intrinsic laryngeal muscle that primarily controls pitch

crista ampularis thickened region of the ear's semicircular canal lining containing sensory cells

criteria-based assessment an assessment model that focuses on obtaining information in a decision tree format; one use is to determine which AAC system to implement

criterion-referenced test nonstandardized probe for study of a language construct in more depth than typically associated with standardized tools

critical period the early years of a child's or animal's life in which the language and vocal patterns of the individual's species are acquired most easily

cross-language study a study conducted with speakers of different languages

cross-modal speech perception the perception of speech through two modalities, such as audition and vision, as in lipreading

crossover frequency the fundamental frequency for which there is an equal probability for perception of two adjacent registers

crown topmost portion of a structure or organ, as the top of the head

crur-, crus combining form, meaning cross: leg-like part

crux cross

cryo- prefix: cold

crypt pitlike depression or tubular recess

CT scan computed tomography

cue, acoustic acoustic information in a segment of speech that conveys phonetic information

cued speech a system for making all the sounds of speech visible. In English it utilizes eight handshapes, placed in four different locations around the face, to remove any ambiguity about what is seen and heard by the person with a hearing impairment. Invented by physicist R. Orin Cornett of Gallaudet College, it requires only cues to ensure one-time communication. Two of its special strengths are first, that it allows virtually everything to be discussed as it happens around the child who has hearing impairment and thus allows the child to learn much more language than is formally taught. Second, it supports a high likelihood that the child who uses it will be a fluent reader. It has been adapted for use in 53 languages and major dialects

cues, nonlinguistic the persons, objects, events, and relationships in a setting that influence the speaker's verbal behavior

cuff the balloonlike part of an artificial airway (i.e., endotracheal tube, tracheostomy tube) that is inflated in the trachea to provide a seal in the airway; usually used during mechanical ventilatory support or in the presence of copious aspiration

-cule suffix: implies something very small

cultural overlap attributes shared by several cultures

culture allied philosophies, ideas, arts, and customs of a group of people that pass from one generation to the next

-culum, -culus suffix: diminutive form of a noun

cursor a movable marker employed for marking a position; visual cue (as a blinking symbol) on a video (computer monitor) display that marks position

cut- prefix: skin

cycle an interval in which a sequence of recurring events is completed; a 360° rotation; same as a *period* in periodic motion

- cycle of respiration completion of both inspiration and expiration phases of respiration

- cycle of vibration one full return to the point at which a function begins to repeat itself

cycling in speech perception training, returning to a training objective that has been achieved with some success to provide reinforcement and additional learning

-cyst suffix: sac or bladder

cystic fibrosis an inherited metabolic disease characterized by excessive production of tenacious mucus and repeated respiratory infection; autosomal-recessive affecting mostly Whites (in USA approximately 1:2500 live White births; 1:17,000 live Black births); early signs include viscid, foul-smelling stool, chronic cough, and persistent upper respiratory infection; also called fibrocystic disease of the pancreas, mucoviscidosis, and fibrocystic disease of the pancreas

cyto-, cyt- prefix: pertaining to cell

cytology science dealing with structure of cells

cytomegalovirus (CMV) one of many herpes-like viruses causing serious problems for newborns and persons with HIV infection or recipients of immunosuppressive medication, especially following organ transplantation

cytoplasm the protoplasm of a cell, excluding that of the nucleus

D

Dental Arch, Deciduous

the dental arch containing a child's 10 temporary teeth

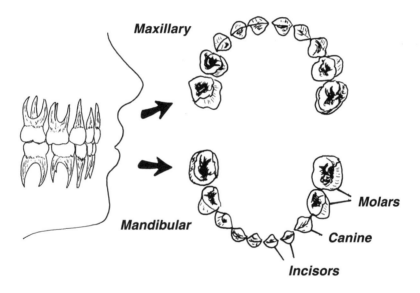

Maxillary

Mandibular

Molars

Canine

Incisors

damp to diminish, suppress, or attenuate an oscillation

damping the rate of absorption of sound energy; related to bandwidth decibel (dB)

de- prefix: away from

dead space, anatomic or physiologic portion of the airway in which gas is only transported (as upper bronchi and trachea) and there is no gas exchange (not alveoli). Mechanical dead space is space created in mechanical ventilation and can cause hypoxemia and hypercarbia

Deaf Culture a subculture that shares a common language (in USA, American Sign Language), beliefs, customs, arts, history, and folklore; primarily composed of individuals who have prelingual deafness

deaf/deafness having minimal or no hearing

- **acoustic trauma deafness** sensorineural hearing loss caused by overexposure to very loud sounds

- **central deafness** deafness from disorder of the auditory mechanisms of the cerebral cortex or brainstem

- **conductive deafness** loss caused by interruption of sound or transmission though the external canal, middle ear, or ossicles

- **cortical deafness** damage from bilateral lesions of the temporal lobe primary receptive area

- **familial deafness** deafness in members of the same family

- **postlingual deafness** loss that occurs after development of speech and language skills

- **prelingual deafness** loss that occurs before speech and language skill development

- **retrocochlear deafness** older term for sensorineural deafness, implies lesion near to cochlea

- **sensorineural deafness** deafness from disorders of the cochlear division of CN IX, the cochlea, or the retrocochlear nerve tracts

decannulation the removal of a cannula or tube that has been placed during surgery

decibel (dB) defined as 10 times the logarithm (base 10) of a ratio of two acoustic powers or intensities or as 20 times the logarithm (base 10) of two acoustic pressures. For example, a 2:1 ratio (log = 0.3) of two intensities is expressed as 3 dB and a 10:1 ratio log = 1.0) is expressed as 10 dB. Correspondingly, a 2:1 ratio of pressures corresponds to 6 dB and a 10:1 ratio of pressures corresponds to 20 dB. Decibels can be used similarly to express the levels of electrical power or electrical voltage. The decibel is one-tenth of a bel.

deciduous shedding, as in the case of the primary dentition

declarative a major sentence type that makes a statement and/or explains

decoding in learning to read, the deciphering of the sounds and meanings of letters, combinations of letters, whole words, and sentences of text; conversion into intelligible form; recognizing and interpreting

decontextualized language utterances about objects, people, events, and relationships outside an immediate context

DECtalk formant-type commercial speech synthesizer offering good intelligibility, variations in speech rate, and varying voices (men, women, children)

decussate to cross over, to intersect

dedicated communication system operates solely for communication

dedicated processing computer hardware system designed for one specific use; technological opposite is general purpose

deductive inferencing reasoning from the general to specific

deep far from the surface

deep structure a component within Chomsky's government-binding theory that contains the sentence structure rules and a language user's lexicon

deformation the result of stress applied to any surface of a deformable continuous medium. Elongation, compression, contraction, and shear are examples; deviation from typical size or shape

degenerative disease disorders with progressive deterioration of tissue or structure function; examples include cancer, arteriosclerosis, osteoarthritis, Alzheimer disease, macular degeneration

deglutition swallowing; movement of nourishment from mouth to stomach; consists of sequential phases, which are subject to a variety of labeling schemes, depending on health care speciality

- **deglutition apnea** required interruption of respiration during swallowing

- **esophageal phase of swallowing** bolus transport down esophagus and into stomach through coordinated contraction of smooth and striated esophageal muscles

- **oral phase of swallowing** early stage of swallowing, in which a bolus is formed and propelled toward the pharynx through repeated contractions of the tongue

- **oral preparatory phase of swallowing** stage of swallowing in which the tongue gathers the food bolus and forms it into a centrally located globular mass ready to be propelled over the back of the tongue

- **oropharyngeal transit time** the time taken between the beginning of swallowing and the time of the bolus passes out of the oropharynx

- **pharyngeal phase of swallowing** bolus passage through the pharynx and into the esophagus in coordination with respiration to assure air supply continuation and aspiration prevention

- **preparatory phase** initial stage of bolus mastication and saliva amalgamation in anticipation of food transport from the mouth and through the pharynx and esophagus

- **squeeze pressure, also contact pressure** pressure exerted during swallowing on a sensor as the lumen is cleared of contents and obliterated. During peristalsis of the pharynx and the esophagus, squeeze pressures typically follow and exceed bolus pressure

degrees of freedom in statistics, the number of independent choices or observations that can be made among sample members; in mechanics, the number of possible movements or movement directions

dehumidifier device removing atmospheric moisture

dehydration excessive fluid loss, especially from body tissues. This can alter the amount and viscosity of vocal fold lubrication and the properties of the vocal fold tissues themselves. Dehydration is also accompanied by imbalance of essential electrolytes

deictic gaze gaze pattern in which visual focus on an object directs a partner's attention to that object

deixis the ability of words and gaze patterns to "point to" objects being referenced in discourse relative to the speaker's current "location" in the discourse. Examples include this in the sentence: You can't top this achievement

de Lange syndrome leads to neurogenically based articulation disorders, along with severely delayed speech production onset; cognitive impairment, microcephaly, seizures, hypertonia, cleft palate, with possible Robin sequence

delayed auditory feedback (DAF) a speaker's speech is fed back to his or her ears through headphones after a delay; most speakers slow their speech down under DAF; technique is used in reducing the speech rate in persons who stutter or clutter and in those who have dysarthria

delirium altered conscious state characterized by confusion, distractibility, disorientation, disordered thinking and memory, illusions, hallucinations, agitation, and disorientation to place and time. A number of toxic structural and metabolic disorders can lead to the condition, including toxic ingestion, drug and alcohol intoxication or withdrawal, nutritional deficiencies, endocrine imbalance, and shock following physical or mental trauma

delusion false perception or belief held with unswerving conviction despite conclusive proof that the conclusions are incorrect

dementia abnormal reduction in memory, thinking, language, and other cognitive functions that results from diffuse brain damage from a variety of disorders, without damage to perception or consciousness; Alzheimer disease is a progressive dementia

- **multi-infarct dementia** progressive organic brain disorder caused by vascular disease and distinguished by rapid, sometimes step-like, decline in intellectual functioning, with disturbances in memory, abstract thinking, impulse control, and judgment

demulcent oily fluid that soothes and decreases irritation, especially of mucous surfaces

demyelination process that selectively damages the myelin sheath (nerve covering); nerve fiber damage may be the primary disorder as in multiple sclerosis or may occur secondary to brain injury or stroke

dendrite branched process of a neuron that transmits information to the cell body and forms a presynaptic connection with another neuron

dendrodendritic synapse synapse between two dendrites

denervation removal of nervous input to a tissue by excision, incision, or blocking; cold, for example, temporarily interrupts nervous input,

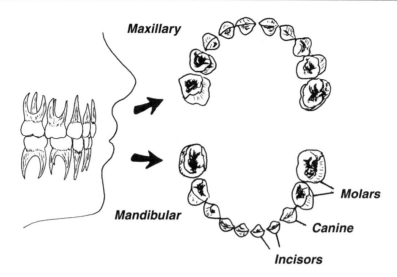

Maxillary

Mandibular

Molars

Canine

Incisors

dental arch, deciduous the dental arch containing a child's 10 temporary teeth

---

with bisection or disease leading to more permanent denervation

dental arch, deciduous the dental arch containing a child's 10 temporary teeth

dentate referring to tooth; notched; tooth-like

dentin calcified portion of tooth situated between the enamel and the pulp chamber

deoxyribonucleic acid (DNA) acid found mainly in the nuclei and mitochondria of animal and vegetable cells, considered as the autoreproducing element of chromosomes and many viruses and repository of hereditary characteristics; known for its double-helix structure

Department of Health and Human Services (DHHS) U. S. government cabinet-level department having responsibility for federal social welfare and health agencies, such as the Food and Drug Administration (FDA); also directs the Social Security Administration, National Institutes of Health, U.S. Office on Consumer Affairs, Office of Civil Rights, Administration on Aging, Public Health Service, and Indian Health Service

dependence, psychological a condition resulting from repeated use of a drug (or other enabling mechanism) in which an individual must continue employing what is depended on to satisfy a strong emotional need; the need for a substance that results from the continuous or periodic use of that substance. This need may be characterized by mental and/or physical changes in users that make it difficult to control or stop dependent usage

depolarization change to an unpolarized condition; in physiology, reversal of the resting potential in excitable cell membranes when stimulated (i.e., the tendency of the cell membrane potential to become positive relative to the potential outside the cell). A positive shift in a cell's resting potential (that is normally negative), thus making it numerically smaller and less polarized

depressant agent that reduces nervous or functional activity, often a drug or anesthetic

depression interim mental state or chronic condition characterized by feelings of sadness, hopelessness, emotional despair, lethargy, and an inability to perform or initiate daily functions. Symptoms include decreased energy, feelings of worthlessness, appetite disturbance, weight change, feelings of inappropriate or excessive guilt, psychomotor agitation or retardation, difficulty thinking or concentrating, recurring thoughts of death or suicide, or suicide attempts; may be physically or psychologically triggered in persons with aphasia

derivational morpheme a type of bound morpheme that changes the grammatical class of the free morpheme to which it is attached (e.g., teacher)

derivative the extent of the ratio of the change in a function to the analogous change in its independent variable as the latter change approaches zero

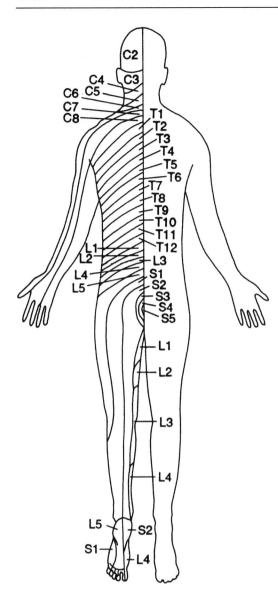

dermatome region of body innervated by a specific spinal nerve

---

-derm- prefix or suffix: skin

dermatologist medical practitioner specializing in diseases of the skin

dermatome region of body innervated by a specific spinal nerve

destructive interference the interference of two or more waves such that full or partial cancellation occurs

detection the ability to recognize the actuality, manner, or fact of something, as in recognizing the presence or absence of sound

determiners words, including articles, adjectives, possessives, quantifiers, and demonstratives, that modify the noun with which they are associated; traditionally called modifiers

detoxification removal or diminishment of poisonous quality; lessening virulence of pathogenic entity; process of withdrawing from dependency on alcohol and/or other drugs

developmental age stage of childhood development determined by such standardized measurements as size, psychologic and social performance, motor skill, plus aptitude and mental assessment; not necessarily the same as the chronological age

developmental apraxia of speech a child's lack of ability to plan or sequence the motor movements of speech, resulting in the impaired production of speech sounds; not attributable to muscle weakness or muscular neurological impairment; sometimes called developmental verbal apraxia

developmental delay inhibited or slowed development relative to peer age-matching

developmental perspective the view that language development is inherently related to concurrent developments in cognition and emotional and social interaction

deviation, standard statistical measure of the degree of variation (dispersion) from the mean; square root of the variance

devoicing assimilation process substitution of a voiceless final sound for a voiced (e.g., /k/ for /g/)

devoicing of final consonants assimilation process substitution of a voiceless final consonant for a voiced (e.g., /t/ for /d/)

dextro- prefix: pertaining to the right side

di- prefix: two, twice

dia-, di- prefix: through, between

diabetes one of several conditions characterized by copious urine excretion. When identified without qualification, the condition is diabetes mellitus, a complicated disorder of protein, carbohydrate, and fat metabolism mainly resulting from poor or no insulin secretion by the pancreas. A less common form is diabetes insipidus, caused by a deficiency of the antidiuretic hormone (ADH)

diacritic (diacritic mark) symbol attached to a phonetic symbol for a sound segment to indicate a particular modification of sound production

diadochokinesia rapid alternating diametrically opposite muscular movements (as flexion and extension or supination and pronation of a limb)

diadochokinesis (DDK) a task involving repetition of movements requiring alternating contraction of agonist and antagonist muscles associated with speech (lips, mandible, tongue)

diagnosis scientific identification of cause or reason for injury, impairment, or disease based patient signs and symptoms, laboratory analysis and other tests, and a health history

dialect a collection of rule-governed consistent or systematic variations in a major language that occur in an identifiable subgroup, distinguished by patterns of phonology, morphology, and/or syntax

- **nonstandard dialect** variation of a major language spoken by an overall population

- **regional dialect** variation used by individuals living in a particular geographic region.

- **social dialect** variation used by a particular social group

- **standard dialect** the generally accepted version of the primary language used in a group

dialogue a series of related verbal exchanges between at least two persons

dialysis method of removing waste-products from the body in the event of kidney failure

diaphoresis sweating, especially excessive sweating

diaphragm musculofibrous partition separating the thoracic and abdominal cavities. It is the primary muscle of inspiration and may be co-activated during singing

diastema a space between two teeth

dichotic influencing or applying to the two ears differently in regard to a conscious aspect (as pitch or loudness) or a physical aspect (as frequency or energy) of sound

dichotic test test in which the listener must identify one or both of two different acoustic signals presented separately and simultaneously, one to each ear

diet habitual nourishment; type and amount of food prescribed for a person for a special purpose

- **elimination diet** diet used to exclude possible cause of an allergy

dietician specialist trained in nutrition

diffusion migration or mixing of one material (e.g., liquid) through another; intermingling

DiGeorge sequence delayed onset of speech production, with global glottal stop substitutions in cases with clefts or VPI; language usually delayed and impaired, with specific deficits in auditory memory and processing; marked also by heart anomalies, facial anomalies (long nose, puffy upper eyelids) small ears with attached lobules and overfolded helices, and learning disabilities

digestive system the complex of organs and glands that prepares (digests) food and liquids in preparation for absorption of nutrients into the bloodstream

digital a signal or message that is represented as discrete values (a sequence of numbers); the signal can only reach certain values on a scale, but no intermediate values. When viewed on an oscilloscope, a digital signal is "squared." This compares with an analog signal, which typically has a continuous appearance. In data communications, digital describes the binary (off/on) output of a computer or terminal

digital signal processing (DSP) computer processing of signals such as sound, video, and other analog material that has been converted to digital form; often used in hearing aids

digitized speech representation or storage of speech in digital form. The speech sounds are recorded by a peripheral device that converts sound input from a stereo system, an instrument, or a microphone into a digitized form that a computer can process, store, and play back

diglossia use in a bilingual community of the two languages determined by social (or other functional) situation; one language or distinct dialect might be for less formal use than another or one language is specified for social interaction and another for religious observance

digraph a symbol formed of two characters, for example, two letters of the alphabet; a group of two consecutive letters with a phonetic value of a single sound (as *ea* in read or *ng* in bring) or whose value is not the sum of a value borne by each in other occurrences (as *ch* in chop where the value is /t/ + /sh/)

dilate to open or expand an orifice

dimensional words words about the physical dimensions of objects

diminuendo in music, to get gradually softer

diphone a segment of speech that represents the interval from the middle of one sound to the middle of a following sound; it begins and ends with a steady-state sound and includes a transition between two given sounds; employed in speech synthesis and speech analysis in general

diphthong sound involving a gradual change in articulatory configuration from an onglide to offglide position. The usual phonetic symbol is a digraph, or combination of two symbols to represent the onglide and offglide portions

dipl- prefix: two

diplegia paralysis of corresponding parts on both sides of the body, typically with greater impairment of legs than arms

diplopia double vision

dis-, di-, dif- prefix: away, negative, apart

disability the inability to perform a function or activity within a "normal" range when compared with typical individuals; World Health Organization defines disability as disablement in activity as part of the ICIDH (International Classification of Impairments, Disabilities, and Handicaps)

disablement term from World Health Organization (WHO) classification for grouping consequences associated with health conditions. Part of the ongoing development of the International Classification of Impairments, Disabilities, and Handicaps (ICIDH)

disappearance early reflexive form in which a child's words indicate that an object is no longer a part of the youngster's immediate experience

discharge in cell biology, electrical signals defined and recorded as action potentials or spikes by electrical recording micropipettes placed within a body cell or near and outside the cell. Neurons and muscles have distinct membranes with channels that open transiently to allow specific ions to move across the membrane into or out of the cell. The movement of ions creates a current that can be measured as a voltage, the action potential. Discharge is the number of action potentials that a neuron or muscle fiber produces; in general electrical science: energy release stored in a battery or a capacitor

discontinuity hypothesis a phonological theory that the sounds in babbling and eventual speech are unrelated

discourse a series of verbal interchanges between speakers on a shared topic

discrimination in speech-perception training, the ability to distinguish one stimulus from another; in speech-recognition testing, sometimes used to refer to word-recognition ability

discrimination score in speech audiometry, percentage of monosyllabic words correctly repeated when presented at an intensity well above the spondee threshold

discrimination task in speech perception, a procedure designed to assess a listener's ability to discriminate, or tell apart, stimuli. Labeling or categorization of stimuli is not required

diskette a semirigid oxide-coated plastic disk enclosed in a plastic jacket that serves as a small, removable disk drive for personal computers

disorder impaired physical or mental state

disorientation mental state produced by lack of awareness of space, time, or person; can be a consequence of drugs, anxiety, or organic disease

displacement weight or volume of a liquid displaced by a floating object of same weight; difference between beginning position of something and any later position

displacement flow air in the glottis that is squeezed out when the vocal folds meet

display, dynamic AAC communication aid or computer displays of symbols that change constantly based on previous system selections

dissonance theory cognitive concept about tendency of individuals to seek a consistent belief system and seek change to eliminate dissonance created by inconsistency. Within the theory, discrepancy between attitudes and behavior most often leads to accommodation of attitude to fit behavior

distal situated away from a point of origin or attachment, such as a bone or a limb; the opposite of proximal. For example, the shoulder is proximal and the hand is distal

distal arthrogryposis syndrome condition in which jaw limitation may lead to late speech production onset, with articulatory impairment from contractures, which usually respond positively to therapeutic management; marked by multiple contractures of limbs and digits, occasional limitation of jaw opening and cleft palate, along with possibility of Robin sequence

distend to swell or stretch out

distinctive features an individual acoustic or articulatory characteristic that distinguishes one class of phonemes from another

distocclusion malocclusion, with the mandibular arch articulating with the maxillary arch that is distal to normal; Class II malocclusion in Angle's classification

distortion adulterated version of an audio or video signal caused by change in the waveform of the original signal

distortion-product evoked otoacoustic emissions (DPOAE) acoustic energy created by stimulating the cochlea with two pure tones (f1 and f2). As a result of cochlear nonlinear processes, energy is created at several frequencies that are combinations of the two stimulating frequencies. The most easily recorded is the 2f1–f2 distortion product (technically, the cubic distortion product)

distoversion tilting of a tooth distal to normal

disyllable two syllables

diuretic a drug that promotes formation and excretion of urine

divergence becoming progressively further apart

divergent for vocal folds, the glottis widens from bottom to top

diverticulum (plural: **diverticula**) pouch or sac that is a deformation (herniation) of an organ wall. In some diverticula, only the mucosal lining herniates through a gap in the wall. In others, all layers of the wall form a permanent bulge. Diverticula are named primarily for their sites: Zenker's (pharyngoesophageal) diverticula form in the hypopharynx just above the upper esophageal sphincter. Midesophageal traction diverticula occur over the tracheal bifurcation and epinephric, or pulsion, diverticula form in the distal esophagus

- **hypopharyngeal diverticula** outpouching of the muscular pharyngeal wall above the cricopharyngeus muscle

divided attention skill aspect of attention enabling a person to appropriately allocate focus and time between a series of activities

dominance state of prevailing

- **dominance of traits** likely physiologic relationship between two or more genes that may occupy the same chromosomal locus (alleles)

- **genetic dominance** autosomal mendelian trait inheritance pattern of consistent phenotypical self-expression

dopamine sympathetic nervous system neurotransmitter that is the precursor to norepinephrine and epinephrine and inhibits movement; dopamine depletion leads to symptoms characteristic of Parkinson disease, such as rigidity, tremors, and bradykinesia

Doppler effect apparent sound or light wave frequency change as the wave source moves toward or away from an observer; frequency rises as the source moves toward the observer and decreases in moving away, as the rise in pitch of an approaching train whistle and the falling pitch as the same locomotive departs

dorsal pertaining to the back of the body or distal

dorsal horns pair of crescent-shaped prominences of gray matter in the spinal cord that contain nuclei for relaying incoming sensory information up the spinal cord

dorsal nucleus of vagus nerve a pool of preganglionic parasympathetic neurons that innervate several internal organs including the heart and those of the gastrointestinal tract. Some of its neurons innervate the smooth muscle of the esophagus sending their axons through the vagus nerve (CN X)

dorsiflexion flexion toward the back as by a muscle, as in flexing the foot with the toes facing the shin

dorsum posterior side, toward the backbone

Down syndrome (also called trisomy 21) a syndrome of mental retardation and a number of abnormalities that vary greatly among those affected; caused by a triplication or translocation of chromosome 21; speech and language develoment can be delayed secondary to cognitive impairment, with possible compensatory articulation secondary to cleft palate and VPI

Dri-aid kit a small package used to keep moisture out of the internal components of listening devices

drill repeated exercises and rote activities

drowning asphyxiation and death caused by immersion in a liquid

duct a tube, especially for the passage of secretions or excretions in the body

dummy forms utterances consisting of a true word combined with an additional sound or syllable that give the appearance of approximating multiword utterances

dyad two individuals interacting as a unit; for example, a caregiver and a child

dynamic assessment approach to evaluation focused on the different ways by which an individual achieves a score rather than the score achieved; approach is characterized by guided learning to determine an individual's potential for change

dynamic range the difference in decibels between an individual's threshold of hearing sensitivity for a sound and the level at which the sound becomes uncomfortably loud; for electroacoustic devices, the range between the least and most intense signals in an analysis or display

dynamics in physics, a branch of mechanics that deals with the study of forces in relation to motion and equilibrium of entities; in music, changes and contrast in force or intensity; processes or systems of change, activity, or growth

dyne a unit of force (in the centimeter-gram-second system); provides a free mass of 1 gram an acceleration of 1 cm per second per second

-dynia suffix: pain

dys- prefix: bad, painful, with difficulty

dysarthria a neurogenic speech disorder that results in weakness, slowness, or incoordination of the muscles of respiration, phonation, articulation, and resonation

- **ataxic dysarthria** neuropathology of damage to the cerebellar system; characterized by slow, inaccurate movement and hypotonia; all aspects of speech may be involved. Specific symptoms include imprecise consonants, excess and equal linguistic stress, and irregular articulatory breakdowns, phonatory disorders, and dysdiadochokinesis

- **flaccid dysarthria** neuropathology of damage to the motor units of cranial or spinal nerves that supply speech muscles (lower motor neuron involvement); speech problems caused mostly by muscle weakness and hypotonia; constellation of speech disorders dependent on the specific nerve that is affected, but includes breathy voice quality, hypernasality, and imprecise production of consonants

- **hyperkinetic dysarthria** neuropathology of damage to basal ganglia (extrapyramidal system), resulting in involuntary movements and variable muscle tone; may affect all aspects of speech, but a dominant symptom is prosodic disturbance; specific problems include prolonged intervals, variable rate, monopitch, loudness variations, inappropriate silences, imprecise consonants, and distorted vowels

- **hypokinetic dysarthria** neuropathology of damage to basal ganglia (extrapyramidal system) resulting in slow movement, limited range of movement, and rigidity; may affect all aspects of speech, but especially voice, articulation, and prosody; specific problems include monopitch, monoloudness, reduced stress, imprecise consonants, inappropriate silences, harsh or breathy voice, and short rushes of speech

- **mixed dysarthrias** a combination of two or more pure dysarthrias; with neuropathology depending on the types of dysarthrias that are mixed; frequent causes include multiple strokes or multiple neurological diseases; speech disorders are varied and dependent on the types of pure dysarthrias that are mixed

- **spastic dysarthria** neuropathology of bilateral damage to the upper motor neuron (direct and indirect motor pathways) resulting in weakness, spastic paralysis, limited range of movement, and slowness of movement; may affect all aspects of speech and usually not confined to one aspect; major speech problems include strained-strangled-harsh voice, hypernasality, slow rate, consonant imprecision, and monopitch and monoloudness

- **unilateral upper motor neuron dysarthria** motor speech disorder caused by damage to the upper motor neurons that supply cranial and spinal nerves involved in speech production; the dominant speech problem is imprecise production of consonants

dyscrasia, blood abnormal condition of the blood, with imbalance of components due to abnormal development or metabolism

dysdiadochokinesis impaired ability to perform rapid alternating movements caused especially by cerebellar lesion but may be observed in other neuropathologies

dysfluency disorder of fluency

dysfunction abnormal or difficult function

dysgraphia loss of proper writing ability when there is no abnormality of a limb and is usually associated with damage to brain language centers. Characterized by spelling errors, reversals, impaired word order, and other manifestations of faulty written language use, such as alexia and aphasia; usually termed agraphia

dyskinesia extrapyramidal disorder of voluntary movement, as in Parkinson disease

- **tardive oral dyskinesia** associated with chronic neuroleptic treatment and characterized by involuntary mouth and tongue movements

dyslalia old term for articulation disorder

dyslexia from the Greek for "difficulty with words or language," dyslexia is a disorder manifested by difficulty in learning to read despite adequate intelligence and sociocultural opportunity; may include other language processing problems

dysmetria deficit in control of the range (distance, power, speed) of movement of a muscular action, as by a limb or the tongue; often describes cerebellar disorder abnormalities

dysmorphology a branch of clinical genetics covering abnormal development of tissue form

dysostosis abnormal condition from defective ossification, especially of fetal cartilage

- **craniofacial dysostosis** widening of skull with high forehead, ocular hypertelorism, maxillary hypoplasia; usually autosomal dominant inheritance; used synonymously for Crouzon disease

- **mandibulofacial dysostosis** primarily malformations of the first branchial arch, manifested in part by cleft palate, malar bone hypoplasia, mandibular hypoplasia; sometimes known as Treacher Collins syndrome or mandibulofacial dysplasia

- **otomandibular dysostosis** mandibular hypoplasia, often accompanied by temporomandibular joint malformation, in addition to eye and/or ear deformation

dyspepsia gastric discomfort, characterized by epigastric pain, nausea, and gas

dysphagia difficulty in swallowing, often in conjunction with esophageal obstructive or motor disorders

- **dysphasia lusoria** difficulty swallowing secondary to an aberrant right subclavian artery

dysphonia any impairment of voice or phonation

- **dysphonia plica ventricularis** phonation using false vocal fold (ventricular band) vibration rather than true vocal fold vibration. Most commonly associated with severe muscular tension dysphonia. Occasionally may be an appropriate compensation for profound true vocal fold dysfunction

- **muscle tension dysphonia** also called muscular tension dysphonia; voice abuse characterized by excessive muscular effort and usually by pressed phonation

- **mutational dysphonia** voice disorder most typically characterized by persistent falsetto voice after puberty in a male; refers to voice with characteristics of the opposite gender

- **spasmodic dysphonia** focal dystonia involving the larynx that can be of adductor, abductor, or mixed type. Adductor spasmodic dysphonia is characterized by strain-strangled interruptions in phonation. Abductor spasmodic dysphonia is characterized by breathy interruptions

- **ventricular dysphonia** disorder caused by use of the ventricular (false) vocal folds; sometimes associated with enlarged ventricular folds; condition is characterized by low pitch, monotone, decreased loudness, harshness, and arrhythmic voicing; diagnosis depends on endoscopy, X ray, or stroboscopy, as condition is very difficult to diagnose from voice sound alone

dysphoria an emotional state characterized by restlessness, anxiety, and depression; an unpleasant mood or a feeling of being ill at ease

dysplasia atypical tissue growth and/or development

- **bronchopulmonary dysplasia** chronic pulmonary insufficiency resulting from long-term artificial pulmonary ventilation; seen most often in premature infants

- **faciodigitogenital dysplasia** x-linked autosomal dominant condition of abnormally wide-set eyes, broad upper lip, anteverted nares, saddlebag scrotum, and lax ligaments; also known as Aarskog-Scott syndrome

dyspnea difficulty or distress in breathing; frequently rapid breathing; can be caused by obstruction to airflow into and out of lungs (asthma or bronchitis) or by various diseases affecting heart and lung tissue

dysprosody impairment of the prosodic aspects of speech, such as stress, rhythm, and intonation

dystonia sustained involuntary movements, such as spasmodic torticollis (turning of the neck)

dystrophy a condition of muscular weakness and degeneration usually caused by genetic myopathies

dystrophy

- **myotonic dystrophy** has both early onset and late onset (adult) forms, with delayed speech and language in early onset type, along with severe articulatory impairment secondary to neuromuscular disease; late onset form leads to articulatory impairment secondary to malocclusion and progressing myotonia

- **oculopharyngeal muscular dystrophy** gradual dysarthria onset after beginning of facial weakness (from condition onset after age 20), with hypernasality following; also marked by pharyngeal muscle weakness

Endoscope

optic instrument employing illumination to view inside a body cavity or organ

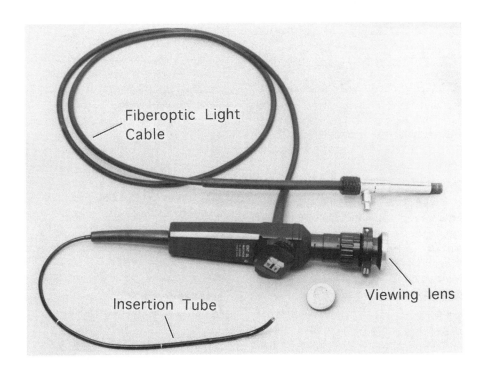

Fiberoptic Light Cable

Viewing lens

Insertion Tube

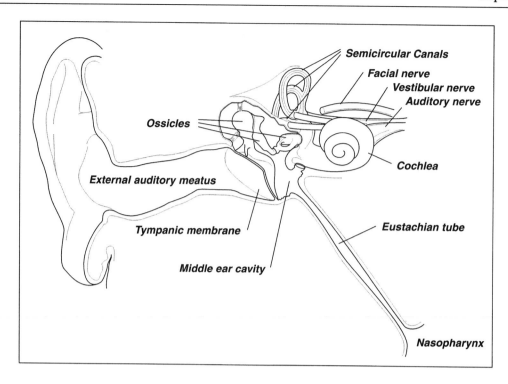

ear organ of hearing and equilibrium; composed of the external ear, which includes the auricle and the external auditory, or acoustic, meatus; the middle ear, or tympanic cavity, houses the ossicles; the internal, or inner, ear, or labyrinth, includes the semicircular canals, vestibule, and cochlea, as well as the organ of Corti

e- prefix: out from

ear organ of hearing and equilibrium; composed of the external ear, which includes the auricle and the external auditory, or acoustic, meatus; the middle ear, or tympanic cavity, houses the ossicles; the internal, or inner, ear, or labyrinth, includes the semicircular canals, vestibule, and cochlea, as well as the organ of Corti

- **inner ear** the structures of the ear that include the cochlea, the semicircular canals, the cochlear and vestibular labyrinths, the organ of Corti, the auditory nerve

eardrum the membranous separation between the outer and middle ears, responsible for initiating the mechanical impedance-matching process of the middle ear; tympanic membrane

earhook the curved apparatus of a behind-the-ear hearing aid and some other types of listening devices that connects the device case to the earmold and hooks over the pinna

early exit/late exit bilingual education programs early exit programs move children from bilingual classes in the first or second year of schooling. Late exit programs provide bilingual classes for 3 or more years of elementary schooling. Both programs exist in transitional bilingual education

earmold a device that fits into the concha and directs sound from the earhook of a listening device to the ear canal

- **earmold acoustics** the influence of the earmold's configuration and structure, such as bore length and venting, on the acoustic properties of the sound delivered to the tympanic membrane by a listening device

- **earmold bore** a hole in the earmold through which an amplified audio signal travels

- **earmold impression** cast made of the concha and ear canal

- **earmold vent** a canal drilled in the earmold for the purpose of aeration or alteration of the audio signal

earmuffs earcups that seal around the ear for protection from sound

earplug material inserted into the ear canal to dampen sound

ear protection hearing preservers such as ear plugs and earmuffs

ear training the same as auditory discrimination training and perceptual training

ec- prefix: out of

echoic a primary verbal operant whose reinforcement is contingent on reproducing the acoustic characteristics of others' speech; the behavioral equivalent of imitation

echolalia the meaningless repetition (usually unintended) of words or phrases (parroted speech) made by others

echo-planar imaging technique using functional magnetic resonance imaging (fMRI) methods and specialized pulse sequences for rapid image acquisition

echopraxia involuntary mimicking of others' movements

ecto- prefix: on the outer side; toward the surface

ectoderm the outermost embryonic germ layer that contributes to various organs, including the nervous system and skin

-ectomy suffix: removal (excision) usually by surgery

ectopic situated away from the normal or expected position

ectrodactyly-ectodermal dysplasia-clefting (EEC) syndrome frequent compensatory articulation secondary to clefting (often bilateral complete); occasional speech and language delay secondary to cognitive impairment; misarticulations secondary to missing or malformed teeth; also marked by sparse hair lacking pigmentation; photophobia

edema, edematous swelling; an accumulation of an excessive amount of fluid in cells, tissues, or serous cavities

- **pulmonary edema** swelling of alveoli in the lung from fluid leaking from the capillaries; can lead to significant respiratory distress

- **Reinke's edema** swelling of Reinke's space from chronic smoking or hypothyroidism

edentulous toothless

efferent directed away from the center, such as arteries, veins, and the neurons that proceed from the central nervous system and innervate a peripheral target organ or such sites as skeletal muscles, smooth muscles, or cardiac muscle

- **general somatic efferent** nerves providing innervation of skeletal muscle

- **general visceral efferent** the autonomic efferent fibers serving viscera and glands

efferent fibers motor fibers that carry impulses from the central nervous system (CNS) to muscles and organs

efficacy effectiveness, efficiency, and effects of treatments; documenting treatment efficacy requires demonstrating that a particular treatment produces the desired outcomes or behavior change in an efficient manner (e.g., is cost effective) as a result of the treatment

effusion in the middle ear, exudation of body fluid from the middle ear membranous walls as a result of inflammation

eighth cranial nerve (CN VIII) one of the pair of cranial nerves conveying impulses of hearing and balance. The vestibular branch connects the sensory structures in the vestibular labyrinth to the vestibular pathways in the brain. The cochlear branch (auditory nerve) connects the sensory structures in the organ of Corti with the auditory pathways in the brain. Also called cranial nerve VIII, vestibulocochlear nerve, acoustic nerve, statoacoustic nerve

elasticity the quality of a material that causes it to return to its original position after being distended or deformed

elastic recoil pressure the alveolar pressure derived from extended (strained) tissue in the lungs, ribcage, and the entire thorax after inspiration (measured in pascals)

elective mutism condition in which an individual chooses not to speak in certain circumstances; the lack of speech is situational and does not appear to reflect an inability to speak

electrical stimulation the membranes of muscle and neurons have ionic channels that are sensitive to changes in electrical voltage. A transient change in voltage across a membrane of these two types of cells results in a progressive and transient change in ionic channels across the cells. Electrical stimulation is an experimental method to depolarize neurons and muscle cells using these ionic channels

electroacoustics science of the transformation of an acoustic signal to an electrical signal or an electrical signal to an acoustic signal

electrocardiography (ECG, EKG) technique for measuring the electrical activity of the heart

electrocochleography (ECoG, EcochG, ECOG) the recording of the synchronous electrical discharge of the compound CN VIII action potential to a click or brief tone burst.

Used initially as a clinical test for deafness, now used primarily to differentiate between various types of inner ear diseases and electrophysiologic monitoring of the inner ear

electrode a terminal in an electrical circuit that transfers current in either direction between a conventional conductor and gas, an electrolyte, a body part, or instrument. It may be a recording electrode or stimulating electrode. Electrodes can be pipettes with specific chemical concentrations or metal with titanium, silver, and stainless steel commonly used. Electrodes can vary in size from a pipette with a tip of 1–2 microns to a large wire 1–2 mm in diameter. Electrodes can be either of surface or penetrating type

- **bipolar electrode** electrode or electrode pair that measures electrical events (action potentials) at two distinct points; in electrophysiology, the resulting signals are usually supplied one to an inverting input, the other to a noninverting input of a differential amplifier; also pairs of electrodes with one negative and one positive charge

- **monopolar electrode** electrode used in a derivation for recording of bioelectric signals, in which the voltage input to the amplifier is measured between a single electrode and a reference electrode

electrode array electrodes placed in pairs on a carrier wire and inserted into the cochlea; a component of a cochlear implant; any arrangement of electrodes, such as used in EEG recordings from the scalp

electroencephalography (EEG) technique for recording brain electric potentials based on information from electrodes attached to the scalp

electroglottography (EGG) technique for recording of electrical conductance of vocal fold contact area versus time; EGG waveforms have been frequently used for voice source analysis

electrolarynx external vibrating tone devices that provide voicing for individuals who are unable to phonate, but have good articulation abilities

electrolyte a solution or liquid containing electically charged particles; compound in a body fluid that can conduct an electric current

electromotility change of shape under electrical stimulation

electromyography (EMG) technique for recording the electric potentials in a muscle,

which can employ either surface or penetrating electrodes, with the latter also termed needle electrode examination

electronystagmography (ENG) technique for registering nystagmus based on information from surface electrodes (nystagmus is involuntary oscillation of the eyeballs occurring normally with dizziness during and after bodily rotation or abnormally after injuries, such as to the cerebellum or the vestibule of the ear)

electrophysiological recording technique of using micropipettes or metal to record inside or outside of neurons and muscle cells. Micropipettes placed in these two types of cells can record action potentials in millivolts. Micropipettes and metal electrodes placed outside this tissue record extracellular signals that are much smaller (in the microvolt range)

electrophysiology the study of electrical phenomena associated with cellular physiology

electrophysiology biological science branch dealing with relationships among electrical phenomena and physiologic function

elision the process by which certain sounds or syllables are deleted when words are produced in sentences or conversation

ellipsis omitting redundant parts of utterances

ellipsoid shaped like a spindle or ellipse

elongation an increase in length

embedding linguistic process of inserting a subordinate clause into an independent main clause

embolism the obstruction of a blood vessel by an object or clot, for example, an embolus

embolus any foreign object within a blood vessel that has been carried by the bloodstream

embryo organism in early developmental stages; in mammals, the stage between the ovum and the fetus, defined typically for humans as between the second and eighth week, inclusive

embryoblast blastocyst inner cell mass that will develop into an embryo

embryology branch of biology pertaining to embryos and their development; features or phenomena connected with the formation and development of embryos

embryonic disc a cluster of cells in embryonic development at about two weeks following conception

-emia suffix: referring to blood

eminence projection or prominence, especially of a bone

emollient substance that soothes or softens the skin or mucous membranes

emphysema pathologic accumulation of air within the lungs due to permanent enlargement of the airspaces distal to the terminal bronchioles; leads to lung elasticity loss and decrease in gas exchange

- **surgical emphysema** the presence of air in subcutaneous tissue from the trauma of surgery or injury

empiricism philosophical view that experience is the source of learning and knowledge

empyema pus accumulation in a body cavity, especially the pleural space, because of bacterial infection

en-, em- prefix: in

enamel the hard outer surface of a tooth

encephalitis inflammation of the brain

encephalo- prefix: pertaining to the brain (literally, within the head)

encephalon the brain, including cerebrum, cerebellum, medulla oblongata, pons, diencephalon, and midbrain

encoding system any system in which an object, sign, sound, or other cue is used as a form of code to produce communication; for example, dots and dashes used for Morse code

encopresis fecal soiling or incontinence

endarterectomy a surgical procedure for removing plaque accumulation on the lining of a major artery

endemic characteristic or uniquely or primarily prevalent in a particular population or geographic area

endo- prefix: toward the interior; within

endocarditis infection of the inner lining of the heart

endocochlear potential the constant positive potential difference between the ear's scala media and the peripheral scalae vestibuli and tympani

endocrine system ductless glands or glands of internal, or hormonal, secretion that help to integrate and control metabolic activity and include the pineal body, pancreas, and paraganglia and the pituitary, thyroid, parathyroid, and adrenal glands as well as the ovaries and testes

endocrine voice disorder abnormal voice production related to disturbances of or changes in the endocrine system; for example, menopausal voice disorder

endoderm innermost embryonic germ layer, which contributes to various organs, including the respiratory and digestive tracts

endogenous originating or produced inside an organism or one of its parts

endolymph fluid in the internal ear's cochlear duct (membranous labyrinth)

endolymphatic duct internal ear duct arising from the saccule of the vestibule and terminating blindly in the petrous portion of the temporal bone

endorphins neuropeptides that reduce pain through influence on the central and peripheral nervous systems

endoscope optic instrument employing illumination to view inside a body cavity or organ (see illustration, p. 76)

- **endoscopic ultrasound (EUS)** (endosonography) use of intraoperative ultrasound to guide endoscope

- **fiberoptic endoscope** extends the instrument's usefulness with flexible glass or plastic fibers, allowing viewing of once inaccessible areas; an abnormal area on the lining of an organ being studied can be directly vizualized and very small samples of tissue can be retrieved with forceps attached to a long cable that runs inside the endoscope

endotracheal intubation/extubation airway management through catheter from the mouth or nose into the trachea; inserted to maintain functioning airway, prevent aspiration, for suctioning of tracheobronchial secretions, or to administer positive pressure ventilation; extubation is removal of the tube

English as a foreign language (EFL) teaching of English to non-native English speakers

English for speakers of other languages (ESOL) teaching of English to non-native English Speakers

enhancement, selective relative benefit of auditory signal arising from resonance of the auditory mechanism

en passant (French) in passing

ensiform with sharp edges and tapering to a slender tip

enteral tube feeding water and nutrients delivered through a gastrointestinal tube

ento- prefix: toward the interior; within

environmental control unit (ECU) AAC hardware device that provides the user with

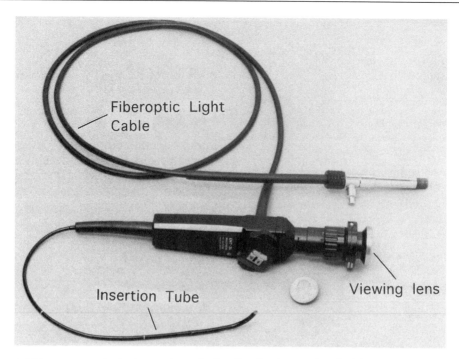

Fiberoptic Light Cable

Insertion Tube

Viewing lens

endoscope optic instrument employing illumination to view inside a body cavity or organ

programmed or spontaneous control over remote, electrically operated appliances (e.g., an electric light or a television set)

enzyme a protein that facilitates a chemical reaction but does not itself undergo permanent change; serves as catalyst

epenthesis sound intrusion process in which a sound element is inserted between consonants in a consonant cluster (e.g., *treat* pronounced tərit)

ep-, epi- prefix: on or above something else

epiglottectomy surgical removal of the epiglottis

epiglottis the leaflike cartilage at the top of the larynx; a diverter valve over the opening to the airway during the swallow; as liquids are swallowed, the epiglottis is erect, but it passively bends over the larynx superior aperture during solid food transit

epilepsy any of several disorders characterized by abnormal electrical rhythms or discharges of the central nervous system; may be manifested as convulsive attacks

epimysium sheath of connective tissue around skeletal muscle

epinephrine hormone secreted by the adrenal medulla from sympathetic nervous system stim-

ulation that leads to physiological manifestations of anxiety and fear; therapeutically employed as a vasoconstrictor; also called adrenaline

epiphyseal plates thin bone cartilage plate forming the boundary of bone shaft growth

episode a part of a narrative that relates a series of events as part of the overall plot

epistaxis nosebleed

epithelium the covering, or most superficial layer, of body surfaces

eponym label for body function, organ, disease, procedure based on a person's name, usually the scientist or physician who made the first identification of the entity. The trend is that eponyms are not possessives, that is, they do not end with apostrophe-s

EPROM acronym for erasable programmable read-only memory. EPROMS are microchips that store binary information indefinitely. They can be used to upgrade and expand the capabilities of a dedicated processor

Epstein-Barr virus (EBV) herpes virus that causes mononucleosis and other lymphoproliferative disorders, notably in patients who have undergone transplantation

equilibrium state of modulation between antagonistic or divergent influences or elements;

the goal of adaptive processes in cognition in which new information is assimilated or accommodated; also, a condition of balance

- **mechanical equilibrium** the state in which all forces acting on a body cancel each other out, leaving a zero net force in all directions

- **stable equilibrium** a unique state to which a system with a restoring force will return after it has been displaced from rest

- **unstable equilibrium** the state in which a disturbance of a mechanical system will cause a drift away from a rest position

equalingual someone who is approximately equally competent in two languages

equipotentiality having equal electrical charge

erythema redness of skin; inflammation

erythrocyte sedimentation rate (ESR) laboratory test used to monitor course of an infection

Escherichia coli **(*E. coli*)** coliform bacteria species of the Enterobacteriaceae family that, although normally found in the intestines, water, milk, and soil, is a frequent cause of urinary tract infection and a serious wound gram-negative pathogen; *E. coli* septicemia can rapidly lead from shock to death

Escobar syndrome impaired articulation secondary to limited mouth opening and poor oral movements, with possible compensatory articulations secondary to cleft palate and/or tongue backing from micrognathia; hypernasality common, along with abnormal oral resonance

esophageal atresia impaired esophagus (often congenital anomaly) ending in a blind pouch or narrow cord preventing passage to the stomach

esophageal dilatation stretching of the walls of the esophagus to recover the lumen at the site of strictures. Devices used for dilatation include mercury-filled bougies, inflatable balloons, metal olives, and firm plastic rods of graded sizes

esophageal phase of swallowing bolus transport down esophagus and into stomach through coordinated contraction of smooth and striated esophageal muscles

esophageal reflux back throw (regurgitation) of gastric juice from the stomach into the pharyngeal region through the esophagus; a leading cause of esophagitis

esophageal speech for persons following laryngectomy and vocal fold excision, speech is produced by taking air in through the mouth, trapping it in the throat, and suddenly releasing it; upper parts of the throat/esophagus vibrate and produce sound in the air release; sound is shaped with lips, tongue, teeth, and other mouth parts in a manner similar to the presurgical method

- **injection method** a method of air intake to produce esophageal speech

esophageal stricture narrowing of the esophageal lumen leading to mechanical obstruction of bolus passage. Strictures may be caused by webs, cancers (malignant strictures), extrinsic compression (enlarged blood vessels, pulmonary tumors, goiters). Ingestion of lye may lead to formation of tight and tortuous fibrotic strictures. Peptic strictures are those occurring in reflux esophagitis that are are short and concentric. Treatment of strictures aims to restore the full size of the lumen, primarily through esophageal dilatation

esophageal web abnormal thin membrane that develops across the esophageal lumen, often near the cricoid cartilage

esophagitis inflammation of the esophagus, most commonly caused by gastroesophageal reflux (reflux esophagitis), ingestion of corrosives (e.g., pill esophagitis), and infections (e.g., fungal or viral esophagitis), or irritation from a nasogastric (NG) tube. Mucosal lesions of typical esophagitis include erosions, exudate, or ulcerations that can lead to heartburn, chest pain, dysphagia, and odynophagia. Severe or chronic esophagitis may be complicated by formation of esophageal strictures or by mucosal metaplasia

esophagospasm Also esophageal spasm or segmental or diffuse esophageal spasm an abnormality characterized by the occurrence of simultaneous powerful contractions predominantly in the smooth muscle segment of the esophagus. Commonly causes chest pain and dysphagia; also called segmental, or diffuse, esophageal spasm

esophagus tube (some 25 cm long) leading from the bottom of the pharynx to the stomach; swallowed food is transported through this structure that consists of three parts: cervical portion from the cricoid cartilage (opposite the sixth cervical vertebra) to the thoracic inlet, thoracic area from the thoracic inlet to the diaphragm, and abdominal part below the diaphragm to the stomach cardiac opening; made up of a fibrous coat, muscular coat, and submucous coat, with a mucous membrane lining

- **lower esophageal sphincter (LES)** specialized muscle that closes the gastroesophageal junction and prevents gastroesophageal reflux by its tonic contraction; relaxes in response to swallowing. Transient LES relaxations in the absence of swallows, or TLESRs. A high-pressure zone in the distal esophagus that relaxes with swallowing

ethnocentrism discriminatory beliefs and behaviors based on the belief that one's personal group is superior

ethnographic pedagogy teaching practices and learning strategies derived from ethnography and conducted in the classroom. An ethnographic researcher becomes involved in a classroom and observes, participates, and helps transform teaching practices

ethnography study and systematic recording of human cultures, with research that is qualitative rather than quantitative (e.g., engages in fieldwork, interviews, and observation), with communicative behaviors being a vital aspect of such studies

ethnolinguistic a set of cultural, ethnic, and linguistic features shared by a social group

etio- prefix: pertaining to cause or origin

etiology science and study of all factors leading to a disease/disorder

e-tran a clear Plexiglas board on which symbols are visible from both sides; used for eye gaze communication

eu- prefix: good

euphoria a state of elation or well-being; an exaggerated sense of physical and emotional well-being not based on reality; referred to by drug users as the "high"

eustachian tube also known as the auditory tube, coursing from the middle ear space to nasopharynx; typically closed, the tube opens during swallowing, chewing, and yawning for equalization of middle ear air pressure with atmospheric pressure

eventcast a type of narrative that relates the characters, roles, and relationships related to a situation

event knowledge a child's accumulated information about familiar routines

event structures sequentially organized, familiar events taken from daily life and routinized to teach language structures to children

eversion turning outward

evocative utterances assertions by toddlers that appear to anticipate affirmation or feedback from a caregiver

evoked otoacoustic emissions (evoked OAE) faint sounds generated by nonlinear cochlear processes in response to acoustic stimulation. They can be detected by placing sensitive recording equipment within the ear canal

evoked potential electrical activity in the brainstem or cerebral cortex elicited by a specific stimulus; such a stimulus may affect the auditory, somatosensory, or visual pathway, with each producing a characteristic brain wave pattern

- **endogenous evoked potentials** evoked potentials that are relatively invariant to changes in the eliciting physical stimulus, but are highly influenced by subject state and require an internal or mental activity (e.g., perceptual or cognitive process) to generate the potential

ex- prefix: out of, toward the surface, exterior

exaggeration a treatment technique employing overemphasis of a selected prosodic behavior or articulatory movement

executive function set of general control processes that coordinate knowledge (i.e., cognition) and metacognitive knowledge, transforming such knowledge into behavioral strategies that ensure an individual's behavior is adaptive and consistent with some goal, as well as being beneficial to the person; a component of metacognition

existence language development term for early reflexive relation in which a word indicates that an object is present

exocrine multicellular glands opening onto the skin surface, such as sweat and sebaceous glands

exophora pronominal form used in a sentence requiring an extralinguistic context to supply the reference for the pronoun; contrasts with anaphora in which the reference is supplied linguistically

expanded speech recorded speech that is altered by duplicating small segments of the signal so that the speech sounds as if it were produced with a slow speaking rate; no additional spectral information is introduced

expansions in language development, caregiver utterances that reproduce a child's utterance and include additional grammatical elements. Also, preschoolers' inclusion of additional elements in a noun phrase that expands the length of their utterances

expectorant agent that promotes mucous and/ or bronchial secretion and facilitates secretion expulsion

expiration process of evacuating air from the lungs during respiration; also called exhalation

expiratory board prosthetic device for improving respiratory muscle strength for speech; person in a wheelchair pulls the board (which is tethered to the chair) toward his or her abdomen and leans against it to stabilize the muscles needed for speech

exposition discourse for conveying information or providing explanation

expressive aphasia a common descriptor for people with aphasia who struggle to talk, yet understand most of what is said to them; also called Broca's aphasia

expressive words words that effectively convey meaning or feeling; in language development, early words whose apparent purpose is to engage others in social exchanges

exsufflation dynamic expulsion of air from a cavity by artificial means, such as use of a mechanical exsufflation to simulate a cough and clear secretions from the distal airways

extension physiologic straightening or moving out of the flexed position, the opposite of flexion; in language development, caregiver utterances that repeat and build on a child's utterance, providing related semantic information

external being on the outside

external auditory meatus the canal that leads from the auricle to the tympanic membrane

exteroreceptor skin or mucous membrane peripheral end organ that responds to external agent stimulation

extra- prefix: outside of, without

extracorporeal located or occurring outside the body

extraction, full mouth removal of all the teeth

extralinguistic the nonlinguistic elements of communication (gestures, intonation, etc.) that supplement or alter a message expressed by words and phrases

extrapyramidal motor system all brain elements influencing body (somatic) movement, excluding the motor neurons, motor cortex, and the pyramidal (corticobulbar and corticospinal) tract. The term is generally taken to principally mean the basal ganglia (striate body) and associated structures, along with descending connections with the midbrain

extrapyramidal syndrome constellation of motor impairments attributable to motor pathway injury other than to the pyramidal tracts

extubation the removal of a tube from a body cavity or orifice

eye gaze AAC method in which an individual directs his or her eyes toward a symbol or object to indicate choice

eyeglass hearing aid style of hearing aid in which the hearing aid is housed in the temple piece of a pair of eyeglasses

E

F

FM Auditory Trainer

classroom assistive listening device in which the teacher wears
a microphone and the signal is transmitted to the student(s)
by means of frequency modulated (FM) radio waves

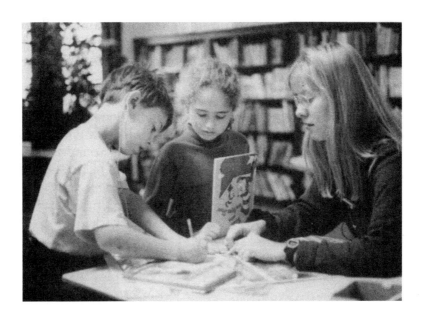

facet a small surface

Fach (German) voice classification, job classification. For example, lyric soprano and dramatic soprano are different Fachs

facilitation act of enabling or assisting a natural process, such as speaking

faciodigitogenital dysplasia x-linked autosomal dominant condition of abnormally wide-set eyes, broad upper lip, anteverted nares, saddlebag scrotum, and lax ligaments

fading treatment technique in which cues or prompts are gradually withdrawn to encourage independent response to the presented stimulus

Fallot's tetralogy congenital heart disease of four defects: pulmonic stenosis, ventricular septal defect, aortic malposition, and right ventricular hypertrophy

falsetto high, light register, applied primarily to men's voices singing in the soprano or alto range. Can also be applied to women's voices. Falsetto voice has relatively few harmonics compared to vocal sound produced with normal voice (in the modal register)

- **mutational falsetto** a psychogenic voice disorder associated with puberty in which the patient uses a falsetto voice

false vocal folds folds of tissue located slightly higher than and parallel to the actual vocal folds

familial deafness deafness in members of the same family

family-centered attitudes and actions that support the family of someone in treatment, enhance family members' competencies, and maintain family autonomy in decision making. Often used in conjunction with the treatment model required by federal law when providing services to infants and toddlers with disabilities and their families and that includes an individualized family service plan (IFSP)

family therapy simultaneous treatment of more than one member of a family; may be supportive, directive, or interpretive

fascia fibrous tissue sheet that envelops the body beneath the external skin, as well as enclosing muscles and groups of muscles. Superficial fascia are sheets of loose connective tissue just beneath skin, with deep fascia surrounding muscles and forming or strengthening ligaments and enveloping and binding various organ and glands

fasciculation involuntary contractions or twitches in a group of muscle fibers innervated by a solitary motor nerve fiber, that can be palpated and seen under the skin; fasciculation of the cardiac muscle is known as fibrillation

fasciculus a small bundle of muscle, nerve, or tendon fibers enveloped by a connective tissue layer

fast adapting sensory fiber some sensory fibers discharge action potentials for a short time when the stimulus is placed or removed and will cease discharging while the stimulus remains on the receptive field. These sensory fibers indicate when a stimulus has arrived and been removed

faucial arches (faucial pillars) the anterior and posterior pillars at the posterior portion of the oral cavity, referred to as the fauces (i.e., the opening into the pharynx). The anterior faucial arches are usually the site for application of thermal stimulation during dysphagia treatment

feature matching ACC assessment process that matches the skills of a nonspeaking individual to the features of a given AAC system

features in phonetics, distinctive properties of sounds

febrile convulsion/seizure fits or seizures caused by a sudden rise in body temperature

febrile state notable body temperature increase, usually accompanied by high pulse and respiration rates

feedback a signal that is returned from the periphery to a central controller; often used to increase stability in a system or a communication exchange

- **acoustic** sound produced when the amplified sound from a device receiver is picked up again by the microphone and reamplified; a high-pitched squeal

- **delayed auditory feedback (DAF)** a speaker's speech is fed back to his or her ears through headphones after a delay; most speakers slow their speech under DAF; the technique is used in reducing the speech rate in persons who stutter or clutter and those who have dysarthria

fenestration an opening or window. Fenestrations are placed in tracheostomy tubes to aid in passage of air through the cannula

festinating gait walking characterized by involuntary hastening or acceleration; frequently occurs in Parkinson disease

fetal alcohol syndrome (FAS) syndrome of children whose mothers were chronic alcohol abusers while the child was in utero; children who have the syndrome may have speech and language delay, articulatory impairment secondary to poor motor skills, compensatory articulation secondary to clefting, growth deficiency, low birth weight, unusual eye spacing, chronic otitis media, sensorineural hearing loss, and mental retardation after infancy; it is now unknown if there is a lower (safe) level of alcohol use during gestation; there is some evidence that less alcohol consumption can lead to malformations less serious than FAS; a less severe form of the syndrome is known as fetal alcohol effect (FAE)

fetal hydantoin syndrome speech delay secondary to cognitive impairment and compensatory articulation secondary to clefting, with language delay and impairment secondary to cognitive limitations; marked also by growth deficiency

fetus the developing unborn child from the end of the eighth week of gestation until birth. The fetal period of development follows the embryonic stage. Unborn offspring of any viviparous animal after it is in a specie-recognizable form

FG syndrome speech delay secondary to cognitive impairment and compensatory articulation secondary to clefting, with language delay and impairment secondary to cognitive limitations; also marked by macrocephaly, strabismus, micrognathia, hearing loss

fiberoptic bronchoscope a type of small diameter (typically 3–6 mm) flexible endoscope used to examine the bronchi

fiberoptics the conduction of light from a source through a bundle of glass or plastic fibers; in wide use for illumination of endoscopic systems to view body cavities and organs

fiberscope flexible fiberoptic viewing instrument with flexibility of shaft allowing viewing of previously inaccessible body areas; specialized instruments include bronchoscope, endoscope, and gastroscope

fibroblast germinal cell of connective tissue; responsible, in part, for the formation of scar in response to tissue injury

fibrosis normal formation of fibrous tissue for repair or replacement, including that of scarring; also atypical situation of the spreading of fibrous connective tissue to replace healthy smooth tissue, most commonly in the lungs, heart, peritoneum, and kidneys

- **interstitial pulmonary fibrosis** scarring and abnormal deposition of collagen within alveolar walls, leading to increased stiffness of lungs and impaired oxygenation. May be caused by autoimmunity, drug hypersensitivity, infection, irradiation, or occupational exposures

figurative language language that conveys meaning through analogy based on stimulus generalization rather than through literal interpretation of words and phrases; expression through analogy

figure and ground psychology of perception concept in which an object has perceptual prominence (figure) against a background or context (ground)

filled pause a pause or gap between utterances that is associated with a vocalization, such as a hesitation sound involving a prolonged vowel or nasal: "I think that his name was . . . mmmmmmm . . . John"

fill-in toddler language development prompting device used by caregivers to encourage a child to complete a statement by supplying the correct word or label left silent (blank) by a caregiver

filter a hardware device or software program that provides a frequency-dependent transmission of energy. Commonly, a filter is used to exclude energy at certain frequencies while passing the energy of other frequencies. A low-pass filter passes the frequencies below a certain cutoff frequency; a high-pass filter passes the frequencies above a certain cutoff frequency; and a band-pass filter passes the energy between a lower and upper cutoff frequency, with a band-reject filter attenuating signal frequencies within a specified frequency band between high and low extremes

- **band-pass filter** filter that allows frequencies only within a certain frequency range to pass

- **band-reject filter** electrical device that attenuates signal frequencies within a specified frequency band between high and low extremes

- **heat moisture exchange filter (HME)** humidification plugged into the tubing of mechanical ventilators that collects warmth and humidity from a patient's breaths, which are then used to moisten the next breath on inspiration

- **high-pass filter** filter that only allows frequencies above a certain cutoff frequency to pass; the cutoff is generally not abrupt but, rather, gentle and is given in terms of a roll-off value, for example, 24 dB/octave

- **low pass filter** filter which allows only frequencies below a certain frequency to pass; the cutoff is generally not abrupt but gentle and is given in terms of a roll-off value, for example, 24 dB/octave

- **notch filter** a filter that attenuates a given frequency band of the input signal

- **source-filter theory** a theory of the acoustic production of speech that states that the energy from a sound source is modified by a filter or set of filters. For example, for vowels, the vibrating vocal folds usually are the source of sound energy and the vocal tract resonances (formants) are the filters

filtered speech speech that has been passed through filter banks to remove or amplify frequency bands in the signal

- **low-pass filtered speech** speech that has been passed through filter banks, leaving the lower, but not the higher, frequencies

filtering frequency-selective modifications of a sound source resulting from the resonating characteristics of the vocal tract

- **inverse filtering** method used for recovering the transglottal airflow during phonation; the technique implies that the voice is fed through a computer filter that compensates for the resonance effects of the supraglottic vocal tract, especially the lowest formants

- **preemphasis** in speech analysis, a filtering that boosts high-frequency energy relative to low-frequency energy. Because speech normally contains its strongest energy in the low frequencies, these frequencies would dominate analysis results if preemphasis were not performed

final consonant deletion a phonological error pattern in which a child omits the consonant at the end of a word

fingerspelling a kind of manual communication, in which words are spelled letter-by-letter using standard hand configurations

first words is the initial milestone in acquiring language and consists of the first use of a meaningful, conventional word at least two different times

fis phenomenon refusal of a child to accept an adult's imitation of the child's misarticulated version of a word; derived from a report of a child who produced the target word [fiʃ] as [fis]

but rejected the adult imitation [fis] as a correct pronunciation of [fiʃ]. The phenomenon appears to demonstrate that the child's productive limitation is not accompanied by a perceptual limitation in evaluating the speech of others

fissure deep groove, furrow, or cleft in an organ surface, such as lung fissures, which delineates the actual lobes; brain fissures more commonly termed sulci/sulcus

fistula atypical tubular opening from a normal cavity or tube to a free (epithelial) surface or to another cavity; may result from congenital incomplete closure of body sections or from abscesses, trauma, or inflammation

- **bronchoesophageal fistula** opening between esophagus and a bronchus, usually secondary to infection or a tumor

- **fistula auris congenita** results from a defect in the formation of the ear's auricle

- **orofacial fistula** opening between oral cavity and facial cutaneous surface

- **oronasal fistula** opening between the nasal and oral cavities

- **tracheoesophageal fistula (TEF)** congenital abnormality, with an opening between the trachea and esophagus often in conjunction with esophageal atresia; can be acquired

Fitzgerald key a left-to-right organization for AAC communication displays. Question words and people are typically found on the left of the display, followed on the right by action words, descriptors, and object nouns

5-dB rule noise protection rule that specifies that the intensity level of a sound can be increased by 5 dB for every 50% reduction in the sound's timed length

flaccid dysarthria motor speech disorder with a neuropathology of damage to the motor units of cranial or spinal nerves that supply speech muscles (lower motor neuron involvement); speech problems caused mostly by muscle weakness and hypotonia; constellation of speech disorders dependent on the specific nerve that is affected, but include breathy voice quality, hypernasality, and imprecise production of consonants

flaccidity absence or reduction of muscle tone typically resulting in a floppy nonfunctional limb or extremity

flange rim or collar of an object that projects beyond the object; the portion of a tracheostomy

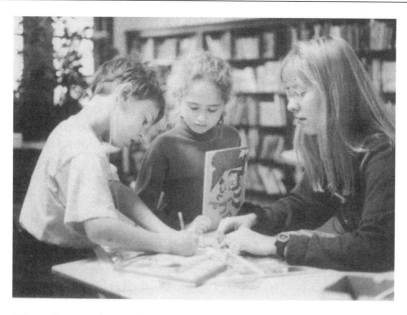

FM auditory trainer   classroom assistive listening device in which the teacher wears a microphone and the signal is transmitted to the student(s) by means of frequency modulated (FM) radio waves

tube that allows for fastening the tube around the neck; may be rigid or flexible

flexion bending a joint to decrease the angle between adjoining bones, as bending the elbow places the ulna near to the humerus; opposite of extension

flora bacteria that live in or on the body; also vegetation, in general

flow the volume of fluid passing through a given cross section of a tube or duct per second; also called volume velocity (measured in liters per second)

flow resistance the ratio of pressure to flow

fluency the flow of speech that is free of abnormal interruptions or disfluencies; seeming to be effortlessly polished; for adults has been specified as an average of 15 sounds per second

fluency inducing conditions situations that almost uniformly eliminate the occurrence of stuttering; for example, choral speaking and speaking to the beat of a metronome

fluent aphasia a category of aphasia characterized by a near normal flow of spoken words, although such utterances may not be clear or understandable

fluid mechanics study of behavior and properties of liquids and gases; subdivided into flu-

id dynamics (fluids in motion) and aerodynamics (gases in motion)

fluoroscopy radiographic procedure in which the internal structure of an object (e.g., the body) is projected as an image on a fluorescent screen for viewing)

flutter modulation in the 10–12 Hz range

FM auditory trainer classroom assistive listening device in which the teacher wears a microphone and the signal is transmitted to the student(s) by means of frequency modulated (FM) radio waves

FM boot a small bootlike device worn on the bottom of a user's hearing aid that contains an FM receiver; used as part of an FM assistive listening device

FM system an assistive listening device that conveys sound from a sound source to a listener by a sinusoidally varying carrier wave; designed to enhance signal-to-noise ratio

focal lesion lesion with damage concentrated in one small area

fontanelle gap between the bones of an infant's cranium covered by sturdy membranes that usually closes around 14 months postpartum

Food and Drug Administration (FDA) U.S. government agency that oversees food, cosmet-

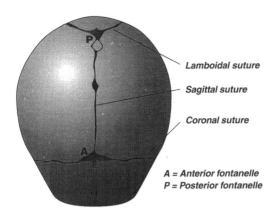

Lamboidal suture

Sagittal suture

Coronal suture

A = Anterior fontanelle
P = Posterior fontanelle

fontanelle gap between the bones of an infant's cranium covered by sturdy membranes that usually closes around 14 months postpartum

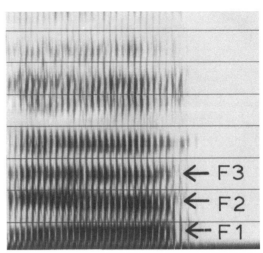

← F3

← F2

← F1

formant a resonance of the vocal tract determined by vocal tract physical parameters and factors including tongue and cheek position, jaw opening, and nasal cavities. A formant is specified by its center frequency (commonly called formant frequency) and bandwidth. Formants are denoted by integers that increase with the relative frequency location of the formants. F_1 is the lowest frequency formant, F_2 is the next highest, and so on. Traditionally, the numbers are subscript to a capital F, but some identify formants with full-size numerals (F1, F2) and others with an italic lowercase f and subscripts (f_1, f_2). Shown is spectrogram of vowel lael

ics, medicines, medical devices, and radiation-emitting consumer products as well as other public health areas designated by Congress, including the regulation of devices such as hearing aids and cochlear implants

foramen magnum the large opening in the base of the skull (occipital bone) through which the spinal cord enters the spinal column; forms the boundary between the brain and spinal cord

force a push or pull; the physical quantity imparted to an object to change its momentum

formant a resonance of the vocal tract determined by vocal tract physical parameters and factors including tongue and cheek position, jaw opening, and nasal cavities. A formant is specified by its center frequency (commonly called formant frequency) and bandwidth. Formants are denoted by integers that increase with the relative frequency location of the formants. F_1 is the lowest frequency formant, F_2 is the next highest, and so on. Traditionally, the numbers are subscript to a capital F, but some identify formants with full-size numerals (F1, F2) and others with an italic lowercase f and subscripts (f_1, f_2)

- **formant frequency** center frequency of a formant

- **formant synthesis** a type of speech synthesis (machine-generated speech) in which resonators are controlled to produce formant-like patterns

- **nasal formant** the low-frequency resonance associated with the nasal tract. For men's

speech, the nasal formant has a frequency of less than 500 Hz

- **singer's formant** a high spectrum peak occurring between about 2.3 and 3.5 kHz in voiced sounds in Western opera and concert singing. This acoustic phenomenon is associated with "ring" in a voice and with a voice's capacity to project over background sound, such as a choir or an orchestra; a similar phenomenon of speaking voice, especially in actors, is the speaker's formant

formant synthesizer a synthesizer that attempts to recreate the changing formants of speech. Typically, a formant synthesizer specifies the frequencies and bandwidths of a small number of formants at small intervals of time

formant transition a change in formant frequency, especially in relation to consonant-vowel or vowel-consonant sequences; occurs over 50–100 ms typically associated with a phonetic boundary; for example, the CV formant

Formant frequencies (in Hz) of the first three formants (F1, F2, F3) of 10 vowels produced by 76 speakers including men, women, and children. Based on data reported by Peterson and Barney (1952). Values for F2 and F3 have been rounded to 50s. The vowel means may be taken to define the approximate formant frequencies of a neutral vowel for each group. Mean F2/F1 and F3/F2 ratios are shown at the bottom of the table.

Vowel	Men			Women			Children		
	F1	F2	F3	F1	F2	F3	F1	F2	F3
[i]	270	2300	3000	300	2800	3300	370	3200	3700
[ɪ]	400	2000	2550	430	2500	3100	530	2750	3600
[ɛ]	530	1850	2500	600	2350	3000	700	2600	3550
[æ]	660	1700	2400	860	2050	2850	1000	2300	3300
[a]	730	1100	2450	850	1200	2800	1030	1350	3200
[ɔ]	570	850	2400	590	900	2700	680	1050	3200
[ʊ]	440	1000	2250	470	1150	2700	560	1400	3300
[u]	300	850	2250	370	950	2650	430	1150	3250
[ʌ]	640	1200	2400	760	1400	2800	850	1600	3350
[ɝ]	490	1350	1700	500	1650	1950	560	1650	2150
Mean	500	1420	2400	575	1700	2800	670	1900	3250
F2/F1	2.84			2.96			2.84		
F3/F2		1.69			1.65			1.71	

formant frequency   center frequency of a formant

---

transition refers to formant pattern changes associated with the consonant-vowel transition

formant tuning a boosting of vocal intensity when F_0 or one of its harmonics coincides exactly with a formant frequency

form of language inventory of elements—sounds and gestures—and the rules for combining them to form words and sentences

- **dummy forms** utterances consisting of a true word combined with an additional sound or syllable that give the appearance of approximating multiword utterances

- **empty forms** forms that are consistent, but do not represent conventional words are combined with a true word and appear to approximate multiword utterances

- **logical form rules** the component of Chomsky's linguistic government-binding theory dealing with the logic of sentences

- **phonetic form rules** the underlying universal rules that generate the basic syntactic relationships in the deep structure of a sentence

fortis sound produced with emphatic expiration and relatively strong articulatory tautness

fossa a depression or hollow, groove, or furrow often on a bone tip

Fourier transform a mathematical procedure that converts a series of values in the time domain (waveform) to a set of values in the frequency domain (spectrum). The spectrum is the Fourier transform of the waveform

- **discrete Fourier transform (DFT)** Fourier transform that operates on digital (discrete) data, that is, sequences of numbers

- **fast Fourier transform (FFT)** an algorithm commonly used in microcomputer programs to calculate a Fourier spectrum. The FFT is a special type of DFT in which the number of points transformed is a power of 2. The number of points expresses the bandwidth of analysis; the higher the value, the narrower the bandwidth

fovea a pit-shaped shallow depression

fractal a geometric figure in which an identical pattern or motif repeats itself over and over on

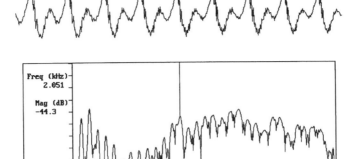

Fourier transform a mathematical procedure that converts a series of values in the time domain (waveform) to a set of values in the frequency domain (spectrum). The spectrum is the Fourier transform of the waveform

an ever-diminishing scale. Self-similarity is an essential characteristic

fractal dimension fractal dimensions are measures of fractal objects that can be used to determine how alike or different the objects are. Box-counting algorithms and mass-radius measurement are two common approaches to determining fractal dimension. The fractal dimension represents the way a set of points fills a given area of space. It may be defined as the slope of the function relating the number of points contained in a given radius (or its magnification) to the radius itself. For example, an object can be assessed under many magnifications. The coast of Britain can be measured, for example, with a meter stick or a millimeter stick, but the latter will yield a larger measure. As magnification is increased (smaller measuring sticks), a point will be reached at which small changes in magnification no longer significantly affect length. That is, a plot of coastline length versus magnification reaches a plateau. That plateau corresponds to fractal dimension. The more irregular the figure (e.g., coastline), the more complex and the more space it occupies, hence, the higher its fractal dimension. A perfect line has a fractal dimension of 1. A figure that fills a plane has a fractal dimension of 2. Fractal dimension cannot be used alone to determine the presence or absence of chaotic behavior. In general, a fractal dimension can be calculated as the quotient of the logarithm of an object's size and the logarithm of the measuring scale

fragile X syndrome leading cause of inherited mental retardation, marked by an X chromo-some with a fragile site on the tip of the long arm, appearing as if the arm of the chromosome is broken

fragmentation, verbal (or uncertainty behavior) excessive interjections and filler sometimes heard in utterances of aging individuals

frame a set of points taken as a single unit of analysis. Software that performs multiple operations over an extended set of data often performs the operations on successive frames, or blocks, of data. In speech analysis systems, the frame is the temporal interval in which operations are performed

Freeman-Sheldon syndrome impaired articulation secondary to limited oral opening and compensatory articulation secondary to clefting and VPI; also marked by a whistling face and appearance of keel-shaped forehead, micrognathia, and Robin sequence

frenulum a little frenum (derives from bridle)

- **frenulum epiglottidis** median glossoepi-glottic fold

- **frenulum of upper lip, frenulum of lower lip** folds of mucous membrane linking the lips to the gums

- **lingual frenulum** fold of mucous membrane from the tongue's underside midline to the floor of the mouth (lack of or minimal lingual frenulum characterizes ankyloglossia)

frenum band of tissue connecting two structures, one of which is mobile; also, a fold of skin or mucous membrane that restricts the range of movement of a structure

frequency the speed with which a given motion repeats itself. In connection with electromagnetics, usually expressed in hertz (Hz), a unit of one cycle per second. Thus a 512 Hz tone is one whose primary components repeat themselves 512 times per second; 512 Hz is roughly middle C on the piano. Four hundred and forty (440) Hz is the tone to which European symphony orchestras adjust the tuning of all instruments. Thus a tone of 2000 Hz sounds much higher in pitch than a tone of 500 Hz, although pitch and frequency are not the same phenomena

- **best frequency** frequency of sound stimulation to which a neuron responds most vigorously; also known as characteristic frequency

- **component frequency** mathematically, a sinusoid; perceptually, a pure tone; also called a partial

- **critical flicker fusion frequency** the least number of flashes of light per second for a pulsing light source to stop stimulating a sensation of a continuous visual image

- **crossover frequency** the fundamental frequency for which there is an equal probability for perception of two adjacent registers

- **dominant frequency** encephalographic frequency that occurs most often

- **frequency domain** aspect of a function defined by amplitude and phase at each frequency component; usually determined by Fourier analysis

- **frequency encoding** in magnetic resonance imaging (MRI), a way to vary magnetic field strength

- **frequency response** a function or functions that specify the relation between amplitude response and frequency characteristics, showing the manner in which the gain and phase of a system vary with the frequency of a stimulus

- **frequency tremor** a periodic (regular) pitch modulation of the voice (an element of vibrato)

- **fundamental frequency (F_0, f_0, F0)** the lowest frequency (first harmonic) of a periodic signal. In speech, the fundamental frequency is the first harmonic of the voice. Fundamental frequency is the reciprocal of the fundamental period. Ideally, fundamental frequency is a physical measure of the lowest periodic component of the vocal fold vibration. Pitch should be used to indicate the perceptual phenomenon in which stimuli

can be rated along a continuum of low to high

- **resonant frequency** in magnetic resonance imaging (MRI), frequency at which discrete magnetic nuclei emit or absorb radiofrequency energy

frequency analysis analysis of a signal showing its partials

frequency-domain operation an operation that is performed in the frequency domain, for example, with a fast Fourier transform (FFT) or linear predictive coding (LPC) spectrum

frequency modulation (FM) modulating frequency in accordance with an input signal to encode a carrier wave

frequency of occurrence the relative number of occurrences of an event or structure in a language sample; for example, the relative number of occurrences of a phoneme or word

frequency of usage (word) a measure indicating how often a particular word occurs during everyday conversation

frication generation of noise through the turbulent flow of air through a constricted region

fricative a speech sound characterized by a long interval of turbulence noise. Fricatives are often classified as stridents or nonstridents, depending on the degree of noise energy; fricative consonants are produced by a constriction of the vocal tract, particularly by directing the airstream against a hard surface, producing noisy air turbulence. Examples include s produced with the teeth, s produced with the lower lip and upper incisors, and th produced with the tongue tip and upper incisors

fringe vocabulary words and expression that are typically content-rich, topic-related, and specific to particular individuals, activities, or environments

frontal anterior; pertaining to the front, about the frontal (coronal) plane, frontal bone, or forehead

function one of a set of related acts advancing a larger action; notably a specific typical action of a body part within a living organism; behaviors or activities expected of a person or thing; generally means a definite end or purpose that someone or something serves or a particular task expected to be accomplished

functional in treatment, an objective that typically is the ability of an individual being treated to be independent; also a skill category for purposeful activities in daily life such as eating,

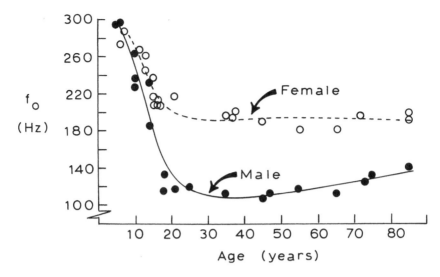

fundamental frequency (F_0, f_0, F0) the lowest frequency (first harmonic) of a periodic signal. In speech, the fundamental frequency is the first harmonic of the voice. Fundamental frequency is the reciprocal of the fundamental period. Ideally, fundamental frequency is a physical measure of the lowest periodic component of the vocal fold vibration. Pitch should be used to indicate the perceptual phenomenon in which stimuli can be rated along a continuum of low to high

dressing, walking, or speaking; pragmatic or practical purposes served by utterances

functional analysis experimentally determining which variables influence the occurrence or nonoccurrence of a behavior

functional independence measure (FIM) an objective measure of independent functioning, developed by a national rehabilitation task force, that is used to monitor recovery and outcome in rehabilitation; it consists of 18 areas of functioning including ambulation, self-care, communication, and cognitive skills, each rated on a scale of 1 (fully dependent) to 7 (fully independent)

functional language disorders language disorders with no apparent organic basis

functional magnetic resonance imaging (fMRI) image of function is created from signals generated by the hemodynamics within the structure of interest, allowing observation of which body structures are active in specific functions; high-resolution images of neural activity are achieved through depictions of oxygen level and flow

functional residual capacity (FRC) lung volume at which the elastic inspiratory forces

equal the elastic expiratory forces; in spontaneous quiet breathing, exhalation stops at FRC

functional voice disorder an abnormality in voice sound and function in the absence of an anatomic or physiologic organic abnormality

fundamental the sinusoidal component of a complex wave whose frequency is equal to the repetition frequency of the waveform. The fundamental frequency is sometimes called the first harmonic

fundamental frequency (F_0, f_0, F0) the lowest frequency (first harmonic) of a periodic signal. In speech, the fundamental frequency is the first harmonic of the voice. Fundamental frequency is the reciprocal of the fundamental period. Ideally, fundamental frequency is a physical measure of the lowest periodic component of the vocal fold vibration. Pitch should be used to indicate the perceptual phenomenon in which stimuli can be rated along a continuum of low to high

- **coefficient of fundamental frequency variation** this measure, expressed in percentage, computes the relative standard deviation of the fundamental frequency. It is the ratio of the standard deviation of the period-to-period variation to the average fundamental frequency

- **crossover frequency** the fundamental frequency for which there is an equal probability for perception of two adjacent registers

- **F_0-tremor frequency** this measure is expressed in hertz and shows the frequency of the most intensive low-frequency F_0 modulating component in the specified F_0 tremor analysis range

- **F_0-tremor intensity index** the average ratio of the frequency magnitude of the most intensive low frequency modulating component (F_0 tremor) to the total frequency magnitude of the analyzed sample. The algorithm for tremor analysis determines the strongest periodic frequency modulation of the voice. This measure is expressed in percentage

fundoplication, Nissen fundoplication surgical procedure used to treat gastroesophageal reflux; procedure involves wrapping of the fundus of the stomach around the gastroesophageal junction

funiculus small, cordlike structure

fusiform spindle-shaped

F

G

Gyrus (pl., gyri)

convolution (fold) of the cerebral hemispheres (denoted by g.)

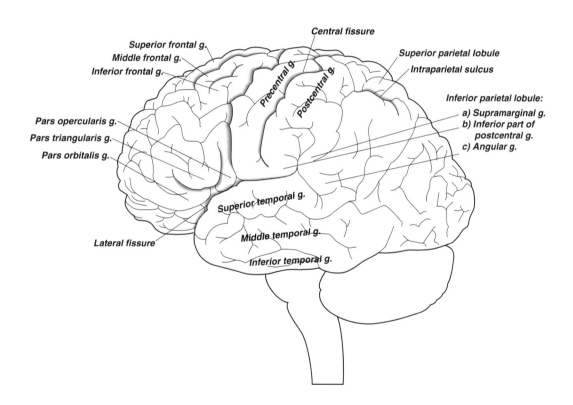

GABA (gamma-aminobutyric acid, (ɡ-aminobutryic acid) neurotransmitter responsible for postsynaptic neuronal inhibition in the brain, lungs, heart, and kidney

gag reflex normal neural reflex activated through touch of the posterior pharynx or soft palate; employed to check the integrity of the vagus and glossopharyngeal nerves

gain in hearing aids, the difference in decibels between the input level of an acoustic signal and the output level

- **automatic gain control (AGC)** nonlinear hearing aid compression circuitry that changes gain as signal level changes and/or limits the output of the hearing aid when the level reaches a specified value

- **effective gain** difference in decibels between a patient's aided and unaided thresholds

- **full-on gain** hearing aid setting that results in the maximum acoustic output

- **functional gain** difference in decibels between unaided and aided thresholds

- **insertion gain** hearing aid gain

- **prescribed gain** gain and frequency response of a hearing aid that are determined by use of a prescriptive formula

- **real-ear gain** gain of a hearing aid at the tympanic membrane, measured with a probe-microphone; the difference between the SPL in the external ear canal and the SPL at the field reference point for a specified sound field

- **target gain** in hearing-aid fitting, the prescribed gain for each frequency against which the actual hearing-aid output is compared

- **use gain** amount of gain provided by a hearing aid when the volume control is set where it is commonly used

gait method of walking or moving by foot; a pattern of foot movements

gamete mature sexual germ cell, either the female ovum or male sperm cell

gamma-aminobutyric acid (GABA) inhibitory neurotransmitter found in brain, heart, lungs, and kidneys

gamma camera nuclear medicine imaging device that records gamma-ray photons produced by radionuclide decay; used for diagnostic scanning of an injected radioactive substance

gangli-, ganglio- prefix: knotlike

ganglion mass of nerve cell bodies mostly outside of the central nervous system

- **inferior ganglion of the vagus nerve** containing cell bodies concerned with special sensation and general afferents from the viscera

gas a fluid (such as air) without inherent shape or volume with a tendency to indefinitely expand unless kept in a container or compressed in a cold environment, when it can become liquid and, in extreme conditions, a solid

- **alveolar gas** pulmonary gas at point of O_2–CO_2 exchange with pulmonary capillary blood

- **blood gases** clinical terminology for determining partial pressures of O_2 and CO_2 in blood

gas sterilization sterilization of medical devices by gas, typically used for devices that could be damaged by heat and moisture sterilization equipment

gastric pertaining to the stomach

gastric juice stomach digestive secretions, primarily consisting of pepsin, hydrochloric acid, rennin, and mucin; pH strongly acid (0.9 to 1.5)

gastroesophageal reflux (GER) retrograde passage of gastric juice from the stomach into the esophagus, capable of reaching the larynx or oral cavity and being aspirated into the lungs; heartburn is among the most common symptoms/complaints

gastroesophageal reflux disorder (GERD) chronic reflux of gastric contents into the esophagus, resulting in damage and/or disease

gastrostomy creation of surgical opening into the stomach through the abdominal wall, generally to provide nutrition for patients with esophageal cancer, tracheoesophageal fistula, or long-term consciousness loss from a stroke or other disorder

- **percutaneous endoscopic gastrostomy (PEG)** artificial means of providing nutrition and hydration via a tube placed through the esophagus into the stomach via endoscopy, with the tube connected to nutrition source though an opening in the stomach. This type of tube is generally more comfortable for a patient than a nasogastric tube. It appears to carry the same risk of aspiration, especially if aspiration precautions (i.e., elevation of the head during feeding) are not allowed

gavage feeding by means of a nasogastric tube; for newborns, the tube may originate in the mouth

gaze coupling a gaze pattern in which caregivers and infants maintain eye contact in long, alternating intervals

-gen suffix: that which generates

genderlect the communication styles that appear to be characteristic of each gender

gene a unique sequence of nucleotides in DNA or RNA located in the germ plasm, usually on a chromosome, and that is the operative unit of inheritance, controlling transmission and expression of one or more traits by specifying the structure of a particular polypeptide (particularly a protein) or by controlling the function of other genetic material

generalization application of what has been learned in treatment to new words, more complex speech, new situations, and new communicative partners; addition of new stimuli or environmental factors to elicit the same response as obtained in a controlled setting

generative grammar attempt to define rules that can generate an unlimited number of acceptable sentences in a language; linked to transformational grammar, which tries to identify rules governing relations among sentence aspects

generic drug name official, common, or public name designating a specific drug by its principal active ingredients, as opposed to a proprietary business brand name; generics, as a rule, are less expensive than brand-name drugs and may be, but not always are, identical to a prescribed brand-name drug

genetic inherited; concerning origin, reproduction, or birth; also, pertaining to the science of genetics or heredity

- **clinical genetics** the science of studying human beings and diagnosing genetic disease

- **inheritance mode** the pattern with which a genetic trait is inherited in a family

- **molecular genetics** the science of studying the structure and function of genes to determine how human disease is caused and how genes function

genetic counseling process of determining and providing information to prospective parents about the likelihood of an inherited condition or disorder in their children

-genic suffix: producing

geniculate referring to the facial nerve geniculum (kneelike or knotted structure)

- **lateral geniculate body** thalamic nucleus that receives optic nerve impulses from the retina en route to the visual cortex

- **medial geniculate body** thalamic nucleus area relaying auditory impulses to the auditory cortex from the lateral lemniscus

genitive word form indicating possession

genome all of a chromosome set derived from one parent; complete gene complement of a set of chromosomes in each cell of a given organism

genotype all of the hereditary information in an organism; pair of genes needed for a particular characteristic or protein

genres categories of discourse for various circumstances

genu knee

ger- prefix: old or aged

geriatric concerning the aging process

gerontology study of aging and its associated phenomena

gestation the carrying of viviparous animals' offspring in the uterus from conception to birth; for humans, the average length, as calculated from the first day of the last typical menstrual period, is 280 days, with a normal range of 259 days (37 weeks) to 287 days (41 weeks). Infants born before the 37th week are usually given the label premature and those born after the 41st week, postmature

gestational age age computed from first day of the mother's last menstrual period to any point thereafter, usually not calculated beyond the first few months of life after birth

gesture unaided communication in which body movements are used to express or emphasize a belief, emotion, or perception; head and arm movements, plus facial display are examples

gingiva gum tissue

gland organized cell group functioning as an organ of secretion or excretion

- **accessory gland** small accumulation of glandular structure, separated from but being near another more sizeable gland, which is similar in structure and likely contributes to the latter's functioning

- **arytenoid glands** large number of laryngeal mucous membrane mixed glands

- **bronchial glands** mucous and seromucous glands with secretory aspects outside the bronchi muscle

- **buccal glands** numerous mixed and racemose (clustered) glands in cheek submucous tissue

- **endocrine glands** ductless glands, with hormone secretions directly transferred into the blood

- **esophageal glands** mucous glands in the esophageal submucosa

- **gastric glands** tubular branched glands in the mucosa of the stomach fundus and body, with parietal cells secreting hydrochloric acid, pepsin-producing zymogen cells, and mucous cells

- **labial glands** lip submucous tissue mucous glands

- **mixed glands** delivering both serous and mucous secretions

- **palatine glands** racemose (clustered) glands in posterior portion of hard palate submucous tissue

- **parathyroid glands** small paired endocrine glands usually embedded on posterior surface of the thyroid gland that secrete a hormone that regulates calcium and phosphorus metabolism

- **parotid gland** largest salivary gland, one of two compound glands inferior and anterior to each ear, discharging through the parotid duct

- **pharyngeal glands** racemose (clustered) glands beneath pharyngeal mucous membrane

- **salivary glands** sublingual and submandibular glands, considered as one; discharging through sublingual ducts

- **sublingual gland** one of two salivary glands beneath the tongue on the mouth floor; mostly secretes mucus

- **submandibular gland** one of two salivary glands in the neck, located between the digastric muscle bellies and mandibular angle; largely serous secretions

- **thyroid gland** ductless gland lying in the front and to the sides of the upper trachea that secretes thyroid hormone (several metabolically active substances)

- **tracheal glands** numerous mixed glands in the tracheal submucosa that open through short ducts into the tracheal lumen

glaucoma condition in which pressure inside the eye is raised and includes atrophy and excavation of the optic nerve; field of vision defects can result

glia supporting or connective tissue of the central nervous system performing less specialized functions of the network of nerves; also known as neuroglia; types include astrocytes, oligodendroglia, microglia, and ependymal cells

glial cells cells that support and nourish neurons in the central nervous system

glide a consonant sound that has a gradual (gliding) change in articulation reflected by a relatively long interval of formant frequency shift

gliding a phonological error pattern in which a child substitutes a glide (e.g., "w") for another sound (e.g., "r")

glioblastoma multiforme aggressive type of brain tumor that grows rapidly

glioma term frequently encompassing all central nervous system (CNS) tumors, including astrocytomas, oligodendrogliomas, and medulloblastomas

glissando a singing "slide" including all possible pitches between the initial and final pitch sounded; similar to portamento and slur

global aphasia the most severe of aphasias; suggestive of severe impairment in comprehension and use of language; a common occurrence in the beginning hours and days of injury but not necessarily indicative of long-term impairment

globus round body, ball

- **globus hystericus** difficulty in swallowing; temporary sensation of a lump in the throat that cannot be coughed up or swallowed; might be caused by emotional conflict or a functional malfunction of CN IX and spasm of the lower throat-encircling inferior constrictor muscle; physical examination and barium studies tend to show typical structures and function

- **globus pallidus** light gray inner portion of the brain's lentiform nucleus, part of the basal ganglia

glossectomy surgical resection of the tongue

- **total glossectomy** surgical resection that includes removal of the tongue-based musculature from the hyoid, glossopharyngeus, and styloglossus

glosso-, gloss- combining form: pertaining to the tongue

glossolalia copious and often emotionally fraught speech that has the impression of lucid speech, but is usually unintelligible to a listener

glossopharyngeal breathing method of breathing than can possibly decrease an individual's dependence on mechanical ventilatory support; also called "frog breathing," it utilizes air injected into the lungs through the "gulping" action of the oral, laryngeal, and pharyngeal muscles

glossopharyngeal nerve ninth cranial nerve (CN IX) fundamental to sensation of taste and also innervating some viscera and glandular secretion, with both sensory and motor fibers of tongue, parotid gland, and pharynx; connects with the vagus nerve (CN X)

glottal referring to the glottis

- **convergent glottal shape** glottal narrowing, from bottom to top
- **glottal attack, hard** abrupt voice initiation with too much stress on individual words, with words in a sentence sounding too separated; a vocally abusive behavior
- **glottal attack, harsh** initiating phonation of a word or sound with a glottal plosive
- **glottal attack, soft** gentle glottal approximation, often obtained using an imaginary /h/
- **glottal chink** opening in the glottis during vocal fold adduction, most commonly posteriorly; may be a normal variant in some cases
- **glottal closure response** the adduction of the vocal folds in response to the entry of foreign material into the larynx; a protective mechanism that may become less effective during periods of chronic airflow redirection, as in conjunction with tracheostomy
- **glottal contact ulcer** benign lesions on the posterior third of the glottal margin; possibly due to trauma, reflux, or vocally abusive behaviors; voice symptoms include low pitch, effortful phonation, and vocal fatigue
- **glottal control** a learned technique in which the vocal folds are kept adducted to assist in controlling airflow through the glottis and upper airway; can be employed by individuals who are ventilator dependent during cuff deflation
- **glottal fry (vocal fry)** a normal voice register that may occur at the end of sentences; very low-pitched vocalization that may sound like the popping of popcorn; also

called vocal fry or pulse register; the vocal register is characterized by low fundamental frequency, with syncopated vibration of vocal folds with a pattern of short glottal waves alternating with larger and longer ones and with a long closed phase

- **glottal resistance** ratio between transglottal airflow and subglottal pressure; mainly reflects the degree of glottal adduction
- **glottal stop (or click)** an abnormality of articulation (for English) where consonants are produced by hard contact of the vocal folds causing a stoppage of air and sudden release; an articulatory error common in individuals with cleft palate
- **glottal volume velocity** the flow of air through the glottis during phonation

glottis the air channel opening between the vocal folds through which air escapes for phonation (voice production) and through which air passes during normal respiration; also called rima glottidis

- **glottis respiratoria** cartilaginous portion of the glottis
- **glottis vocalis** membranous portion of the glottis

glottogram, flow (FGG) recording of the transglottal airflow versus time, that is, of the sound of the voice source; generally obtained from inverse filtering; acoustical representation of the voice source

glue ear ear fluid becomes hyperviscous

glycosuria abnormal amount of sugar, especially glucose, in the urine, routinely associated with diabetes mellitus

gnatho-, gnath- prefix: pertaining to the jaw

gnomic having the same shape under changes in size; characterized by aphorism (concise adage)

goblet cells mucus secreting cells in the airway

goiter chronic thyroid gland enlargement; rarely of size to obstruct bolus passage in swallowing

Golabi-Rosen syndrome speech and language delayed and impaired common and variable depending on degree of cognitive deficiency, with articulation impairment cause by large tongue; also noted by macrostomia

Goldberg-Shprintzen syndrome impaired speech secondary to cognitive impairment and cleft palate, with language delayed and impaired secondary to cognitive impairment and hypernasality secondary to cleft palate; also marked by lower lip pit or mount, short stature, long curled eyelashes

Goldenhar syndrome marked by misarticulation secondary to tongue motion asymmetry, malocclusion, and possible compensatory articulation secondary to clefting, with hypernasality common and hoarseness caused by unilateral vocal cord paresis; language is delayed and impaired in presence of cognitive impairment

Goltz syndrome dental anomalies can lead to articulation problems and oral mucosal lesions, cognitive impairment can lead to speech delay, along with delayed and impaired language; also marked by syndactyly, small eyes, strabismus

gooseflesh autonomic skin response to chilly environment, emotional stimulus, or skin irritation resulting in erection of skin hairs caused by involuntary muscles

government-binding theory linguistic theory of Noam Chomsky presuming innate human disposition to language acquisition that is internalized and has universal aspects

- **deep structure** component within government-binding theory that contains the sentence structure rules and a language user's lexicon

- **logical form rules** component of government-binding theory dealing with the logic of sentences

- **S-structures** abstract surface structure portion of government-binding linguistic theory

grace days former contractual arrangement, especially in European opera houses, in which female performers were permitted to refrain from singing during the premenstrual and early menstrual portions of their cycles, at their discretion

grammar the collection of rules that characterize the regularities or patterns of a language

- **case grammar** a generative grammar that emphasizes the cases or semantic roles assumed by nouns in relationship to the verb of a sentence

- **descriptive grammar** a set of linguistic rules that describes the regularities present in a set of utterances

- **descriptive patterns** syntactic devices found in text grammar that signal a topic is being described

- **formal grammar** the collective set of written rules that describe the conventional regularities in a language

- **generative grammar** a grammar naming a limited number of rules capable of generating an unlimited number of acceptable sentences in a language

- **intuitive grammar** implicit, underlying knowledge of the acceptable patterns and regularities in a given language

- **pivot grammar** a description of children's early grammar that describes a limited number of words (pivots) occurring only in certain positions and a larger set of words (open) combined with them to form simple sequences of two or three words

- **prescriptive grammar** a collection of rules that purports to dictate correct grammatical structures to the speakers of a language

- **story grammar** the structure of narratives that may be treatment targets for children with language disorders

- **text grammar** characteristic styles associated with language found in textbooks

- **transformational generative grammar** a linguistic theory proposing that universal rules generate underlying structures that may be transformed by rules to derive the specific sentence forms and internal relationships of each language

grammatical structure rules information stored in the brain about the way sentences are parsed in one's native language

grammatical verbs verbs that play a grammatic role without conveying specific action; compare with lexical verbs

grammatic closure the ability to complete phrases or sentences despite missing words or morphemes (e.g., filling in the verb form *are* versus *is* to conjugate with the subject *they*)

grammatic complexity measure of the number of transformational rules related to the production or comprehension of a grammatical structure

grammatic ellipsis linguistic device in which speakers eliminate information expected to be apparent to listeners from the context

grand mal seizure obsolete term for generalized tonic-clonic seizure, characterized by a sudden onset of muscle contraction often with cry or moan and a fall to the ground, giving way to clonic convulsive movements; term is in disfavor

granuloma inflammatory mass, usually following repeated irritation. May occur, for example, at a tracheotomy stoma site or on the vocal

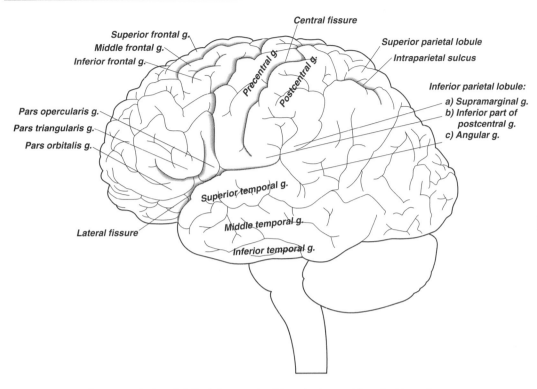

Superior frontal g.
Middle frontal g.
Inferior frontal g.

Central fissure

Precentral g.
Postcentral g.

Superior parietal lobule
Intraparietal sulcus

Inferior parietal lobule:
a) Supramarginal g.
b) Inferior part of postcentral g.
c) Angular g.

Pars opercularis g.
Pars triangularis g.
Pars orbitalis g.

Superior temporal g.

Lateral fissure

Middle temporal g.

Inferior temporal g.

gyrus (pl., gyri)   convolution (fold) of the cerebral hemispheres (denoted by g.)

folds after intubation (i.e., intubation granuloma). Also is a raised lesion generally covered with mucosa, most commonly in the region of the vocal process or medial surface of the arytenoid; often caused by reflux and/or muscle tension dysphonia

grapheme letter or letter combination that represents the phonemes of a language

graphology the way a language is written; study of handwriting, often for personality study

grave accent grave (`), usually over a vowel

gray matter gray tissue found in cortex of the cerebrum, cerebellum, and spinal cord core, and internal nuclei (e.g., basal ganglia; the dark or gray color is imparted by aggregates of neuronal cell bodies)

GRBAS scale scale for describing the degree and nature of voice dysfunction; G = overall grade, R = rough, B = breathy, A = asthenic, S = strained

groove in phonetics, a narrow groove formed in an articulator, especially the tongue, with groove sounds including the fricative /s/ in

which air is channeled through a groove in the apex of the tongue

grooving, central movement of the tongue to form a central depressed area where the food bolus is gathered and shaped into a globular mass before it is propelled posteriorly on a swallowing path

groping patterns in language development, early attempts at true two-word utterances produced with effort and hesitation; in speech disorders, a difficult, labored pattern of articulation

ground electrical conductor connected to the electrical return in a power system, for example, earth, or to a large conductor conventionally used as a reference potential (zero), for example, the steel frame of a car; also, the background against which an object or image appears, as in figure-ground pattern

guest workers people who are recruited to work in a society or nation other than their homeland

gustation sense of taste

gyrus (pl., gyri) convolution (fold) of the cerebral hemispheres

H

hair cells

hair cells in the cochlea's organ of Corti provide the link between mechanical movement of the basilar membrane and excitation of auditory nerve fibers. Small hair-like structures (cilia) protrude from the upper surfaces of the cells. Nerve fibers terminate on the cell bodies. There are three rows of outer hair cells. They are innervated, in complex fashion, by only a small percentage of the total available nerve fibers. There is one row of inner hair cells. They are innervated, in relatively point-to-point fashion, by the vast majority (about 95%) of auditory nerve fibers; there are similar hair cells in the inner ear's sensory epithelium of the membranous labyrinth (vestibular hair cells) as well as in the tongue's taste buds

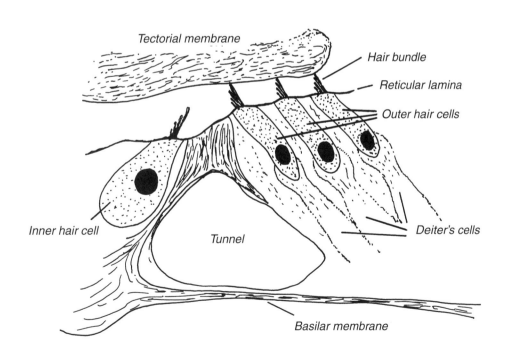

H₂ receptor blocker histamine mediates its effects through several different receptors. Acid secretion by gastric mucosa is mediated by H_2, the type 2 histamine receptors. H_2 receptor blocking drugs interfere with H_2 reception, reducing gastric acid secretion

habilitation program or intervention aimed at the initial development of an individual's skills and abilities for functioning in the community

hair cells hair cells in the cochlea's organ of Corti provide the link between mechanical movement of the basilar membrane and excitation of auditory nerve fibers. Small hair-like structures (cilia) protrude from the upper surfaces of the cells. Nerve fibers terminate on the cell bodies. There are three rows of outer hair cells. They are innervated, in complex fashion, by only a small percentage of the total available nerve fibers. There is one row of inner hair cells. They are innervated, in relatively point-to-point fashion, by the vast majority (about 95%) of auditory nerve fibers; there are similar hair cells in the inner ear's sensory epithelium of the membranous labyrinth (vestibular hair cells) as well as in the tongue's taste buds

- **inner hair cells** the inner row of about 3,500 hair cells that play a primary role in auditory signal transduction
- **outer hair cells** outer three rows of some 12,000 hair cells

half-life time required by living tissue, an organ, or an organism to eliminate by biological processes half the quantity of a substance that has been ingested

halitosis bad breath

Hallermann-Streiff syndrome severe micrognathia leads to articulation impairment from problems with tongue manipulation; also marked by obstructive apnea, microphthalmia, cataracts, nystagmus

hallucination false perception; belief that non-existent thing is real; may be visual, auditory, tactile, or of taste or smell and may be provoked by psychological illness (i.e., schizophrenia) or by brain-affected physical disorders such as temporal lobe epilepsy or stroke; may be caused by drugs or sensory deprivation

hallucinogens a broad group of drugs that excite the central nervous system and cause dis-

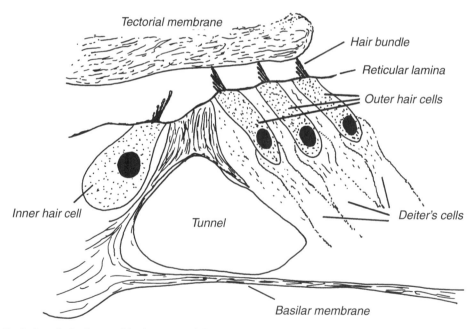

hair cells hair cells in the cochlea's organ of Corti provide the link between mechanical movement of the basilar membrane and excitation of auditory nerve fibers. Small hair-like structures (cilia) protrude from the upper surfaces of the cells. Nerve fibers terminate on the cell bodies. There are three rows of outer hair cells. They are innervated, in complex fashion, by only a small percentage of the total available nerve fibers. There is one row of inner hair cells. They are innervated, in relatively point-to-point fashion, by the vast majority (about 95%) of auditory nerve fibers; there are similar hair cells in the inner ear's sensory epithelium of the membranous labyrinth (vestibular hair cells) as well as in the tongue's taste buds

tortions of sensory perception; examples include lysergic acid diethylamide (LSD), mescaline, psilocybin

hamulus a hook-shaped structure

handicap personal or social ramifications felt or encountered from having sustained an injury or disability; it entails the perceived disadvantages of being injured

hard disk computer data storage medium made up of a rigid electromagnetic-coated disk allowing information to be recorded on it and retrieved from it; usually permanently installed, as compared with a removable diskette

hard glottal attack abrupt voice initiation with too much stress on individual words, with words in a sentence sounding too separated; a vocally abusive behavior

hard of hearing having a hearing loss; usually not used to refer to a profound hearing loss

hard palate the bony portion of the roof of the mouth made up of the palatal processes of the maxillae and the horizontal plates of the palatine bones

hard-wired property of an electronic circuit that is determined by the wiring of the hardware, as opposed to being programmable by software or controlled by a switch; also, referring to brain connections that are believed to be innate (inborn), especially for neural pathways

harmonic an integer multiple of the fundamental frequency in voiced sounds. Ideally, the voice source can be conceptualized as a line spectrum in which energy appears as a series of harmonics; also, a frequency that is an integer multiple of a given fundamental. Harmonics of a fundamental are equally spaced in frequency. Partial in a spectrum in which the frequency of each partial equals n times the fundamental frequency, n being the number of the harmonic

- **simple harmonic motion** sinusoidal motion; the smoothest back and forth motion possible

- **subharmonic** a frequency obtained by dividing a fundamental frequency by an integer greater than zero

harsh glottal attack initiating phonation of a word or sound with a glottal plosive

head proximal portion of a bone

headphone earphone

head pointer a device worn on the individual's head that allows the user to use head motion to point toward a symbol or object

head shadow attenuation of sound to one ear because of the presence of the head between the ear and the sound source

head-turn conditioning a technique used to test infants' discrimination of speech sounds between the ages of 6 and 12 months of age. Infants sit on a parent's lap and watch an assistant located on their right play with silent toys. At the same time a loudspeaker located on the infant's left plays a background sound over and over. The infant is trained to produce a head-turn response when the background sound is changed to a comparison sound. If the infant does so when the sound changes, he or she is reinforced with a visual stimulus (a toy animal located in a black box is lighted and animated for a 6-second period). Two kinds of trials are run: *change trials* during which the sound is changed, the infant's head-turn responses are monitored, and a head-turn response results in the presentation of the visual reinforcer; and *control trials* during which the sound is not changed, but the infant's head-turn responses are still monitored, and head-turn responses that occur are scored as false alarms. If infants produce significantly more head-turns on *change trials* then *control trials*, they are assumed capable of discriminating the two sounds

heaps an early form of children's narrative in which unrelated elements are told in unorganized collections

hearing aid an electronic listening device designed to amplify and deliver sound from the environment to the listener; includes a microphone, amplifier, and receiver

- **behind-the-ear (BTE) hearing aid** a hearing aid that is worn over the pinna and is coupled to the ear canal by means of an earmold

- **body hearing aid** a hearing aid worn on the body; includes a box worn on the torso and a cord connecting to an ear-level receiver

- **compression** nonlinear amplifier gain used to determine and limit output gain as a function of input gain; compression ratio is the ratio in decibels between the acoustic input to a hearing-aid amplifier and its auditory output

- **digital hearing aid** hearing aid that utilizes digital technology to process the signal

- **direct audio input (DAI)** hard-wired connection that leads directly from a sound source to a hearing aid or other listening device

- **DSP hearing aid** hearing aid that utilizes digital signal processing; signal is converted from an analog to digital signal, the signal is manipulated according to a processing algorithm, and then the signal is converted back into an analog signal

- **eyeglass hearing aid** style of hearing aid in which the hearing aid is housed in the temple piece of a pair of eyeglasses

- **in-the-canal (ITC) hearing aid** fits in the external ear canal, with only a partial filling of the concha

- **in-the-ear (ITE) hearing aid** fits into the concha of the ear

- **maximum power output (MPO)** maximum level intensity that a hearing aid can produce; SSPL (saturation sound pressure level) is an MPO measure beyond which an aid does not amplify

- **multiple-memory hearing aid** a hearing aid that can be programmed to process the speech signal in more than one way, so that the user can adjust the processing strategy for different listening environments

- **programmable hearing aid** hearing aid in which several parameters of the instrument, such as gain, are under computer control

- **vibrotactile hearing aid** an assistive listening device that converts acoustic energy into vibratory patterns that are delivered to the skin

hearing aid evaluation (HAE) procedure in which appropriate hearing aid is selected for an individual

hearing aid linear amplification hearing aid amplification system in which there is a one-to-one correspondence between the input and output until the maximum output level is reached

hearing aid orientation (HAO) process of instructing a patient (and a patient's family member) to handle, use, and maintain a new hearing aid

hearing conservation prevention or reduction of hearing loss through a program of identifying and minimizing risk, monitoring hearing sensitivity, educating, and providing protection from noise exposure

hearing disability functional limitations imposed on an individual as a result of hearing loss

hearing disorder a disturbance of the auditory structures and/or auditory functioning

hearing handicap perceived difficulties in everyday functioning that arise as a result of hearing loss

hearing impairment abnormal or reduced hearing sensitivity; hearing loss that has adverse effects on communication

hearing level a decibel scale of sound intensity in which the reference, or zero point, is the intensity corresponding to average normal hearing for the particular acoustic signal under consideration. Usually defined by the mode of the distribution of hearing threshold levels in a sample of the general population of young adults

hearing loss abnormal or reduced hearing sensitivity; hearing impairment

- **acquired** hearing loss contracted after birth

- **adventitious** hearing loss occurring after birth

- **central hearing loss** damage to the eighth nerve (CN VIII), in brainstem, or cortex

- **conductive hearing loss** hearing loss caused by obstruction to the normal sound-conducting mechanism of the outer and/or middle ears. Usually treatable by medicine or surgery. Relatively easy to manage with hearing aids, as direct amplification usually is successful

- **congenital hearing loss** hearing loss that exists at or dates from birth; reduced hearing sensitivity related to pre- or perinatal causes

- **dominant hereditary hearing loss** hearing loss that stems from a genetic characteristic on at least one gene of a pair of traits

- **fluctuating hearing loss** hearing loss that varies in magnitude over time

- **hard of hearing** having a hearing loss; usually not used to refer to a profound hearing loss

- **mild hearing loss** hearing thresholds between 25 and 40 dB HL

- **mixed hearing loss** a hearing loss that has a conductive and a sensorineural component

- **moderate hearing loss** hearing thresholds between 40 and 55 dB HL

- **moderate to severe hearing loss** hearing thresholds between 55 and 70 dB HL

- **noise-induced hearing loss (NIHL)** sensorineural hearing loss that is the result of exposure to excessive levels of sound; auditory trauma caused by loud sound and resulting in permanent hearing loss

- **occupational hearing loss** noise-induced hearing loss incurred on the job

- **perilingual hearing loss** loss acquired during the stage of spoken language acquisition

- **postlingual hearing loss** deficit incurred after the acquisition of spoken language

- **prelingual hearing loss** loss incurred before the acquisition of spoken language

- **profound hearing loss** hearing loss greater than 90 dB HL

- **sensorineural hearing loss (SNHL)** deafness from disorders of the cochlear division of CN VIII, the cochlea, or the retrocochlear nerve tracts; the loss can be identified as mild, moderate, severe, or profound, measured in decibels

- **severe hearing loss** hearing thresholds between 70 and 90 dB HL

- **traumatic hearing loss** hearing loss that is incurred suddenly; acute and rapid onset

hearing protection devices designed to minimize the risk of noise-induced hearing loss; includes in-the-ear plugs and headset-type over-the-ear protectors

hearing threshold level of intensity at which a sound is just audible to an individual

heartburn burning painful feeling in the esophagus; generally from reflux of gastric contents

heart failure, congestive a chronic failure of the heart to pump enough blood to support body metabolism; congestion and fluid accumulation in various organs in the body (such as the lungs) result

heat moisture exchange filter (HME) humidification plugged into the tubing of mechanical ventilators that collects warmth and humidity from a patient's breaths, which is then used to moisten the next breath on inspiration

hegemony domination; the ascendancy of one group over another, expecting compliance and subservience by the subordinate group

helical computed tomography (CT) scans produced by moving a patient at a constant rate through the bore of a CT scanner while the scanning tube is rotated around the patient. This produces a true volumetric dataset and allows standard transverse views, as well as images in any plane desired

helicotrema hooklike region of the cochlea, forming the minute union of the scala vestibuli and scala tympani at the apical end of the cochlea

hematocrit the percentage of red blood cells in whole blood

hematuria abnormal blood in the urine

hemi- prefix: half

hemianesthesia sensation absence on either side of the body

hemianopia the loss of half of the visual field in one or both eyes

- **homonymous hemianopia** loss of the same visual field (right or left) in both eyes

hemiballismus hyperkinetic condition involving involuntary and uncontrollable flailing of extremities of the right or left half of the body

hemilaryngectomy, standard surgical resection of half of the laryngeal cartilage, the true and false vocal fold, and one arytenoid

hemiparesis a partial loss of movement on one side of the body due to muscle weakness from a brain injury; loss involves face, body, arm, and/or leg

hemiplegia a total loss of movement on one side of the body. Usually involves the lower and upper extremities

hemisensory impairment reduction or loss of sensory functions on one side of the body. May result in reduced appreciation of touch, hot and cold, or pain sensation

hemispheric specialization the concept that one cerebral hemisphere is more highly specialized for a given task or function (e.g., language) than the other hemisphere

hemi-walker a broad-based walker-cane combination designed to stabilize the gait of people with marked hemiparesis

hemo-, hema- prefix: pertaining to blood

hemodynamics study of functional aspects of blood circulation

hemoglobin substance in red blood cells carrying oxygen; iron-containing respiratory pigment of vertebrate red blood cells that primarily transports oxygen from the lungs to the tissues of the body and consists of four polypeptide chains designated alpha, beta, gamma, and delta, each of which is linked to a heme molecule, that combines loosely and reversibly with oxygen in the lungs or gills to form oxyhemoglobin and with carbon dioxide in the tissues to form carbaminohemoglobin

hemoptysis coughing up of blood from respiratory tract

hemorrhage external or internal loss of blood in a short time; can be from cut or rupture of veins, arteries, or capillaries

hepatitis inflammation of the liver, with accompanying liver cell damage and risk of death; may be short-term or chronic; may be caused by viral infection, as well as by chronic exposure to poisons, chemicals, or abused drugs, such as by alcohol

hepatoxicity (hepatotoxic reaction) damage to or destruction of liver cells, which can be caused by certain drugs

hernia bulge of an organ through a weakened or otherwise atypical muscle wall of the cavity that surrounds it; may be congenital or acquired

- **hiatal hernia** protrusion of part of the stomach through the diaphragm into the thorax. This is an anatomical term and should not necessarily be equated with symptoms or a diseased state, although it is commonly associated with gastroesophageal reflux (GER); also called hiatus hernia

herpes skin inflammation caused by herpes viruses characterized by groups of small blisters

- **herpes simplex** variety of infections noted for outbreaks on the lips, external nares, and genitalia

- **herpes zoster** caused by varicella zoster virus, with pain and vesicles along the distribution of a nerve

hertz (Hz) wave frequency measurement of 1 cycle per second; named after the physicist Heinrich Hertz (1857–1894)

Heschl's gyrus temporal lobe area generally defined as Broadmann area 41 and considered the primary reception area for auditory sense; also called transverse temporal gyri; named for Richard L. Heschl (1824–1881)

hetero-, heter- prefix: other, different

heterogeneous grouping the use of mixed ability and/or mixed groups, including language groups or classes. The opposite is homogeneous grouping, or tracking

hiatal hernia protrusion of part of the stomach through the diaphragm into the thorax. This is an anatomical term and should not necessarily be equated with symptoms or a diseased state, although it is commonly associated with gastroesophageal reflux (GER); also called hiatus hernia

hiatus opening, aperture, or gap

hidden Markov model (HMM) a mathematical model that can be used in speech recognition consisting of a finite set of states; transition probabilities between the states; a finite set of possible outcomes; and a probability distribution over the set of outcomes associated with each state. Similar to a Markov model, except that in a hidden Markov model, the states are not directly associated with outcomes, but rather with possibilities, because the most likely dynamic systems can be inferred, along with models for underlying processes

high-amplitude sucking (HAS) a technique used to test infants' discrimination of speech sounds between the ages of birth and 4 months. Infants suck on a pacifier and the strength of each sucking response is measured using a pressure transducer

high spontaneous rate auditory nerve fibers demonstrating a high rate of spontaneous discharge and low threshold of stimulation

hirsutism in females, coarse hair on the face, chest, upper back, or abdomen as an adverse effect of certain drugs; more generally, profuse or unusual hair distribution

Hispanics Spanish speakers in the United States.

histamine compound in all cells released in inflammatory allergic reactions, causing capillary dilation, blood pressure decrease, gastric juice secretion increase, and contraction of the bronchi and uterus smooth muscles

histochemical relating to the branch of histology that applies chemical techniques to identify components of cells and tissues

histogram display of data arrayed by frequency of occurrence; graph showing the occurrence of a parameter value; thus, a fundamental frequency histogram shows the occurrence of different fundamental frequency values, for example, in fluent speech or in a song; or a medical patient's course can be plotted through a histogram of progression of body temperature, pulse, and respiration

- **interspike interval histogram** neural response histograms providing detail of the timing between individual responses of nerve fibers

histology science of microscopic identification of cells and tissues

hoarseness voice quality that results from leakage of air and aperiodic vibration of the vocal folds; pitch may be too low; any condition that changes the mass and size of the vocal folds, including vocal nodules, may cause vocal hoarseness

holistic health care treatment approaches that emphasize an array of functionally related behaviors, providing care relating to an individual's physical, social, emotional, economic, and spiritual response to illness

homeo- prefix: sameness or similarity

homeostasis a tendency of biological systems to maintain stability while continually adjusting to conditions that are optimal for survival

hominids any of a family (*hominidae*) of bipedal primate mammals including modern humans and immediate ancestors

homophenes words that look identical on the mouth (as mouthed)

homophony relationship in which two or more words are pronounced alike, but have different meanings; for example, to, too, and two

homorganic sounds having the same place of production; for example, /b/ and /m/ are homorganic, because they are both bilabials

homotypic sounds having the same manner of production; for example, /m/ and /n/ are homotypic because they are both nasal consonants

Hooke's law stress of an elastic solid is proportional to the strain responsible for it

horizontal plane divides body or part into upper and lower regions; with upright stature, any plane parallel to the horizon or perpendicular to the axis of the body

hormone product of living cells circulating in body fluids and producing a specific effect on the activity of cells remote from its point of origin; synthetic product that acts like a hormone

hotspot the acoustic location of the best instances of a phonetic category

human immunodeficiency virus (HIV-1) a retrovirus that is the causative agent of the acquired immunodeficiency syndrome (AIDS)

human papilloma virus (HPV) cause of common warts of hands and feet, in addition to mucous membranes

humming speech treatment technique involving the production of a single continuing speech sound such as /m/ or /n/

Huntington's chorea rare inherited disease of the central nervous system characterized by progressive dementia and involuntary choreic movements, resulting from degeneration of the caudate and putamen nuclei

Hurler-Scheie syndrome late articulatory problems from chronic mucous secretion and thickening of the tongue and lips; mucopolysaccharidosis I–H; marked by growth deficiency and congestive heart failure

hyaline cartilage smooth cartilage covering the ends of bones at articulations; nonvascular connective tissue that calcifies with advancing age

hydramnios excess amniotic fluid

hydrocephalus abnormal accumulation of cerebrospinal fluid within the cranial vault, usually accompanied by increased pressure; generally caused by infection, developmental anomalies, trauma, or brain tumors

hydrodynamics the study of fluids under pressure

hydrostat a fluid-filled muscular organ that forms its own skeletal support by the selective contraction of certain muscle fibers; device for regulating water level

hydrotherapy scientific application of water in treating disease

hyoid bone a horseshoe-shaped bone known as the "tongue bone"; attached to muscles of the tongue and related structures, as well as to the larynx and related structures

hyper- prefix: above; increased, or too much of something

hyperactivity extreme activity; abnormally increased motor activity or function

hyperadduction of the vocal folds overly strong adduction of muscles that causes the vocal folds to be pressed at midline

hypercapnia excessively high levels of CO_2 in the blood

hyperextension movement of a joint to a position of more extension than natural alignment

hyperfunction excessive muscle effort: for example, pressed voice, muscular tension dysphonia

hyperkinetic dysarthria a type of motor speech disorder; its neuropathology is damage to basal ganglia (extrapyramidal system) resulting in slow or rapid involuntary movements and variable muscle tone; may affect all aspects of speech, but a dominant symptom is prosodic disturbance; specific problems include prolonged intervals, variable rate, monopitch, loudness variations, inappropriate silences, imprecise consonants, and distorted vowels

hyperlexia a precocious ability to recognize written words significantly above an individual's language or cognitive skill level

hypernasal excessive nasal resonance

hyperpolarization an electrical charge across the membrane of a neuron or muscle cell in which the inside of the membrane becomes more negative. It makes the cell less able to depolarize and decreases the likelihood that action potentials will be generated

hyperreflexia an exaggerated response of deep tendon reflexes that indicates that the nervous system is in an excited state. May occur during withdrawal from sedative-hypnotic agents or alcohol

hypersensitivity, drug overresponsiveness to drug action; can be intolerance to even small doses; some individuals with demonstrated adverse reaction to a particular drug will also be sensitive to medications with closely related chemical composition

hypertension abnormally high blood pressure levels; may relate to pulmonary pathology. The latter occurs when resistance to blood flow by constriction of blood vessels in the lungs increases pressures in the right cardiac ventricle

hyperthermia unusually high fever; body temperature beyond typical

hyperthyroidism hyperactivity of the thyroid gland, which is usually enlarged; marked by weight loss, tremor, fatigue, heat intolerance

hypertonic increased muscular tone (tension or spasticity); with greater osmotic pressure than typical blood plasma or interstitial fluid (liquid in which cells shrink)

hypertrophy excess growth of a particular tissue

hyperventilation ventilation that exceeds the needs of the body. Reflected in abnormally low CO_2 pressure in blood

hypnotic, sedative drug that depresses the central nervous system (CNS); includes barbiturates and benzodiazepines

hypo- prefix: below; decreased, or too little of something

hypoadduction of the vocal folds reduced vocal fold adduction resulting in disordered voice (flaccid or hypokinetic); usually of neurological origin

hypocalcemia low levels of calcium in the blood

hypoflexia abnormally low response on reflex stimulation

hypofunction low muscular effort, for example, soft breathy voice

hypoglossal nerve CN XII, the cranial nerve essential for swallowing and tongue movement

hypoglycemia low blood sugar, often from too much insulin; may lead to hunger, headache, ataxia, weakness, anxiety

hypokinetic dysarthria a type of motor speech disorder resulting from damage to the basal ganglia (extrapyramidal system) resulting in slow movement, limited range of movement, and rigidity; may affect all aspects of speech, but especially voice, articulation, and prosody; specific problems include monopitch, monoloudness, reduced stress, imprecise consonants, inappropriate silences, harsh and breathy voice, and short rushes of speech

hyponasal deficient nasal resonance

hyponymy the semantic relationship of a meaning-inclusion between class, property, or action, with one word, the hyponym (e.g., chair), including the meaning of another word, the superordinate (e.g., furniture)

hypopharyngeal diverticula outpouching of the muscular pharyngeal wall above the cricopharyngeus muscle

hypoplasia uncompleted or underdeveloped structures

- **mandibular hypoplasia** underdevelopment of the mandible as seen in some children with craniofacial anomalies (e.g., Robin sequence, hemifacial microsomias, Treacher Collins syndrome)

hypopnea very slow and shallow respiration; in well-conditioned athletes can be considered normal; elsewise can be a significant sign of brainstem damage

hypotension abnormally low blood pressure levels; blood circulation may be inadequate to circulate oxygen throughout the body

hypothermia lowering of body temperature below the normal range with no typical reflex actions, such as shivering; most often seen with infants and older persons; can be adverse effect of some drugs

hypothesis premise made to elicit a response to its credible or empirical consequences; statement based on a theory to predict the interrelationship between variables

hypothesis testing in language development, utterances by toddlers produced with rising intonation as an apparent request for confirmation or feedback from the caregiver

hypothyroidism under-activity of the thyroid gland; marked by weight gain, lethargy, arthritis

hypotonia low or lessened muscle tone, as with flaccid paralysis

hypoventilation ventilation that is inadequate to meet the needs of the body; reflected by increased levels of CO_2 in the arterial blood

hypoxemia a decreased amount of oxygen in the arterial blood; symptoms include cyanosis, restlessness, stupor

hypoxia a decreased amount of oxygen in inspired gases, blood, or tissues; characterized by hypertension, tachycardia, mental confusion, dizziness, vasoconstriction

hypsarhythmia chaotic abnormal electroencephalogram reading typically seen with infantile spasm

H

I

intubation, endotracheal

airway management through catheter inserted from the mouth or nose into the trachea; inserted to maintain functioning airway, prevent aspiration, for suctioning of tracheobronchial secretions, or to administer positive pressure ventilation; extubation is removal of the tube

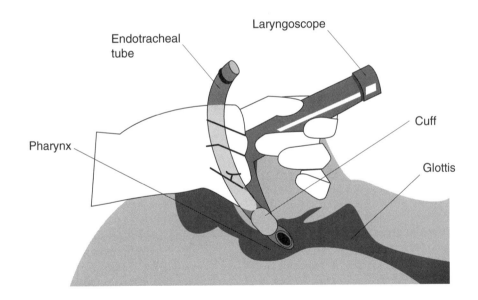

Endotracheal tube

Laryngoscope

Pharynx

Cuff

Glottis

iatrogenic illness or adverse affect resulting from a medical or surgical test or treatment

icon an image that represents an object, concept, or message

iconic the resemblance of a sign (an icon) to its referent

icon prediction AAC picture-based prediction method

identification the ability to label auditory stimuli

identification task in speech perception, a procedure designed to assess a listener's ability to label, or identify, speech sounds

ideographs pictures representing ideas and concepts, such as symbols for *first, under,* and *lonely*

idio- prefix: peculiar

idiolect language variations unique to an individual speaker

idiom expressive form common to groups, eras, or movements; a structured syntactical or grammatical aspect of a particular subgroup of language

idiopathic cause unknown

ilium uppermost of the three bones composing the hipbone

illocutionary the component of a speech act that includes the outcome or effect intended by a speaker; the social stage of communication development in which a child is interactive and communication is intentional; may be nonverbal

- **illocutionary force** a speaker's dispositions or attitudes toward one's own utterances

- **illocutionary stage** the stage in communication development beginning at approximately 6 months when an infant begins to signal intentions through gesture and vocalization

illusion a mental impression derived from the misinterpretation of sensory stimuli

-ilos suffix: diminutive form of noun

imagery a treatment technique employing visualization to facilitate the production of the target behavior

imaging techniques procedures that produce pictures of internal structures or functions of the body

imitation the relatively immediate reproduction of a significant portion of someone's preceding behavior

- **elicited imitation** language imitation by a child specifically prompted by a caregiver

- **selective imitation** children's partial imitations of adult utterances

immersion bilingual education schooling in which some or most subject content is taught through a second, majority language

- **double immersion** schooling in which subject content is taught through a second and third language (e.g., Hebrew and French for first-language English speakers)

immittance general audiological term describing measures of tympanic membrane admittance, impedance, or compliance

immune resistant to infections; protected by antibodies and related factors

- **immune response** body's mechanism to produce antibodies to combat invading malignancies and antigens

immunization procedures inducing or helping a response in the body that protects against possible future infections

immunodeficiency defective immune response ability

immunosuppression the inability of the body to produce antibodies to fight off infections; stoppage or interruption of immunologic response; procedure for suppressing immune system with drugs

impairment the physical or psychological result of injury or disease of an organ or body function

impedance measured in ohms, impedance is the opposition to an electrical current flow and consists of the vector sum of resistance and reactance; an analogous quantity is defined in other domains, for example, acoustics

- **input impedance** the impedance presented by an electric circuit to its signal source; for example, the reactance of the differential amplifier input capacitance considered in parallel with the amplifier input resistance

impedance audiometry battery of measures designed to assess middle ear functioning, including tympanometry and acoustic reflex threshold determination

imperative a major sentence type that expresses a command

impression cast made for a prosthetic device, such as of the concha and/or ear canal for the purpose of creating an earmold for a hearing aid

improvement documented positive changes in an individual being treated compared to initial assessment or baseline performance; not the same as effectiveness of treatment, which requires controlled evidence

impulse a stimulus carried by a nerve fiber; wave of depolarization; electrochemical neural transmitting process; sudden irresistible, often irrational, impulse, want, craving, or action

impulse noise a burst of sound, such as produced by a gunshot or an explosion; having an instantaneous rise time and short duration

impulsivity neurological inability to sustain inhibition

in-, im- prefix: in, into, not

incidence the rate of new occurrences of a disease or condition within a defined population at risk during a specified time span; can be expressed as a ratio with the number of cases as the numerator and possible population size as denominator; a number of specified new events

incisors anterior four teeth of dental arch

inclusion educating students with disabilities alongside typically developing peers within the regular classrooms

incompatible behaviors actions that cannot be produced simultaneously, such as sitting and walking; used to reduce certain undesirable behaviors

incompressibility incapable of being reduced in volume by pressure

incontinence the inability to control urination or defecation; can be caused by a loss of sphincter control following a stroke (CVA, or brain attack)

incubation time between exposure to an infection and the onset of symptoms

incudostapedial joint point of union of incus and stapes in the middle ear

incus second of the three small bones constituting the ossicular chain; named incus (Latin for anvil) because of its anvil-like shape

indicating caregivers' use of their infants' line of sight to locate an object of interest

individualized educational plan (IEP) an education plan required by federal law and developed by the local school team and parents that outlines educational objectives for children with disabilities, updated once a year

individualized family service plan (IFSP) federally mandated plan for the education of preschool children with an emphasis on family involvement, updated annually

Individuals With Disabilities Education Act (IDEA) U.S. Public Laws 94-142 and 99-457, which mandate free and appropriate education for all children with disabilities over the age of 3 years and encourages services for children below 3 years of age

induction discovery learning; a three-step process through which a student recognizes a pattern or relationship, explains the pattern or relationship, and hypothesizes the rule governing the pattern or relationship; drawing a generalized conclusion by inferring from particular instances

induction loop loop of wire in the ceiling of the portion or all of a room designated as an assistive listening area; sound is transmitted by electromagnetic (inductive) energy, along with an amplifier and a microphone for the primary speaker(s); speech signals are amplified and circulated through the loop wire, with the resulting signal adapted by telecoil circuits of many hearing aids, vibrotactile devices, cochlear implant systems, or headphone induction loop receivers; magnetic loop

inertia the tendency for a body at rest to remain at rest, and for a body in motion to remain in motion; descriptive term for the property of a body that resists change in its motion

infantile/primitive reflexes automatic responses that produce change in muscle tone and movement of the limbs; typically present in newborns; examples include the asymmetrical and symmetrical tonic neck reflexes

- **asymmetric tonic neck reflex (ATNR)** can be elicited by turning an infant's head laterally in a supine position. Visible evidence includes extension of the extremities on the chin side or flexion on the occiput side. The ATNR is commonly persistent in children with severe motor deficits related to cerebral palsy

- **Moro reflex (startle reflex)** elicited with infant in supine position. The head is allowed to drop back suddenly from at least 3 cm off a padded surface. On extension of the neck, there is a quick symmetrical abduction and upward movement of the arms followed by opening of the hands. Adduction and flexion of the arms can then be noted

- **positive support reflex** can be elicited by suspending an infant around the trunk or axillae with the head in neutral or midline flexed position. The infant is bounced five times on the balls of the feet. The balls of the feet are then taken into contact with the table surface. Co-contraction of opposing muscle groups of the legs occur, resulting in a position capable of supporting weight

- **tonic labyrinthine reflex** can be evaluated in supine or prone position. In supine, infant's head is extended 45° below the horizontal and then flexed 45° above the horizontal. While the neck is extended 45° the limbs extend. With the neck flexed 45°, the limbs flex

infarct an area of necrosis or dead tissue resulting from an insufficient blood supply (tissue anoxia)

infarction sudden stoppage of blood supply that leads to a large necrotic area in tissue or an organ

- **myocardial infarction (MI)** heart muscle necrosis due to blockage of blood (by arterial obstruction, arteriosclerosis, or thrombus); a type of heart attack

infection disease-causing parasitic organism multiplication in the body

- **airborne infection** transmission by dust, particles, or droplets suspended in air
- **anaerobic infection** infection caused by anaerobic bacteria, those that do not require (and in most cases cannot tolerate) the presence of oxygen and that usually are found in deep puncture wounds; examples include tetanus and gangrene
- **droplet infection** spread of infection from minute drops of secretions in a person's breath
- **endogenous infection** caused by agent harbored in the body, likely from an asymptomatic previous infection

inferencing reaching a conclusion on the basis of facts or evidence

- **deductive inferencing** reasoning from the general to specific

inferior the lower point; nearer the feet

infinitive a phrase in the form of the word *to* and a verb that can be a noun, adjective, or adverb (e.g., to err is human . . .)

inflammation response to body injury or abnormal stimulation noted by redness, swelling, and pain, sometimes with accompanying function loss

- **inflammatory neuropathies** disorders of peripheral nerves mediated by cellular and humoral products of inflammation, typically triggered by autoimmunity

inflection word form change for marking characteristics such as case, gender, number, tense, person, mood, or voice; form, suffix, prefix, or element involved in such variation; change in vocal loudness, pitch, or rhythm

information processing the hypothetical concept of mental stages or processes that organize and access information. Also, assigning meaning to sensory input based on the extraction of cues or constraints through various processes or stages of cognition, including encoding, organizing, storing, retrieving, comparing, and generating or reconstructing information; these stages involve the interaction between sensory (e.g., auditory processes) and central processes (e.g., cognitive and linguistic processes) through feedback and feedforward loops

infra prefix: below the part named by the word to which it is attached

infraglottic below the level of the glottis (space between the vocal folds); region includes the trachea, thorax, and related structures

infrahyoid muscle group a collection of extrinsic laryngeal muscles including the sternohyoid, sternothyroid, omohyoid, and thyroid muscles

infrared system assistive listening device that broadcasts from the sound source to a receiver/amplifier by means of infrared light waves

infraverted in dentition, an inadequately erupted tooth

inguinal pertaining to the groin

inhalant a volatile substance that is introduced into the body via the nasal passages from a high-vapor device; also group of finely powered or liquid drugs delivered to the respiratory passages by such mechanisms as low pressure aerosol containers

inhalation method a method of air intake to produce esophageal speech

inhalation phonation a technique of voice therapy to evoke true vocal fold vibration in clients who are aphonic

inhaler specialized equipment used to introduce medication into the lungs

inheritance mode, genetic the pattern with which a trait is inherited in a family

- **autosomal dominant inheritance** a 50% probability of inheriting a trait because of the presence of the dominant gene on one of the autosomes from one parent; dominant genes can be expressed in an offspring, even if only one parent codes for the trait

- **autosomal recessive inheritance** a 25% probability of inheriting a trait because of the presence of a recessive gene on one of the autosomes in both parents; both halves of a gene must be the same copy of the gene to be expressed. If only one copy is provided in a gene pair, the offspring will not manifest the trait but could be a carrier of the recessive trait, because he or she has one copy of the allele

- **inheritance mode** the pattern with which a trait is inherited in a family

- **multifactorial inheritance** genetic expression of an abnormal trait caused by several or many genes at various locations, plus environmental influences

inhibit to arrest or repress

inhibition, neurological synaptic inputs to neurons or cardiac or smooth muscle cells that open channels causing cell membrane to retreat from depolarization, with that cell less likely to open its voltage sensitive sodium channels and conduct action potentials

injection method a method of air intake to produce esophageal speech

in-migrants encompasses immigrants, migrants, refugees

innate inborn, or genetic; presumably not requiring experience, learning, or developmental mechanisms; relating to fundamental nature

innervation stimulation by means of a nerve; route of neural regulation

- **adrenergic innervation** characterized by synapses that release the neurotransmitter norepinephrine and are found particularly in the sympathetic division of the autonomic nervous system

- **autonomic innervation** the nervous system that innervates the visceral organs. It has two divisions, the sympathetic and parasympathetic

- **cholinergic innervation** neurons that secrete acetylcholine (ACh) at their terminals. These include neurons in the central nervous system, all of the alpha motor neurons that innervate skeletal muscle fibers, neurons in the autonomic nervous system between pre- and postganglionic nerve fibers, and the postganglionic neurons that innervate car-

diac and smooth muscle. Although ACh is the same transmitter released at all cholinergic synapses, the receptor on the postsynaptic membrane will differ for the type of synapse (i.e., muscarinic or nicotinic)

innominate nameless

input information transferred into a computer from some external source by the keyboard, the mouse, a disk drive, switch, or alternative keyboard

input impedance the impedance presented by an electric circuit to its signal source, for example, the reactance of the differential amplifier input capacitance considered in parallel with the amplifier input resistance

input/output (I/O) means by which information is exchanged between a computer control circuit and its peripheral devices; in medicine, measuring of fluid intake and output

input signal acoustic signal that enters a listening device

insertion the relatively mobile point of attachment of a muscle, typically to the bone it moves

in situ in typical or natural position; tumor that has not invaded or metastasized neighboring tissues

inspiration inhalation; drawing air into the respiratory system

inspiratory capacity the maximum inspiratory volume possible to be exhaled from the closure of a resting exhalation

inspiratory cycle the respiratory phase in which air is inhaled into the lungs, where oxygen is exchanged for carbon dioxide (end product of tissue metabolism)

inspiratory/expiratory ratio the relationship in the breath cycle of the length of the inspiratory phase to the length of the expiratory phase during mechanical ventilatory support. It is expressed as a numeric ratio (e.g., 1:4)

inspiratory pressure, peak the highest measured airway pressure during the inspiratory phase of mechanical ventilatory support; pressure significantly exceeding this level causes the high pressure alarm on the ventilator to sound

inspiratory reserve volume the volume of air that can be inhaled beyond a typical resting inspiration

instruction, process an emphasis on "doing" in the classroom rather than on creating a product; focusing on procedures and techniques rather than on learning outcomes; teaching "how to" through inquiry rather than teaching through the transmission and memorization of knowledge

integration in mathematics, the process or technique of finding a function (integral) of a given variable, of which a given function is the derivative with respect to the same variable

- **sensory integration** organization and interpretation of input from the body's various sensory systems

intelligibility the degree to which an individual's speech can be understood by familiar or unfamiliar listeners

intensity magnitude of sound expressed as the relationship between two pressures or powers; measure of energy flow per unit of area per unit of time

intentionality behavior that exhibits a conscious attempt to achieve some goal by influencing others' behavior

inter- prefix: between

interactionism a philosophical perspective that emphasizes the mutual influence of cognitive processes or social contexts on language development

interarytenoid muscle an intrinsic laryngeal muscle that connects the two arytenoid cartilages

interaural intensity difference the difference between signal intensity arriving at left and right ears of a listener

interaural phase difference the difference in arrival time of an auditory signal arriving at left and right ears of a listener

interaural timing behavioral task requiring the subject to determine the order of two acoustic events presented to each ear separately at slightly different times

intercostal between the ribs

interdisciplinary team model team members perform only those tasks specific to their respective disciplines, but share information with each other and attempt to unify their findings for optimal assessment and treatment

interference the observation that features or rules of one language conflict with learning another language; a point of connection between two processes or operations, as in two sound waves meeting and producing alternating loud and soft sounds

interference pattern record of action potentials summing the simultaneous electrical

activity of several different signal sources or different motor units in electromyography

interference signal extraneous signal superimposed on a signal of interest; for example, in EMG of a given muscle it may be a 60 Hz (or its integral multiple) signal of an electrocardiogram or a signal from a distant muscle

interlanguage language integrating aspects of the first and second language used by a second-language learner while learning the second language

interleave to interweave patterns of signals; alternating the sending of blocks of data to two or more stations on a multipoint circuit

interleave processing a cochlear implant processing strategy in which trains of pulses are delivered across electrodes in the electrode array in a nonsimultaneous fashion

interlocking verbal behavior paradigm B. F. Skinner's model illustrating the interactive nature of verbal exchanges between speaking partners

intermediate care a rehabilitation center other than a hospital (where intensive treatment might be provided over a brief period) or a long-term setting (where minimal health care and daily life assistance are provided); intermediate care is designed for persons who are disabled or have chronic illness

intermittent mandatory ventilation (IMV) a mode of cycled ventilation in which the patient may breathe spontaneously between timed mandatory breaths

internal within the body

International Phonetic Alphabet (IPA) an alphabet designed to provide universal symbols to represent all the known speech sounds used in human languages

interneuron neuron with cell body and axon entirely in the central nervous system (CNS); interneurons have either excitatory or inhibitory synapses and are important to relaying initial sensory input throughout the CNS and synaptically effecting motor neurons

internuncial neuron a connecting or intervening neuron in a neural pathway

intero- prefix: aimed inward or farther from the surface

interoceptor sensory receptor of the viscera activated by stimuli from within the body

interpretation method, rich analyzing children's utterances considering the linguistic and nonlinguistic context

THE INTERNATIONAL PHONETIC ALPHABET (revised to 1993)

CONSONANTS (PULMONIC)

	Bilabial	Labiodental	Dental	Alveolar	Postalveolar	Retroflex	Palatal.	Velar	Uvular	Pharyngeal	Glottal
Plosive	p b			t d		ʈ ɖ	c ɟ	k g	q ɢ		ʔ
Nasal	m	ɱ		n		ɳ	ɲ	ŋ	N		
Trill	B			r					R		
Tap or Flap				ɾ		ɽ					
Fricative	ɸ β	f v	θ ð	s z	ʃ ʒ	ʂ ʐ	ç ʝ	x ɣ	χ ʁ	ħ ʕ	h ɦ
Lateral fricative				ɬ ɮ							
Approximant		ʋ		ɹ		ɻ	j	ɰ			
Lateral approximant				l		ɭ	ʎ	L			

Where symbols appear in pairs, the one to the right represents a voiced consonant. Shaded areas denote articulations judged impossible.

International Phonetic Alphabet (IPA) an alphabet designed to provide universal symbols to represent all the known speech sounds used in human languages

interpreter person translating to allow persons speaking different languages to communicate

- **interpreter, oral** trained individual who silently repeats a talker's message as it is spoken, so that a person who is hard of hearing may lipread the message

interrogative sentence category for questions; a form of intonation characterized by a terminal pitch rise used for questions

interstitial pertaining to the space between cells and organs

- **interstitial pulmonary fibrosis** scarring and abnormal deposition of collagen within alveolar walls, leading to increased stiffness of lungs and impaired oxygenation. May be caused by autoimmunity, drug hypersensitivity, infection, irradiation, or occupational exposures
- **interstitial tissue** supportive and connective tissue covering and within major elements or an organ

intersystemic reorganization a treatment strategy that pairs speaking with a rhythmic activity such as pushing a button or squeezing a ball

interval the difference between two pitches expressed in terms of musical scale; distance between two notes in oscillations per second

intervention arranging treatment to facilitate learning and/or healing; acting to effect change

interview assessment procedure to assess conversational fluency and communication handicap in which individuals talk about their conversational problems and consider possible reasons as to why communication breakdowns happen; a form of discourse characterized by questions and answers

intervocalic a consonant that occupies a position between two vowels; for example, the second [p] in the word *paper* is intervocalic

in-the-ear (ITE) hearing aid style of aid in which receiver, microphone and body of aid fit within the user's ear canal and concha (see illustration, p. 118)

intonation the melody of speech provided by variation of fundamental frequency during speech

- **intonation contour** perceived pattern of fundamental frequency change over time; also acoustic pattern of fundamental frequency change;
- **overall intonation contour** pitch or F_0 configuration from the initiation to the end of an utterance
- **intonation question** question that is signaled by change in intonation rather than

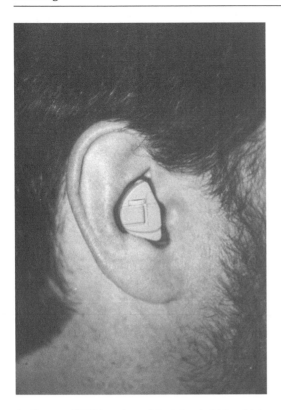

in-the-ear (ITE) hearing aid style of aid in which receiver, microphone and body of aid fit within the user's ear canal and concha

by change in syntax; for example, You came home?

intoning a treatment technique of vocalizing or verbalizing while maintaining a simple intonation contour

intra- prefix: within

intracellular within a cell

intracultural variation the tendency for cultural groups to reflect internal variation as a function of such factors as age, gender, socioeconomic status, education, exposure to other cultures, and so on

intrafusal applies to elements within muscle spindles

intransitive verb lexical verb that carries or contains a direct object

intraoral within the mouth or oral cavity

intraosseous eruption eruption of tooth through bone

intrapleural pressure pressure measured within the pleural linings of the lungs

intraural between the two ears

intraverbal a primary verbal operant in which a speaker's verbal behavior is influenced by his or her previous verbal behavior; the behavioral equivalent of chains, as in recitation, alliteration, tongue twisters, and cliches

intrinsic inherent, situated within

intro- prefix: into or within

intubation the insertion of a tube into the body

- **endotracheal intubation** airway management through catheter inserted from the mouth or nose into the trachea; inserted to maintain functioning airway, prevent aspiration, for suctioning of tracheobronchial secretions, or to administer positive pressure ventilation; extubation is removal of the tube

inventory in phonology, a list of sounds used by a particular individual speaker, sometimes referenced to a particular situation; also called sound inventory

inverse filtering analysis method used for recovering the transglottal airflow during phonation; the technique implies that the voice is fed through a computer filter that compensates for the resonance effects of the supraglottic vocal tract, especially the lowest formants

inverse square law principle that the amount of measured radiation and the intensity of such waves as sound is inversely proportional to the square of the distance from the wave source

inversion the turning inward of a structure or part

in vitro process or activity happening within an artificial environment, as in a culture media or test tube; outside the body

in vivo in the living body

ion an atom or group of atoms carrying positive or negative charge

ionizing radiation high-energy electromagnetic waves (such as X rays, gamma rays) and particulate rays (i.e., electrons, neutrons, alpha particles, beta rays, heavy nuclei) that dissociate material in their paths into ions; directly affects living organisms by retarding development or destroying cells, also leading to gene mutations and chromosome breaks; animal tissues with high atomic weights, such as calcium, soak up higher doses from a given radiating source than does soft tissue

ipsi- prefix: same; self

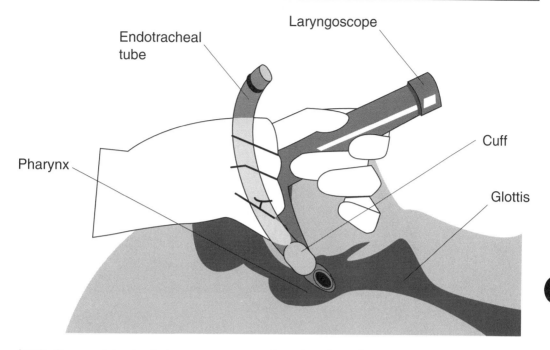

Endotracheal tube

Laryngoscope

Pharynx

Cuff

Glottis

intubation, endotracheal airway management through catheter inserted from the mouth or nose into the trachea; inserted to maintain functioning airway, prevent aspiration, for suctioning of tracheo-bronchial secretions, or to administer positive pressure ventilation; extubation is removal of the tube

ipsilateral same side of the body

iris colored part of the eye

irregular form form of a word, phrase, or other construction that is an exception to the general rules of the grammar; e.g., most words form plurals by adding /s/, /z/, or /ɪz/, but irregular plural forms include words such as women, geese, oxen, and children

ischemia a deficient supply of oxygenated blood to a part or an organ of the body; causes disorders ranging from arterial embolism and atherosclerosis to thrombosis and vasoconstriction

iso- prefix: equal

isolation point a real-time word recognition processing event that occurs when a listener initially identifies a target word, often using only a portion of the acoustic information

isometric constant muscle length during contraction

isomorphism similarity in form between two or more body parts or organisms; mathematical concept of behavioral patterns repeated in subsystems of a larger system, such as generations of a family; also used to refer to similar elements of different views of a situation as distinguished from elements that are dissimilar

isthmus a narrow passageway between cavities; slenderest aspect of the brainstem at the confluence of the mid- and hindbrain

iteration in mathematics, the repetitive process of substituting the solution to an equation back into the same equation to obtain the next solution

-itis adjectival suffix for nouns; informally means inflammation or irritation

J

temporomandibular joint (TMJ)

Synovial jaw articulation between the mandibular head, mandibular fossa, and temporal bone articular tubercle; joint is divided into two cavities by a fibrocartilaginous articular disk.

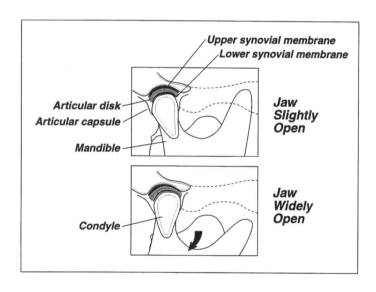

jargon specialized vocabulary or distinctive idiom of an activity or group; in language development, infant sound production of syllable strings produced with adultlike intonation; spoken words may or may not contain real words; even when parts are recognizable, strings may be incomprehensible; unintelligible fluent utterances produced by individuals with aphasia

jargon aphasia aphasia type noted by lack of use of proper function words such as articles and prepositions and appropriate endings to words such as plurals, tenses, and possessives; may be seen in written and/or spoken language; inability to create sentence because of syntactic, morphological, and semantic deficits; can result from lesion in dominant temporal lobe; also known as agrammatism

jaundice yellowness of skin, sclera, and excretions from a high amount of bilirubin in the blood; a symptom of one of a number of different diseases and disorders of the liver, gallbladder, and blood

jaw in humans, the massive unpaired mandible (lower jaw) plus the paired maxillae (upper-jaw) that provide movement for food ingestion and speech

jejunostomy surgery to create opening to the jejunum through the abdominal wall

- **percutaneous endoscopic jejunostomy** artificial means of providing nutrition and hydration via a tube placed through the esophagus into the jejunum via endoscopy, with the tube connected to nutrition source though an opening in the stomach

jitter an index of instability in the laryngeal waveform, usually measured as the cycle-to-cycle variation in the fundamental period; often perceived as hoarseness

jitter, absolute a discrete measure of very short term (cycle-to-cycle) variation of the pitch periods expressed in microseconds. This parameter is dependent on the fundamental frequency of the voicing sample. Therefore, normative data differs significantly for men and women. Higher pitch results in lower values

jitter percentage a relative measure of very short term (cycle-to-cycle) variation of the pitch periods expressed in percent. The influence of the average fundamental frequency is significantly reduced. This parameter is very sensitive to pitch variations

joint anatomically, the location of union, generally more or less movable, between two bones

- **cochlear joint** the spiral joint of the ear, providing hinges of opposing articular surfaces, providing flexion and lateral deviation

- **cricoarytenoid joint** synovial laryngeal joint from the base of each arytenoid cartilage and the top border of the cricoid cartilage lamina

- **cricothyroid joint** synovial laryngeal articulation between the thyroid cartilage inferior horn and the side of the cricoid cartilage

- **temporomandibular joint (TMJ)** synovial jaw articulation between the mandibular head, mandibular fossa, and temporal bone articular tubercle; joint is divided into two cavities by a fibrocartilaginous articular disk. (see illustration, p. 121)

joystick a peripheral device with a moveable stick used to provide two-dimensional control to computers for applications ranging from games to graphics software

juncture boundary between linguistic elements, including words, phrases, and sentences

just noticeable difference (JND) the smallest increment of stimulus change in which the stimulus can be perceived as different; difference limen

K

karyotype

chromosomal characteristics of an individual cell or a species (cell line), usually shown as a display of metaphase chromosomes from a photomicrograph of a single cell nucleus displayed in pairs.

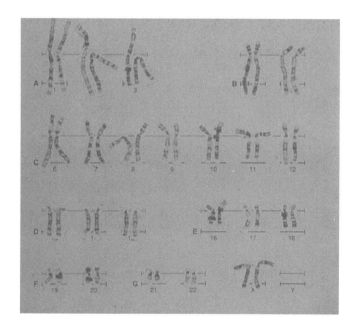

k (from *kilo-*) symbol for 1,000, as in 1 kHz for 1000 Hz

Kabuchi makeup syndrome speech delay and compensatory articulation secondary to clefting is common, with language delay and impairment secondary to cognitive impairment; also marked by protuberant large ears, scoliosis, heart anomalies

K-AMP circuit hearing-aid circuit designed to provide more gain for moderate-level sound, no gain for high-intensity sound, and compression limiting for the highest level sound; also often more amplification for high frequencies

Kartagener's syndrome a subset of the immotile cilia syndrome, characterized by the triad of bronchiectasis, nasal polyps or sinusitis, and situs inversus totalis

karyotype chromosomal characteristics of an individual cell or a species (cell line), usually shown as a display of metaphase chromosomes from a photomicrograph of a single cell nucleus displayed in pairs (see illustration, p. 123)

Kb, kbyte kilobyte; one thousand bytes

keratinized possessing a horny layer of flattened cells containing keratin

keratosis skin lesion composed of a buildup of keratin (a tough, fibrous protein), including on the surface of the vocal folds

kernicterus atypical toxic bilirubin accumulation in central nervous system (CNS) tissues; a condition of infantile jaundice in which brain tissue can be affected by a yellow pigment and degenerative lesions

keyboard grouping of systematically arranged keys by which a machine or device is operated; the best known contemporary keyboards are the common typing interfaces for computers

- **alternative keyboard** a computer hardware device that replaces or works in conjunction with the standard keyboard

- **emulator** AAC keyboard interface with a CPU

- **membrane keyboard** keyboard of two electrically conductive flat surfaces separated by nonconductive flat surfaces separated by nonconductive spacers. Touching the top alphanumeric printed keyboard lightly forces the two surfaces together, which sends an electronic signal to a CPU in the same manner as a conventional keyboard; often used in AAC systems

- **overlay** AAC keyboard cover to define or illustrate the layout of particular or special keys

- **WUERTY** conventional keyboard layout, named after the successive left-hand keys in second row from top

keyguard a plastic or Plexiglas overlay device that covers a standard or alternative keyboard, with holes cut out for each key. Keyguards allow the user to slide a pointer over the surface without accidentally activating keys

kilo- prefix: thousand

kinematics study of the motion of particles and bodies without reference to the forces associated with that motion

kinesthesia self-awareness of movement; including sense of one's own body parts, direction, and weight

kinetic energy the energy of matter in motion; work needed from an external force to bring a mass from rest to a particular state of motion

kinocilium protoplasmic tendril on a cell surface, notably on hair cells of the ear's vestibular mechanism

kneepoint point on an input-output function of a hearing aid where compression is activated

Koplik spots spots on the inside of cheeks in the early stages of measles

Korsakoff syndrome an organic brain syndrome associated with prolonged, heavy ingestion of alcohol, characterized by amnesia for recent events, an inability to form new memories, confabulation, and sometimes hallucinations and agitation

kyphosis bending of the spine in an anterior-posterior manner; extensive flexion

Limbic System

the central nervous system structures responsible for mediation of motivation and arousal, memory, and some aspects of attention, including the hippocampus, amygdala, dentate gyrus, cingulate gyrus, and fornix; influences the autonomic motor and endocrine systems

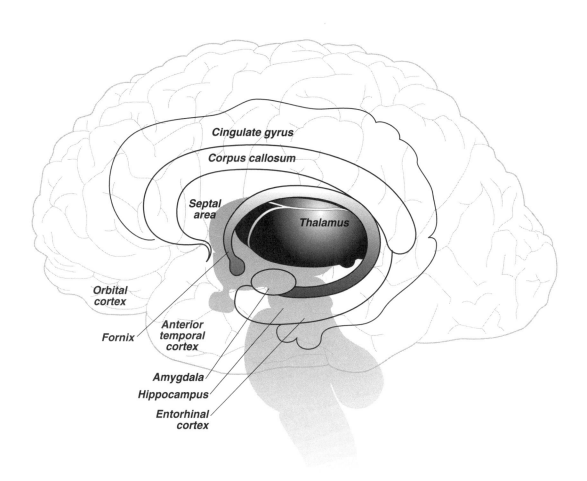

L1/L2 first language, second language

labeling a language-stimulation technique in which an adult provides names to objects, actions, and events

labial bilabial and labiodental consonants, with American English labial consonants being [p], [b], [m], [w], [f], [v]

labial assimilation phonological error pattern substitution of a labial sound for a nonlabial (e.g., /b/ for /d/), consonants assimilate to the place of production of labials

lability in psychiatry: characterized by rapidly changing emotions, from laughing to crying, not necessarily appropriate situational reaction

labio- prefix: pertaining to lips

labiodental pertaining to lips and teeth; a place of articulation for consonants

labioglossolaryngeal related to lips, tongue, and larynx; a description of bulbar paralysis with involvement of these parts

labioverted tilted toward the lip

labyrinth complex maze of passages; the inner ear including the cochlea, semicircular ducts, and vestibular system

- **bony labyrinth** linked cavities within the petrous portion of the temporal bone otic capsule (cochlea, vestibule, semicircular canals) filled with perilymph, in which the membranous labyrinth is suspended; also called osseous labyrinth

- **cochlear labyrinth** cochlea's content, including spiral organ (cochlear duct) and perilymphatic channels (scalae)

- **membranous labyrinth** complex structure of linked membranous canaliculi and sacs suspended within the bony labyrinth, which is primarily divided into the cochlear labyrinth and the vestibular labyrinth

- **vestibular labyrinth** portion of membranous labyrinth within the semicircular canals and the bony labyrinth vestibule

labyrinthitis inflammation (chronic or acute) of structures inside the ears; symptoms can include vertigo, vomiting, nystagmus; etiology includes infection, trauma, influenza complication, otitis media, or meningitis

lacri- prefix: pertaining to tears

lacto- prefix: pertaining to milk or lactic acid

lacuna a small cavity or pit; gap, as in the vision field

lag a difference in time between one point and another

lal-, lala-, lalia, lalo- combining forms: pertaining to speech, babbling, or speech disorder

lamella thin plate or scale

lamina thin plate or layer

- **lamina of cartilaginous auditory tube** narrow lateral and medial aspects of the auditory tube cartilaginous portion

- **lamina of cricoid cartilage** quadrate plate making up the posterior part of the cricoid cartilage

- **lamina of semicircular duct** connective tissue between the ear's semicircular duct and the bony semicircular canal, enclosing the perilymph

- **lamina of thyroid cartilage** paired quadrilateral plates of the thyroid cartilage forming a posterior open angle and being closed anteriorly

- **lamina propria** laryngeal tissue layers below the epithelium; in adult humans, the lamina propria has superficial, intermediate, and deep layers

- **osseous serial lamina** bony plate in the ear along the surface of the modiolus, forming the separation of the scalae vestibuli and tympani

laminal sound produced with the blade, or lamina, of the tongue

laminar smooth or layered; in fluid mechanics, indicating parallel flow lines

laminar flow a type of airflow in which the air moves in smooth layers; contrasts with **turbulence**

language system of arbitrary sounds, gestures, or marks arranged in a conventional code employed as a social tool of mutual understanding to communicate ideas and or feelings within a specific group or community; useful sound delivered by the vocal mechanisms; means by which nonhumans communicate; language study as an educational subject

- **aided language stimulation** interactive, receptive, and expressive communication training that uses picture communication displays to model language skills

- **American Sign Language (ASL)** a manual system of communication used by members of the Deaf Culture in the United States; sometimes referred to with the term Ameslan. Having a distinct grammar and syntax, ASL is a separate language

- **cognitive academic language proficiency (CALP)** skill with the language taught in schools, which in the United States is usually English. CALP is the foundation of academic, analytical conversation and of independent acquisition of factual information. CALP is employed to use acquired information to find relationships, make inferences, and draw conclusions

- **contextualized language** utterances that relate to the context in which they occur

- **creole language** a language created by children from a pidgin language

- **decontextualized language** utterances about objects, people, events, and relationships outside an immediate context

- **figurative language** language that conveys meaning through analogy based on stimulus generalization rather than through literal interpretation of words and phrases; expression through analogy

- **interlanguage** language integrating aspects of the first and second language used by a second-language learner while learning a second language

- **language dominance** the language or dialect that an individual prefers and uses most often or in which he or she has a greater or greatest proficiency

- **language families** groups of languages that share historical roots

- **language minority** a person or a group speaking a language of low prestige or having low numbers in a society

- **language parameters** aspects of language that form the foundation for linguistic functioning

- **language proficiency** the competence with which an individual speaks, comprehends, reads, writes, and uses a particular language or dialect

- **language universals** features that are considered to be part of most, if not all, human language

- **language variations** structural or phonological differences in individuals' or subgroups' production of a major language

- **marked language** a minority language distinct from a majority one and usually not highly valued in society

- **native language magnet (NLM)** theory a theory of the development of speech perception in the first year of life that accounts for the change from a language-general mode of speech perception to one that is language-specific

- **pidgin language** a simplified hybridization of two language systems, typically used for trading purposes or in conducting business; has no native speakers

- **presymbolic language** communication stage preceding use of gestures, words, and actions to denote specific language concepts or words

- **primary language** the major language spoken and understood by a population

- **receptive language ability** an individual's skill in understanding language

- **second language extension** an option in a secondary school, with the second language allotted extra time on the curriculum. Other students choose different subject options or more time on their first language

- **second language learning** developing facility with a second language by an adult who was previously exposed only to a single language

- **sign language system** of manual communication in which hand configurations, positions, and movements are used to express concepts and linguistic information

- **spoken language** processing an interactive system of peripheral and central functions used to recognize and understand real-world transitory utterances as meaningful speech

- **standard language** the primary language expected by most speakers in formal contexts

- **target language** the language being learned or taught

- **whole language** a professional theory incorporating teaching strategies and experiences to promote children learning to read, write, speak, and listen in more natural language situations. Instruction under a whole language approach runs more to the informal, the transactional, and follows the psychosociolinguistic approach. Also, an amorphous cluster of ideas about language development in the classroom. The approach does not use (is opposed to) basal readers and phonics in learning to read. Generally, the approach supports a holistic and integrated teaching of reading, writing, spelling, and oracy. The language used must have relevance and meaning to the child. Language development engages cooperative sharing and cultivates empowerment. The use of language for communication is stressed: function matters more than the form of language

language acquisition device (LAD) the hypothetical innate mental structure that allows a child to process incoming linguistic signals and generate a grammar for the resulting language

language-based classroom model a model of service delivery in which a speech-language pathologist is in charge of a class organized specially for students with communication disorders, although some typically speaking children also may be involved; the clinician teaches these children all day or part of the day

language delay acquisition of normal language competencies at a slower rate than would be expected, given a child's chronological age and other levels of functioning

language disorder language behaviors that exhibit slower than expected development or variations in development that significantly interfere with an individual's communication abilities; unrelated to primary intellectual, sensory, or emotional deficits

- **mixed language disorder** a language impairment resulting from both organic and environmental factors

- **organic language disorder** language disorder associated with physiological causes such as brain damage or hearing loss

- **specific language impairment (SLI)** language disorders that appear unrelated to organic causes or any other general disability

language-specific listening and/or speaking in a way that is unique to a particular language

laryngeal about the larynx

- **laryngeal cleft** a cleft in the larynx that may present with cough during feeding; stridor may be present at rest or increased with feeds; an anatomic abnormality resulting from incomplete closure of the tracheoesophageal septum or cricoid cartilage or both in the 6th to 7th week of fetal life

- **laryngeal diversion procedures** also known as subglottic closures, designed to separate the lower respiratory tract from the upper digestive tract without affecting the glottic or supraglottic parts of the larynx

- **laryngeal height** vertical position of the larynx; mostly measured in relation to the rest position

- **laryngeal leukoplakia** appearance of white patches on the laryngeal mucosa; voice may be hoarse; may be premalignant; reduction in or elimination of smoking is recommended

- **laryngeal stoma** an opening made into the front of the neck through the trachea to allow for breathing in patients with laryngectomy

- **laryngeal suspension procedure** to elevate suspension of the larynx to a position under the tongue to remove the throat from the bolus pathway and prevent aspiration during swallowing

- **laryngeal tube cavity** formed by the vocal folds and the arytenoid, epiglottis, and thyroid cartilages and the structures joining them

- **laryngeal ventricle** cavity formed by the gap between the true and false vocal folds

- **laryngeal vestibule** the structures of the endolarynx, bounded by the rim of the epiglottis, superior edge of the aryepiglottic folds, tips of the arytenoid cartilages, and superior edge of the interarytenoid space

- **laryngeal web** an abnormal tissue connection attaching the vocal folds to each other that can cause breathing problems or an abnormal production of voice

- **longitudinal tension** stretching the vocal folds

- **muscles, extrinsic laryngeal** the strap muscles in the neck, responsible for adjusting laryngeal height and for stabilizing the larynx

- **muscles, intrinsic laryngeal** muscles within the larynx responsible for abduction, adduction, and longitudinal tension of the vocal folds; the cricothyroid, lateral cricoarytenoid, transverse and oblique arytenoid, posterior cricoarytenoid, thyroarytenoid muscles, which control the area of the glottic aperture

laryngectomee person whose larynx has been removed

laryngectomy removal of the larynx, either partial or total; in both, a surgical tracheostomy is performed that creates a stoma for air to enter and leave the trachea; a partial laryngectomy preserves the voice, with only part of the vocal mechanism excised; the entire vocal apparatus is removed in a total procedure and the stoma becomes permanent

- **standard hemilaryngectomy** resection of half of the laryngeal cartilage, the true and false vocal fold, and one arytenoid

- **supracricoid laryngectomy** resection of the entire laryngeal cartilage, true and false

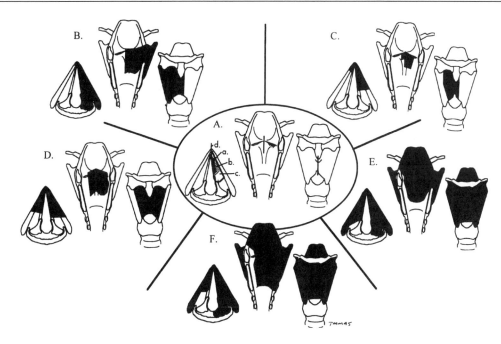

laryngectomy removal of the larynx, either partial or total; in both, a surgical tracheostomy is performed that creates a stoma for air to enter and leave the trachea; a partial laryngectomy preserves the voice, with only part of the vocal mechanism excised; the entire vocal apparatus is removed in a total procedure and the stoma becomes permanent

vocal folds, preepiglottic fat, and the paraglottic space bilaterally; a portion of the epiglottis may or may not be preserved

- **total laryngectomy** removal of the entire cricoid and thyroid cartilages as well as the epiglottis, with resection extending from the upper tracheal rings to hyoid bone

laryngectomy tube an artificial airway utilized only after laryngectomy to assist in maintaining stoma opening

laryngitis inflammation of laryngeal mucous membrane, with concurrent vocal fold edema (swelling) and hoarseness or loss of voice

- **laryngitis sicca** dry voice
- **reflux laryngitis** inflammation of the larynx due to irritation from gastric juice

laryngo- combining form: pertaining to larynx

laryngocele atypical air-filled cavity adjoining the laryngeal ventricle caused by evagination of the ventricle mucous membrane; may displace and cause enlargement of the false vocal fold, leading to airway obstruction and hoarseness

laryngologist physician specializing in disorders of the larynx and voice in most countries; in some areas of Europe, the laryngologist is primarily responsible for surgery, with diagnosis performed by phoniatricians, which is not a physician category in the USA

laryngomalacia/chondromalacia of the larynx a condition in which the laryngeal cartilages are excessively soft and may collapse in response to inspiratory pressures, obstructing the airway; often seen in epiglottis of young children

laryngopathia gravidarium voice changes common with pregnancy, associated with edema of the lamina propria

laryngopathia premenstrualis voice changes associated with the menstrual cycle, noted by decreased vocal efficiency, loss of highest singing notes, vocal fatigue, slight hoarseness, and some muffling of the voice; submucosal laryngeal hemorrhage is common

laryngopharyngeal reflux (LPR) a form of gastroesophageal reflux (GER) in which gastric juice affects the larynx and adjacent structures; commonly associated with hoarseness, frequent throat clearing, granulomas, and other laryngeal problems, even in the absence of heartburn

laryngoplasty surgical treatment to improve phonation in people with vocal fold paralysis or weakness; involves medial displacement of

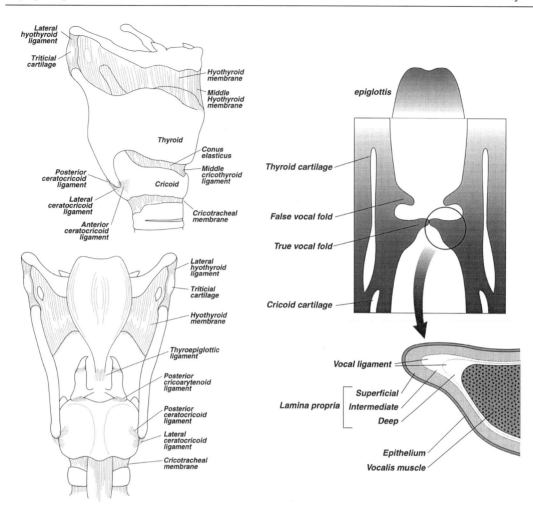

larynx part of the cartilaginous air passage structure, located above the trachea and below the pharynx, that houses the vocal folds and the muscles serving laryngeal vocal mechanisms; used to generate voiced sound and whisper during speech production; composed of three single cartilages and three paired cartilages, all linked by ligaments; single cartilages are the thyroid, cricoid, and epiglottis; paired cartilages are the arytenoid, corniculate, and cuneiform

vocal folds with the help of implant materials to promote better approximation

laryngoscope lighted hollow tube instrument to visualize and operate on the interior of the larynx through the mouth; also used for directly viewing the larynx and glottis for proper placement of an endotracheal tube

laryngospasm involuntary muscular contraction of the larynx; usually includes tight closure of the glottis and may occur during a procedure such as a fiberoptic examination of the larynx, if the scope touches the false vocal folds, arytenoid cartilages, or true vocal folds

laryngotracheal separation procedure of subglottic closure, where the trachea is brought to the skin as in a tracheotomy, but the proximal segment is left closed as a sling pouch

larynx part of the cartilaginous air passage structure, located above the trachea and below the pharynx, that houses the vocal folds and the muscles serving laryngeal vocal mechanisms; used to generate voiced sound and whisper during speech production; composed of three single cartilages and three paired cartilages, all linked by ligaments; single cartilages are the thyroid, cricoid, and epiglottis; paired cartilages are the arytenoid, corniculate, and cuneiform

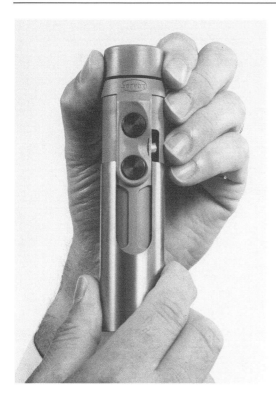

larynx, artificial mechanical voice box for persons who have had a total laryngectomy; electrolarynxes are hand-held battery-powered devices employing various vibration/sound strategies and pneumatic larynxes draw on air from the lungs to create vibration for voice

---

- **larynx, artificial** mechanical voice box for persons who have had a total laryngectomy; electrolarynxes are hand-held battery-powered devices employing various vibration/sound strategies and pneumatic larynxes draw on air from the lungs to create vibration for voice

laser an acronym for *l*ight *a*mplification by *s*timulated *e*mission of *r*adiation, which is concentrated (coherent) monochromatic radiation of the visible, ultraviolet, or infrared spectrum; employed in surgical tools for precise vaporization or cauterization of tissue

latency the time between occurrence of a physiologic event, usually a spike or evoked potential, and a stimulus

latency period gap between electrical stimulation of a neuron or muscle cell and onset of response of that tissue, which for neurons will be the discharge of an action potential, and for muscle can be the discharge of an action poten-

tial or the development of tension; also synonymous with incubation of a pathogen

lateral away from the midline of the body; also, a class of speech sounds produced with a midline obstruction that causes sound to be emitted laterally (to one or both sides)

latero- prefix: pertaining to the side

Latinos Spanish speakers of Latin American extraction; Spanish term often used in English, by U.S. Spanish speakers, themselves, especially in the Southwestern U.S

lax distinctive feature proposed by Roman Jakobson and Morris Halle to describe sounds that are produced with relatively little muscular effort; for example, the vowel /ɪ/ is lax but vowel /i/ is tense

lax vowels vowels with an inherently short duration; [ɪ], [ə], [ʊ]

leak, partial intentional leak maintained in a tracheostomy tube cuff to allow a patient access to airflow through the upper airway for the purposes of speaking, swallowing, and airway clearance

learning disabilities heterogeneous group of disorders, presumed to be caused by central nervous system (CNS) dysfunction, manifested by significant difficulties in the acquisition and use of listening, speaking, reading, writing, reasoning, or mathematical abilities; not a result of sensory, motor, or emotional disorder

learning effect performance on a test improves as a function of familiarity with the test procedures and test items and not because of a change in ability

learning style an individual's characteristic cognitive, affective, modality, and physiological behaviors and preferences employed in perceiving, interacting with, and responding to the learning environment

least restrictive environment (LRE) term appears in the language of the Individuals with Disabilities Education Act (IDEA) formerly known as the Education of All Handicapped Children Act (PL 94-142); applies to the placement of special education-eligible students in the educational environment that least restricts their interactions with typical students; in most cases, this would be an age-appropriate typical classroom

LED displays light-emitting-diode displays used in AAC devices and portable computers, which are easy to read, but require more battery power than other display modes

legato in music, smooth, connected

lemma glossed word or phrase; a proposition employed to demonstrate another proposition; a prephonological form of a word in the mental lexicon

lemniscus a fiber tract of the central nervous system (CNS) ascending from sensory relay nuclei to the thalamus

- **lateral lemniscus** originating in the cochlear and auditory relay nuclei of the rhombencephalon through the thalamus and to the auditory cortex; also called auditory lemmscus

lenis speech sound produced with relatively little air pressure; opposed to *fortis*

lenticular relating to a lens; lentil-shaped

lenticular nucleus forms part of the basal ganglia of the cerebrum, consisting of the globus pallidus and putamen

lepto- prefix: thin, weak, small, delicate, slender

Lesch-Nyhan syndrome later speech production hampered by by dysarthria and athetosis, with associated nasal and oral resonance abnormalities, variable breath support, and delayed language in cases with cognitive impairment; also marked by self-mutilation, mild growth deficiency, gout, high uric acid levels

lesion region of damaged tissue, injury, or wound; infected area of a skin disease

- **focal lesion** lesion with damage concentrated in one small area

leuko-, leuco- prefix: white or white corpuscle

leukocyte white blood cell; primary cells mediating infection and tissue damage by counteracting or quashing organisms. They act as scavengers of damaged cells by phagocytosis to initiate the repair process

leukoplakia a white plaque typically occurring on the mucous membranes, including the vocal folds

levator something that elevates or raises, as a muscle or a surgical instrument

level, sound logarithmic and comparative measure of sound intensity; the unit is normally dB

levo- prefix: left

levodopa antiparkinsonian medication; increases dopamine levels

lexical access process of recognizing and producing words stored in the brain for use in meaningful language; typically an automated process

lexical activation some change in status of a subset of word candidates contained in the mental lexicon

lexical ambiguity uncertainty in meaning of a word because the word has two or more meanings

lexical category a part of speech

lexical competency competence in vocabulary

lexical neighbors words that are phonemically (or visually) similar

lexical-semantic processes language processes that deal with storage and use of word meanings

lexical stress the pattern of the stressed and unstressed syllables at the word level

lexical verbs verbs that express a specific activity

lexicon vocabulary of a language, an individual, or a subject; inventory of a language's morphemes; also called lexis

- **mental lexicon** speaker's knowledge about words, including sounds, meanings, and grammatical roles

lied (German) in music, song, particularly art song

lift vocal production transition point along a pitch scale at which vocalization becomes easier

ligament fibrous connective tissue connecting bones or cartilage or supporting muscles or fasciae

- **phrenoesophageal ligament (or membrane)** an extension of the fascia of the diaphragm that anchors the gastroesophageal junction in the hiatus of the diaphragm. The membrane contains collagen and elastic fibers that allow the gastroesophageal junction to move up into the hiatus on swallowing and then move back down to its resting position. Degeneration and laxity of the membrane is a feature of hiatus hernias, with functioning also related to gastroesophageal reflux (GER)

light pointer AAC device that focuses a beam of light on the surface of a communication system

limbic bordering

limbic system the central nervous system structures responsible for mediation of motivation and arousal, memory, and some aspects of attention, including the hippocampus, amygdala, dentate gyrus, cingulate gyrus, and fornix; influences the autonomic motor and endocrine systems

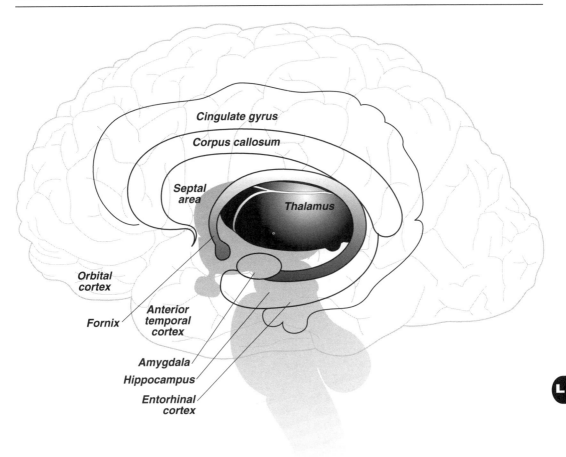

limbic system the central nervous system structures responsible for mediation of motivation and arousal, memory, and some aspects of attention, including the hippocampus, amygdala, dentate gyrus, cingulate gyrus, and fornix; influences the autonomic motor and endocrine systems

limbus the border of a structure

limen, difference (DL) just noticeable difference or smallest detectable change (threshold) in a stimulus, usually pertaining to frequency, intensity, or duration

linear having a straight line with a single dimension; having or being a reaction or output that is directly proportional to the input; relating to, or based on, depending on a sequential process

linear amplification hearing aid amplification system in which there is a one-to-one correspondence between the input and output until the maximum output level is reached

linear predictive coding (LPC) speech spectrum analysis method using a weighted linear sum of samples to predict an upcoming value; the spectrum arrived at represents formant frequencies and amplitudes

linear syntactic relationships in language development, an aspect of children's early grammar describing the additive meaning of words combined in utterances

linear system a system in which the relation between input and output varies in a constant, or linear, fashion

lingua- pertaining to the tongue

Lingua a European Community (EC) program to increase majority language learning across Europe. The program funds scholarships, student exchanges, and teaching materials to improve language learning and teaching in the EC under the umbrella Socrates program to promote transnational cooperation in education

lingua franca a language employed for a mutual or commercial vocabulary among persons of diverse native tongues; like a common language

lingual referring to the tongue

lingual nerve one of the branches of the trigeminal mandibular nerve that innervates the anterior portion of the tongue and carries input of sensory fibers responding to taste, touch, and pressure

linguaverted tilted toward the tongue

linguicism the use of languages to legitimate and reproduce unequal divisions of power and resources in society

linguistic about linguistics

- **linguistic aspects** the dimensions of grammar, semantics, and pragmatics relating to the structure, meaning, and use of language

- **linguistic competence** speaker's underlying knowledge of and idealized skill with the system of rules of the language he or she is using

- **linguistic context** the utterances that precede and contribute to the setting responded to by a speaker

- **linguistic-contextual information** anything that influences the a priori probability of an oncoming utterance or the post hoc, retroactive recognition of an ongoing utterance

- **linguistic experience** the total exposure to a particular language that occurs for an individual

- **linguistic performance** speakers' actualized production of language in daily communication

linguistics the study of language, including phonology, morphology, semantics, and pragmatics; covering the parts, essence, interrelationships, and variation of language; exploring how language works and is used, as well as the interface of language and society

- **comparative linguistics** analysis of the differences and similarities between languages

- **descriptive linguistics** analysis and description of languages

- **developmental linguistics** studies of the linguistic aspects of children's developing language

- **historical linguistics** studies of the changes that occur in languages over time

lingula small tongue-shaped anatomic structure

lipid a fat or fatlike substance that is water insoluble

liquid crystal display (LCD) screens commonly used in AAC devices and other portable computer devices that can be difficult to read without backlighting in bright locations

lipreading recognizing speech using only the visual speech signal, as the shape of the mouth in forming words and other visual cues, such as facial expression

liquid phonological class of consonant sounds made without complete constriction between the tongue and the mouth roof [l] (laterals) and [r] (rhotics); also, a substance that assumes the shape of its container, but preserves its volume and is the intermediate matter state between solid and gas

listening check informal assessment of whether a listening device is functioning appropriately

literacy ability to read and to communicate through written language

- **emergent literacy** children's early reading and writing development

- **skills-based literacy** emphasis placed on the acquisition of phonics and other forms, rather than on ways of using these forms

lobe a division of an organ, usually demarcated by fissures or constrictions; also, one of the five major divisions of the cerebral hemispheres: frontal, parietal, temporal, occipital, and limbic

lobectomy surgical removal of a lobe of the lung; resection of a large portion to the brain

localization the process of identification of a sound source presented in free field; also the principle that focal regions of the brain can be associated with particular functions or behaviors

location relational words in language development, early relational words naming to the location of items of interest

locative action relations spatial relationship or location of actions

locative state relations spatial relationships between entities

locked-in syndrome a condition in which the patient is paralyzed and mute with intact cognitive functioning from an infarct that has caused a pseudocoma, with communication generally limited to eye movements or blinking; often caused by bilateral brainstem stroke

locus specific place

locus theory postulate that the places of articulation are identified with a particular value of a formant frequency

locutionary the component of speech act theory that is the act of speaking

locutionary stage the stage in communication development beginning when the first words are used as speech

loft in music, a suggested term for the highest (loftiest) register; usually referred to as falsetto voice

logarithm the exponent indicating the power to which a base must be raised to equal a given number. Commonly used bases are 10 and the natural number e

log, daily process for assessing conversational fluency and communication handicap in which respondents self-monitor behaviors of interest and provide self-reports; usually completed more than once over a set period of time

logistic map a simple quadratic equation that exhibits chaotic behavior under special initial conditions and parameters. It is the simplest chaotic system

logo- prefix: pertaining to speech or words

logogen in speech perception, a theoretical passive sensing device associated with each word in a mental lexicon. Activation of a logogen is the means to recognition of a particular word

logographics a system of communication in which spoken language is transcribed into a graphic form of written communication with a visual symbol representing each word or morpheme. Chinese script is an example

Lombard effect modification of vocal loudness in response to auditory input. For example, the tendency to speak louder in the presence of background noise

longitudinal along the length of a structure; involving the repeated examination of a group of subjects over time in relation to study variables

long-term average spectrum (LTAS) graph showing a long-time average of the sound intensity in various frequency bands; the appearance of an LTAS is strongly dependent on the filters used

long-term care ongoing care for people with prolonged personal and medical care needs that cannot be provided independently; may be provided in a residential care setting or at home

loop, induction loop of wire in the ceiling of the portion or all of a room designated as an assistive listening area; sound is transmitted by electromagnetic (inductive) energy, along with an amplifier and a microphone for the primary speaker(s); speech signals are amplified and circulated through the loop wire, with the resulting signal adapted by telecoil circuits of many hearing aids, vibrotactile devices, coch-

lear implant systems, or headphone induction loop receivers; magnetic loop

lordosis abnormal anterior-posterior (concave) curve of spine in the lower back

loudness the amount of sound perceived by a listener; a perceptual quantity that can only be assessed with an auditory system. Loudness corresponds to intensity and to the amplitude of a sound wave

- **loudness discomfort level (LDL)** level at which sound is perceived to be uncomfortably loud

- **most comfortable loudness (MCL)** level at which sound is most comfortable for a listener, usually measured in dB HL

- **uncomfortable loudness level (ULL, UCL)** intensity level at which a listener judges a sound to be uncomfortably loud; loudness discomfort level

low distinctive feature proposed by Roman Jakobson and Morris Halle to describe sounds that are produced with a lowered or depressed tongue position (relative to a neutral position); vowels /æ/ and /ɑ/ are low

lower esophageal sphincter (LES) specialized muscle that closes the gastroesophageal junction and prevents gastroesophageal reflux by its tonic contraction; relaxes in response to swallowing; transient LES relaxations in the absence of swallowings, or TLESRs. A high-pressure zone in the distal esophagus that relaxes with swallowing

low spontaneous rate auditory nerve fibers with low rate of spontaneous discharge and relatively high threshold of stimulation

Lucite trademarked name of acrylic resin (plastic) often used for constructing hearing aid earmolds

Ludwig's angina cellulitis; painful soft-tissue infection and swelling of the floor of the mouth capable of compromising (blocking) the airway

lumbar pertaining to the loins, body parts of back, and sides between ribs and pelvis

lumbar puncture insertion of aspiration needle into subarachnoid region of lumbar area of spinal cord to collect material for laboratory study, relieve pressure, inject material for radiographic contrast, or inject medication or other therapeutic medium

lumen interior space of a tubular organ; bore of a shaft, as of a catheter or a hollow needle; unit of luminous flux equal to the light emitted in a solid angle by a uniform point source of one candle intensity

L

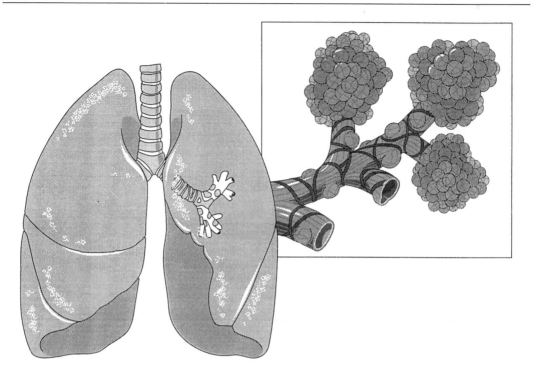

lung   the body's main respiration organ; one of a visceral pair in the pulmonary cavities of the thorax; site of blood aeration

lung the body's main respiration organ; one of a visceral pair in the pulmonary cavities of the thorax; site of blood aeration

- **obstructive lung disease** airway disease classification in which airflow out of the lungs is impeded by narrowing of the small- or medium-sized airways due to spasm, inflammation, or scarring. Overinflation of the lung, prolongation of the expiration, air hunger, dyspnea, and respiratory insufficiency can result

lung capacities volumes contained in the subglottic air system; after a maximum inhalation following a maximum exhalation the lung volume equals the vital capacity; spirometry and manometry measure lung volume and intrapulmonary pressure to provide lung capacity for a given individual

- **functional residual capacity** residual volume plus expiratory reserve volume

- **inspiratory capacity** inspiratory reserve volume and tidal volume

- **total lung capacity** measured at the end of maximum inspiration, is the sum of inspiratory capacity and functional residual capacity

- **vital capacity** expiratory reserve volume, plus tidal volume, plus inspiratory reserve volume

Lyme disease a systemic illness resulting from infection with the spirochete *Borrelia burgdorferi* spread by deer ticks

lymph a transparent yellow liquid originating in body tissues and organs

lymph node one of many small bumps in the lymphatic system that filter lymph and deter infection and in which plasma cells, lymphocytes, and monocytes are formed

lymphocytes most common lymph cells; agents of immunity constituting 20% to 30% of the white blood cells of typical human blood

lymphoid tissue tissue of lymphatic organs, including tonsils, thymus, spleen

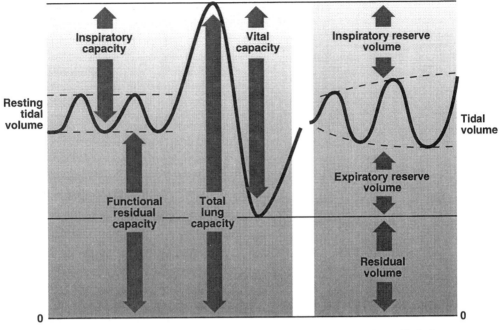

Special Divisions for Pulmonary Function Tests

Primary Subdivisions of Lung Volume

lung capacities   volumes contained in the subglottic air system; after a maximum inhalation following a maximum exhalation the lung volume equals the vital capacity; spirometry and manometry measure lung volume and intrapulmonary pressure to provide lung capacity for a given individual

Mandible

lower jaw

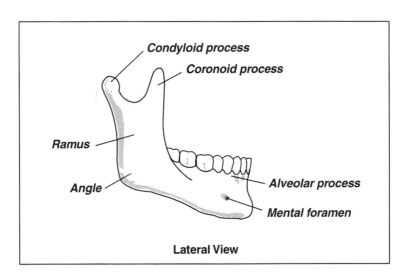

Lateral View

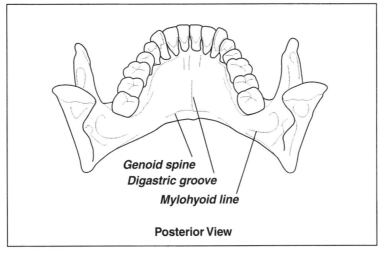

Posterior View

macro- prefix: large or atypically large

macrocephaly congenitally enlarged brain and skull in comparison to the total body size

macroglossia enlarged tongue

macrophage a type of monocyte in body tissue, especially the spleen, lymph nodes, alveoli, and tonsils that assists in the immune response and helps in the body's defense against disease organisms

macula sensory receptor of saccule and utricle; a definable skin area that varies in color from surrounding tissue

Maffucci syndrome articulation and oral resonance may be impaired by oral hemangiomas; also marked by bone deformity, neoplasms

magnetic loop loop of wire in the ceiling of the portion or all of a room designated as an assistive listening area; sound is transmitted by electromagnetic (inductive) energy, along with an amplifier and a microphone for the primary speaker(s); speech signals are amplified and circulated through the loop wire, with the resulting signal adapted by telecoil circuits of many hearing aids, vibrotactile devices, cochlear implant systems, or headphone induction loop receivers; magnetic loop induction loop

magnetic resonance imaging (MRI) scan computerized image technology that uses nuclear magnetic resonance to create cross sectional images, or "slices," of the human body, providing vivid details of internal hard and soft body tissues for specifying the precise region, nature, and extent of an injury, anomaly or anatomical feature

- **functional magnetic resonance imaging (fMRI)** image of function is created from signals generated by the hemodynamics within the structure of interest, allowing observation of which body structures are active in specific functions; high-resolution images of neural activity are achieved through depictions of oxygen level and flow

- **ultrafast magnetic resonance imaging (uMRI)** scanning technique allowing rapid magnetic resonance imaging scans to be performed, with swallowing studies, among others, benefiting

mainstreaming providing the opportunity for students with disabilities to interact with typically developing peers in regular classrooms with special assistance as needed; return of persons recovering from mental illness to the general population

maintenance independent use of skills developed through treatment and/or therapy in an individuals's natural settings

major histocompatibility complex (MHC) a complex of cell-surface proteins that act in differentiating self- and nonself-cells as part of the immunity response

mal- prefix: defective, bad, wrong

maladaptive strategy inappropriate or faulty intrapersonal behavioral mechanisms for coping with difficulties, such as avoidance behavior (as might be seen in ducking out of conversation by a person with a hearing loss)

malaise general uneasy feeling of discomfort, weakness, or distress that can mark the onset of disease

malignant as tumor type, means being locally invasive, with destructive growth and metastasis; tending to worsen, being resistant to treatment

malleus the largest, outermost bone in the ossicular chain of the middle ear that attaches to the tympanic membrane; named malleus (Latin for hammer) because of its hammerlike shape

malocclusion any deviation from a normal or typical occlusion of the teeth

- **Angle's classification of malocclusion** identification of malocclusion, based on the mesiodistal association of the permanent molars and incisors. There are three classes, identified by Roman numerals; see Angle's classification of malocclusion for illustration

- **Class I malocclusion** malocclusion in which there is normal orientation of the molars, but there is an abnormal orientation of the incisors

- **Class II malocclusion** relationship between upper and lower dental arches in which the first mandibular molars are retracted at least one tooth from the first maxillary molars

- **Class III malocclusion** relationship between upper and lower dental arches in which the first mandibular molar is advanced farther than one tooth beyond the first maxillary molar

- **distocclusion** malocclusion, with the mandibular arch articulating with the maxillary arch that is distal to normal; Class II malocclusion in Angle's classification

mamm- prefix: pertaining to the breast, mammary gland

managed care health care reimbursement plan in which an organization intercedes between patient and provider and determines the kind and extent of services that will be provided

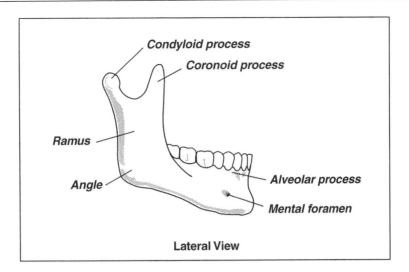

Lateral View

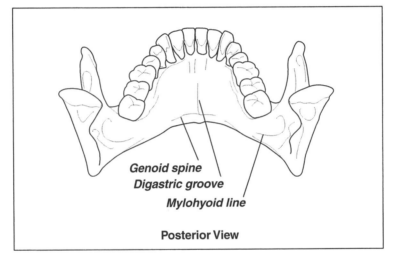

Posterior View

mandible   lower jaw

management intervention to prevent or remediate a disorder or disease, as well compensatory approaches (e.g., strategies, technologies) to reduce harm from deficits resistant to remediation

mand a primary verbal operant that responds to a deprivation state or aversive stimulus and specifies its reinforcer; the behavioral equivalent of commanding, demanding, or requesting

Mandelbrot set a series of two equations containing real and imaginary components that, when iterated and plotted on a two-dimensional graph, depict a very complex and classic fractal pattern; named for Benoit Mandelbrot (1924–)

mandible   lower jaw

mandibulofacial dysplasia abnormal tissue development of the jaw and face

manner of articulation a phonetic feature of speech sounds that specifies the overall manner in which a sound is produced; the manner feature includes specifications such as stop, nasal, fricative, and glide

manometer device for measuring air pressure differences; an instrument used for measuring the pressure exerted by a liquid or a gas in a container, as compared to atmospheric pressure

manual alphabet series of hand configurations that correspond to each letter in the alphabet; used to fingerspell words in manual communication

manual approach educational philosophy for deaf children that emphasizes the use of sign language and fingerspelling for the early development of language skills

manual communication communication modes that entail the use of fingerspelling, signs, and gestures

manual pointing AAC form of direct selection involving pointing with the hand or fingers, with or without a pointing aid

manubrium in ear, process of malleus forming the major attachment to the tympanic membrane; also, the upper portion of the sternum

- **anterior process of manubrium** ear's anterior prominence of manubrium, providing point of attachment for anterior ligament of malleus

- **lateral process of manubrium** superior process of manubrium to which tympanic membrane is attached, forming the anterior and posterior malleolar folds and the pars flaccida of the tympanic membrane

- **lever advantage** the benefit derived through reduction of the length of the long process of stapes relative to the manubrium malli

map, auditory-articulatory knowledge a speaker of a language learns early in life that links specific movements of the person's articulators to the specific sounds caused by those movements

map, cochlear implant specifications of threshold, suprathreshold, and frequency by which the speech processor of a cochlear implant processes the speech signal and delivers it in electrical form to the electrodes in the electrode array

map, logistic a simple quadratic equation that exhibits chaotic behavior under special initial conditions and parameters. It is the simplest chaotic system

mapped, polymodally information that is stored in the brain in a way that is not specific to any one sensory modality

map, perceptual representation stored in memory that indicates the relationships among a variety of stimuli; specifically, the distances from one another

mapping vocabulary acquisition hypothesis that preschoolers first do fast mapping in quickly associating a new word and its referent and then expand and modify meaning of that word through ongoing experiences in a process of extended mapping

map, return similar to phase plane plot, but analyzed data must be digital. This graphic technique represents the relationship between a point and any subsequent point in a time series

marcato in music, each note accented

marked semantic aspect of words that refers to the negative end of a dimension or continuum (e.g., length)

marked language a minority language distinct from a majority one and usually not highly valued in society

marking in language development, caregivers' means of attracting attention to an object by moving or shaking it in their infants' field of view; in professional voice, using the voice gently (typically during rehearsals) to avoid injury or fatigue; in speech production, saying a word with a subtle, unconventional error to make a distinction between it and another, similar-sounding word

Markov model a network model of states and transitions in which the transitions between states are associated with probabilities of occurrence

- **hidden Markov model (HMM)** a mathematical model that can be used in speech recognition consisting of a finite set of states, transition probabilities between the states, a finite set of possible outcomes, and a probability distribution over the set of outcomes associated with each state. Similar to a Markov model, except that in a hidden Markov model, the states are not directly associated with outcomes, but rather with possibilities, because the most likely dynamic systems can be inferred, along with models for underlying processes

masker for tinnitus, an electronic listening device that delivers low-level noise to the ear to screen out tinnitus ringing; any stimulus that interferes with detection of a target signal

masking noise that interferes with the perception of another sound

mass characteristic of a body that is a measure of its inertia commonly understood as a measure of the amount of material the body contains and provides its weight in a gravitational field

mass activity reflex a reflex in which the response is evidenced by the entire body

masseter muscle of mastication that is a primary mover in closing the jaw; innervated by a branch of the trigeminal nerve (CN V)

mass noun nouns that name items perceived as integral wholes that cannot be divided (e.g., milk and sand)

mastication chewing

mastoid process bony projection of skull's temporal bone behind and below the ears

mater coverings of the central nervous system (CNS); mother

matrix basis for the origination of another thing; intercellular material in which tissue cells (i.e., connective tissue cells) are embedded; rectangular display of mathematical elements that can be joined to arrive at sums and products with like displays with a matching numbers of rows and columns; primary grammatical clause that includes a subordinate clause

matrix sentence a form of a sentence before embedding or after embedded sentences have been removed

maxilla bony portion of the upper jaw that contains the palatine, frontal, and alveolar processes

mean length of utterance (MLU) average length of a sample of 50 to 100 child utterances; computed by dividing the total number of words/morphemes in the utterance sample by the number of utterances

means-end analysis cognitive means of applying a scheme or behavior pattern to achieve a desired goal; as in determining the means (or process for) achieving a purpose (end product)

meatus passageway, particularly the opening to the exterior of a canal

- **external acoustic (auditory) meatus** canal coursing laterally from the auricle to the tympanic membrane, consisting of bony inner aspect and a cartilaginous outer portion

- **internal acoustic (auditory) meatus** located on the posterior surface of the petrous portion of the temporal bone

mechanical ventilation mechanical assistance in the breathing process; it may be used to augment the efforts of a patient who has spontaneous, but weak, breaths or for individuals who do not breathe on their own

mechanics physical science branch that explores the effects of energy and forces on objects

mechanoreceptor sensory receptor sensitive to mechanical stimulation such as pressure on or distortion of the skin

meconium ileus blockage of the small intestine in a neonate

medial toward the midline of the body or subpart

median number standing for the middle sum of sample scores

mediastinum the space between the two pleural cavities that contain the lungs within the thorax. It contains the esophagus, trachea, esophagus, thymus, and blood vessels

medio-, medius prefix: middle

medulla inner or central portion of an organ

- **medulla oblongata** the lowest part of the brainstem and extending to the spinal cord containing neuronal pathways controlling respiration, blood pressure, and swallowing

mega-, megalo- prefix: of great size

meiosis a two-stage cell division process, producing egg or sperm cells, each containing half the number of chromosomes in typical cells; with fertilization, the nuclei of the sperm and ovum fuse and produce a zygote with the full number of chromosomes

mel an auditory unit for the measurement of frequency. It follows certain nonlinear properties of the human perception of frequency

melodic intonation therapy (MIT) therapy approach, with utterances spoken in a song-like fashion, emphasizing the melody pattern, rhythm, and points of syllable stress of a spoken model

mel scale a frequency scale that allows for differences in the perceived pitch of a tone

melting pot term for amalgamation of a variety of immigrant ethnic groups in the USA

membrane pliable, thin layer of tissue lining body cavities, dividing spaces, or binding structures

- **basal membrane of semicircular duct** foundation for the semicircular duct epithelium

- **basement membrane** delicate noncellular layer on the bottom of the epithelium

- **basilar membrane** forms most of the cochlear duct floor and separates that duct from the scala tympani, also supporting the organ of Corti

- **cell membrane** boundary of all body cells that controls permeability for cell entry and exit

- **cricothyroid membrane** bilateral membrane between the inferior side and arch of the thyroid lamina: one membrane on each side

- **fibroelastic membrane of the larynx** elastic and fibrous layer that replaces submucosa in the larynx that is divided by the laryngeal ventricle

- **membranous glottis** the anterior three-fifths of the vocal fold margin; the soft tissue of the vocal folds (note that the term "glottis" is loosely used here, because glottis is actually the space between the vocal folds)

- **membranous labyrinth** membranous sac housed within bony labyrinth of inner ear, holding the receptor organs of hearing and vestibular sense

- **mucous membrane** thin sheets of tissue lining body cavities or canals that open to the exterior, such as the mouth, digestive tube, and respiratory passages

- **otolithic membrane** membranous covering of the utricular macula

- **phrenoesophageal membrane (or ligament)** an extension of the fascia of the diaphragm that anchors the gastroesophageal junction in the hiatus of the diaphragm. The membrane contains collagen and elastic fibers that allow the gastroesophageal junction to move up into the hiatus on swallowing and then move back down to its resting position. Degeneration and laxity of the membrane is a feature of hiatus hernias, with functioning also related to gastroesophageal reflux (GER)

- **quadrangular membrane** elastic, mucosa-covered membrane extending from the sides of the epiglottic cartilage to the corniculate and arytenoid cartilages; forming the aryepiglottic fold and the wall between the pyriform sinus and larynx

- **Reissner's membrane** in the ear, membranous separation between scala vestibuli and scala media

- **serous membrane** thin sheet lining body cavities

- **tectorial membrane** gel-like layer within the ear's cochlear partition, with cilia of outer hair cells embedded in the membrane; thus, displacement of hair cells results in shearing movement between upper surface of hair cell and tectorial membrane

- **tympanic membrane** thin, taut membranous separation between the outer and middle ears, responsible for initiating the mechanical impedance-matching process of the middle ear; eardrum

- **vestibular membrane** separation of the cochlear duct from the vestibular canal

membrane channel a protein or glycoprotein that spans the lipid bilayer of a cell membrane and forms a channel between the intracellular and extracellular space. Channels are selective, allowing the passage of particular ionic species. The conduits may be opened or closed by changes in membrane potential, hormones, neurotransmitters, or the ionic milieu of the cytoplasm

memory capacity to encode, process, and retrieve events, knowledge, feelings, and decisions

- **auditory memory** acquisition, storage, and retrieval of auditory sound patterns in both short- and long-term form

- **declarative, or explicit, memory** conscious awareness or recollection of previously acquired information that is retrievable on command

- **episodic memory** cumulative set of experiences that make up an individual's understanding of a concept or event

- **long-term memory** declarative, or explicit, memory, plus procedural, or implicit, memory; long-term memory storage of unlimited capacity; involves both storage and processing of information

- **mental representations** storage in memory of information about the items in a particular category; can take forms ranging from some sort of composite image to a list of individual instances

- **metamemory** knowledge and awareness of one's own memory systems and strategies

- **procedural, or implicit, memory** processing and use of previous experience or knowledge in the absence of conscious awareness or recollection to support learning and guide performance

- **semantic memory** an individual's understanding of a word's meaning, including the words and concepts the person associates with the word

- **short-term memory** brief storage of limited capacity with minimal processing requirements

- **working memory** component of long-term memory that is at a heightened state of activation for a limited time; involves both storage and processing of information (e.g., inference, transformation, executive processing)

memory, computer

- **direct memory access (DMA)** method by which primary memory can be read from or written to without passing through the computer CPU. In speech application, DMA permits a digital signal to be stored to a hard disk during the digitization process

- **random access memory (RAM)** memory in a computer that can be read and altered by the user

- **read-only memory (ROM)** memory in a computer than can be read only, not altered by writing of new information or editing

menarche onset of menstruation at puberty

meninges membranous linings of the brain and spinal cord: dura mater, arachnoid mater, and pia mater

meningitis infection or inflammation of the meninges covering the brain and/or spinal cord; common cause of childhood deafness

meningo- prefix: pertaining to membranes, especially the meninges that serve as coverings in the central nervous system (CNS)

menopause cessation of menstrual cycles and menstruation

menstrual cycle normal cyclical variation of hormones in adult females of child-bearing age and body responses caused by the variation

menstrual period first portion of the menstrual cycle, associated with endometrial shedding and vaginal bleeding

mental age intellectual age

mentalism philosophical perspective that emphasizes that knowledge derives from the organization of the mind

mental lexicon speaker's knowledge about words, including sounds, meanings, and grammatical roles

mental representations storage in memory of information about the items in a particular category; can take forms ranging from some sort of composite image to a list of individual instances

mental retardation intellectual function below normal range

mental rules underlying systems of knowledge reflected in typical consistent behavior patterns

menu-driven computer program that presents a list of commands for user selection

mesencephalic referring to the midbrain, just rostral to the pons

mesencephalon midbrain; one of three brainstem portions, lying below the cerebrum and above the pons; contains nuclei of third and fourth (CN III, CN IV) cranial nerves and part of CN V, as well as nuclei of some auditory and visual reflexes

mesial toward the midline of the body or subpart, especially the dental arch

meso- prefix: middle, mean

mesoderm embryonic middle germ layer that is the origin of connective tissue, muscle, bone, blood, and most circulatory system components

messa di voce traditional exercise in Italian singing tradition consisting of a long prolonged crescendo and diminuendo on a sustained tone

meta- prefix: after; mounted or built upon

metabolism sum of physical and chemical processes in a living organism that are involved in the changing of a substance to another

- **basal metabolism** oxygen employed by a waking individual during minimal physical activity

- **carbohydrate metabolism** breakdown, oxidation, and synthesis of carbohydrates in tissues

- **energy metabolism** metabolic reactions to provide or release energy

- **respiratory metabolism** exchange of gases in the lungs and oxidation of foodstuffs in the tissues, along with water and carbon dioxide production

metacognition awareness and appropriate use of knowledge awareness of the task and strategy variables that affect performance and the use of that knowledge to plan, monitor, and regulate performance, including attention, learning, and the use of language; second phase (following cognition) in the development of knowledge that is active and involves conscious control over knowledge

metalinguistic ability speaker's ability to consciously evaluate his or her language behavior

metalinguistics aspects of language competence that extend beyond unconscious usage for comprehension and production; involves ability to think about language in its abstract form: to reflect on aspects of language apart from its content—to analyze it and make judgments about it; metalinguistic knowledge underlies performance on a number of tasks, including phonological awareness (e.g., segmentation, rhyming), organization and storage of words (e.g., multiple word meanings), and figurative language (e.g., metaphor, idiom, humor); may be considered a subset of metacognition, as using language is one of the goals of metacognitive processes

metamemory knowledge and awareness of one's own memory systems and strategies

metanarrative skill ability to analyze and comprehend a story

M

metaphor figure of speech in which a word or phrase for an individual, object, or idea is used to suggest a likeness or analogy with another individual, object, or idea; figurative language (e.g., He's an ox!)

metaphoric transparency extent of similarity between a figurative expression and its literal referent

metastasis spread of disease from a body part to another location; often used for spread of tumors, especially malignancies

metathesis phonological error pattern in which two sounds in a word are reversed (peek pronounced /kip/)

metencephalon embryonic portion of the brain from which the cerebellum and pons originate

mezza voce half voice; in practice, means singing softly, with proper support

mezzo soprano half soprano; common female range, higher than contralto, but lower than soprano

mho unit of measure of admittance; as reciprocal of impedance; is the word ohm spelled backwards

micro-, micr- prefix: of small size

microcephaly small, underdeveloped cranium and brain

microcomputer relatively small, freestanding computer system based on a microprocessor; commonly known as a personal computer (PC)

micrognathia abnormal smallness of jaws, particularly the lower jaw

micrometer one thousandth of a millimeter, one millionth of a meter

micron former term for micrometer

microphone transducer that converts an audio signal into an electronic signal

- **contact microphone** microphone that directly attaches to a part of the body, for example, the skin of the neck near the larynx

- **directional microphone** microphone that is most sensitive to sound originating from the front of a listener, such as a hearing aid user

- **omnidirectional microphone** microphone sensitive to sound from all possible directions

- **probe microphone** transducer inserted into the external ear canal to measure sound near the tympanic membrane

microprocessor microchip containing all the components of a central processing unit (CPU)

microtia abnormally small and often malformed external ear (auricle)

midbrain uppermost portion of the brainstem

middle (or mixed) in singing, a mixture of qualities from various voice registers, cultivated to allow consistent quality throughout the frequency range

middle C C4 on the piano keyboard, with an international concert pitch frequency of 261.6 Hz

middle ear portion of the ear that contains the ossicles, the opening to the eustachian tube, parts of the facial nerve, tympanic membrane (eardrum) and related structures, stapedius and tensor tympani tendons; tympanic cavity, air-filled space in the temporal bone; three joined ossicles (small bones), malleus, incus, and stapes, extend from the tympanic membrane to the oval window

middle-latency response (MLR) auditory evoked potential characterized by a positive peak in the latency range from 30–35 ms; identified with primary auditory cortex

milk scan radionuclide test for aspiration and gastroesophageal reflux (GER), with a small amount of radionuclide-labeled milk ingested by an infant being monitored; also called scintigraphy

milliliter (ml) one thousandth of a liter

millimeter (mm) millimeter; one thousandth of a meter

mimetic characterized by imitation, mimicry, or copying

minimal distance principle language development comprehension strategy in which the noun closest to the verb is assumed to be the agent

minimal pairs/contrastive sets treatment technique in which a person is exposed to two (minimal pairs) or more (contrastive sets) sets of stimuli that differ in only one dimension; usually the individual is expected to discriminate between the sets of stimuli

minority segment of a population varying from other portions in some characteristics (language, skin coloration, homeland) and often subject to differential treatment; being a legal minor; lesser in number of two groups of a whole

- **involuntary minorities** also known as caste-like minorities; differing from immigrants and "voluntary minorities," in that they have not willingly migrated to a country

- **language minority** person or a group speaking a language of low prestige or having small numbers in a society

Minspeak pictographic encoding system developed by Bruce Baker that relies on the concept of multimeaning symbols

minute ventilation (V$_E$) product of tidal volume and rate, generally about 5 to 10 L/min. Or 100/ml/kg/min; alveolar ventilation may decrease, if there is increased dead space or decreased minute ventilation (decreased respiratory rate or tidal volume)

minute volume volume of air exchanged by an organism in 1 minute

mio- prefix: less

mio-, myelo-, my- prefix: pertaining to muscle

mitochondria cell organelle employing enzymes for cell respiration that provides cellular energy source

mitosis typical cell division that produces self-similar cells

mixed dysarthrias type of motor speech disorder that is a combination of two or more pure dysarthrias; the neuropathology is varied, depending on the types of dysarthrias that are mixed; causes frequently include multiple strokes or neurological diseases; speech disorders are varied and dependent on the types of pure dysarthrias that are mixed

mixed hearing loss loss that has both conductive and sensorineural components

mixed language disorder language impairment resulting from both organic (congenital) and environmental factors

mnemonic mental device used by individuals to help in memorization (e.g., acronyms, rhymes, verbal mediators, visual imagery, drawing)

Möbius syndrome inanimate articulators leads to severe articulation impairment, along with muffled oral resonance and delayed expressive language development; sometimes spelled Moebius syndrome

modal auxiliary verb auxiliary verb that expresses a speaker's attitude or mood about the main verb

modality component of deep structure in case grammar that carries the tense and sentence type; any of the five senses; a means of language expression, such as speech or manual signing

modal register vocal register used during normal conversation (i.e., the register used most frequently)

modeling demonstrating a desired behavior to prompt an imitative response; needed when a clinician cannot evoke a response elsewise; used frequently in treating communicative disorders

modem short term for modulator/demodulator; device that converts signals from one sort of device (as a computer) to a format compatible with another (as a telephone)

modified barium swallow (MBS) dynamic (moving) X-ray examination of oral and pharyngeal swallowing function, with a barium bolus studied through fluoroscopic observation

modiolus cone-shaped core of the bony labyrinth forming the central core of the cochlea

modulate to alter the intensity, frequency, or quality of a stimulus

modulation periodic variation of a signal property; for example, as vibrato corresponds to a regular variation of fundamental frequency, it can be regarded as a modulation of that signal property

- **amplitude modulation (AM)** signal information controls the amplitude of a carrier signal
- **frequency modulation (FM)** signal information controls the frequency of a carrier signal

Mohr syndrome articulatory impairment secondary to lingual anomalies and possible compensatory articulation secondary to cleft palate; also marked by hyperplastic frenulae, maxillary hypoplasia

molars posterior three teeth of the mature dental arch; used for grinding

momentum quantity of motion

- **linear momentum** sum obtained by multiplying the mass of a body by its linear speed

monaural of or relating to sound with a single transmission path; of one ear

monitor display device for video signals from a computer control unit or AAC device

mono- prefix: single

monoamine oxidase (MAO) enzyme that catalyzes amine oxidation

monoamine oxidase (MAO) inhibitor drug group mainly prescribed to treat depression, also having antianxiety effects

M

Order of Acquisition in Brown's 14 Grammatical Morphemes

Rank	Morpheme	Example
1	Present progressive inflection	He eating.
2	Preposition in	Juice in cup.
3	Preposition on	Sleep on bed.
4	Regular plural inflection	My toys.
5	Past Irregular	I ate cookie.
6	Possessive inflection	Mommy's shoe.
7	Uncontractible copula	Here it is! They were nice.
8	Articles	A boy took the ball.
9	Regular past tense	He walked fast.
10	Regular third person singular	She bakes cakes.
11	Irregular third person singular	He has some. She does, too.
12	Uncontractible auxiliary	Is she reading? You were reading.
13	Contractible copula	Tommy's tall! They are all tall?
14	Contractible auxiliary	She's reading. They are reading.

Source: Adapted from *A First Language: The Early Stages*, by R. Brown, 1973. Cambridge, MA: Harvard University Press.

grammatical morpheme   morpheme serving a grammatical function

monologue in language development, private speech in which children talk to themselves during play, often to reflect on their emotional state

- **affect expressive monologue** preschooler self-talk that reflects on the child's emotions

- **associated monologue** play behavior mode in which children share personal monologues on a given topic

- **collective monologue** children playing near each other who speak simultaneously, but not necessarily to each other

monopitch lacking variation in vocal pitch (perception of vocal fundamental frequency)

monoplegia paralysis of one limb

monopolar electrode electrode used for recording bioelectric signals in which the voltage input to the amplifier is measured between a single electrode and a reference electrode

monosyllabic word word of one syllable

morbidity state of illness or disease: ratio of sick to healthy in a geographical area; frequency that complications develop following a medical treatment or procedure

morph an individual particular occurrence of a morpheme

morph-, morpho- prefix: form

morpheme the minimal, meaningful unit of language that contains no smaller meaningful parts; may be a simple word such as "bell" or may be bound to another unit, as in the plural marker for "bells"

- **bound morpheme** subclass of morphemes that are meaningless unless attached to a free morpheme; includes derivational and inflectional morphemes

- **derivational morpheme** type of bound morpheme that changes the grammatical class of the free morpheme to which it is attached (e.g., teacher)

- **free morpheme** morpheme that can occur independently and carry meaning

- **grammatical morpheme** morpheme serving a grammatical function

- **inflectional morpheme** type of bound morpheme that inflects the word it is attached to for tense (play*ed*), plurality (cat*s*), possession (John's), and degree (green*er*)

morphology units of meaning that make up the grammar of a language; rules that modify meaning at the word level; linguistics discipline looking at the internal structure of words composed of more than one meaningful part, dealing primarily with how speakers comprehend complex words and the means language users employ to create new ones

Morse code communication system originally developed for use with telegraph systems that uses a series of short and long pulses (*dits* and *dahs*) to represent letters and numbers

morula solid embryonic cluster of cells formed by the fourth or fifth day following conception

motherese (also parentese or child-directed speech) distinctive style of talking exhibited by caregivers when speaking with their toddlers. When compared to the speech directed toward adults, motherese has exaggerated intonation contours, slower tempo, and higher overall fundamental frequency

motilin polypeptide secreted by cells within the duodenum that causes contraction of intestinal smooth muscle

motor physiology/anatomy: relating to neural generation and transmission of impulses causing muscle fibers to contract or glands to secrete; compare efferent

motor area precentral gyrus of the brain's frontal lobe; the point at which execution of voluntary motor acts is initiated

motor endplate point of contact between motor neuron and muscle fiber; formation through which a motor neuron makes a synaptic contact with a striated muscle cell; also called myoneuronal junction

motor neuron efferent nerve cell that relays nerve impulses from the spinal cord or brain to muscles or glands; older term is motoneuron

• **motor neuron pool** closely knit alpha motor neurons that innervate one muscle

motor neuron disease overall term for group of neurological pathologies, including spinal muscular atrophy, amyotrophic lateral sclerosis, progressive bulbar paralysis, and primary lateral sclerosis; often familial

motor speech areas cerebral hemispheric regions associated with motor control of speech, for example, Broca's area and orofacial motor cortex

motor theory speech perception theory based on the premise that speech is perceived in relation to the motor processes (articulation) by which it is produced

motor trigeminal nucleus cranial motor nucleus with motor neurons that innervate several muscles of the mandible, such as the jaw-closing muscles (i.e., masseter) and a jaw-opening muscle (i.e., anterior digastric), as well as muscles of the mouth floor

mouse input device for a computer; usually is a small hand-held box moved on a horizontal surface, with its relative position echoed on the computer monitor screen

mouse emulator alternative access method avoiding the physical movement required for mouse usage; can include alternative keyboards, touch tablets, or switches; alternative keyboards usually employ arrow keys to indicate cursor movement; switches usually require an indirect selection method

mouth stick adaptive pointer that attaches to a mouth guard that is held by the teeth

muco, muc- prefix: pertaining to mucus or mucous membrane

mucocele mucous cyst; cystic anomaly of the cranial bones' air cavities

mucociliary clearance expulsion from the tracheobronchial tree of inspired material, cellular debris, and excessive secretions by action of ciliated cells in the respiratory tract; mucus and debris are propelled upward by the beating of the cilia; important respiratory tract defense

mucolytic pharmaceutical agent used to loosen mucus for easier physiologic removal from the airway

mucopolysaccharidosis one of several lysosomal storage diseases with disordered metabolism of mucopolysaccharides (a protein-polysaccharide complex) with defects of bone, cartilage, and connective tissue

mucosa membraneous covering of the respiratory tract surfaces, such as the oral and nasal cavities, as well as the pharynx, larynx, and lower airways, plus other canals opening to the body exterior; synonymous with mucous membrane

mucosal tear vocal fold surface disruption; usually caused by trauma, as well as by vocal abuse, smoking, alcohol

mucosal wave undulation along the vocal fold surface traveling in the direction of airflow

mucous pertaining to tissue that secretes mucus

mucus viscous fluid secreted by mucous tissue and glands

multi- prefix: many or much

M

multichannel more than one channel of information; often used to describe cochlear implants that present various channels of information to different regions of the cochlea

multidisciplinary team model team members from many disciplines provide services in isolation from one another and perform only tasks specific to their respective disciplines; results and recommendations are discussed at team meetings

multifactorial inheritance genetic expression of an abnormal trait caused by several or many genes at various locations, plus environmental influences

multiinfarct dementia progressive organic brain disorder caused by vascular disease and distinguished by rapid intellectual functioning decline, with disturbances in memory, abstract thinking, impulse control, and judgment

multiple-memory hearing aid hearing aid that can be programmed to process the speech signal in more than one way, so that a user can adjust the processing strategy for various listening environments

multiple sclerosis (MS) central nervous system demyelinating disorder that is fairly common; leads to plaques (sclerotic patches) in the brain and spinal cord; generally first appears in early adulthood; symptoms include dysarthria, visual loss, diplopia, nystagmus, weakness, paresthesias, and mood alteration

multipolar neuron neuron with one axon and many dendrites; the typical neuron form of internuncial neurons and motor neurons

multisensory approach educational approach for deaf children that emphasizes the use of vision, residual hearing, and touch to enhance communication

mumps infectious inflammation and swelling of the parotid gland

muscarinic having influence on the nervous system that appears like parasympathetic postganglionic stimulation

muscle tissue of contractible fiber (generally grouped as smooth, skeletal, cardiac) that cause movement of organs and body parts

- **auxiliary respiratory muscles** accessory muscles of breathing that assist in the expansion or compression of the rib cage by fixing, elevating, or depressing the ribs; include muscles of the thoracic cavity, abdominal wall, and back; contraction allows for deep inhalation, forced exhalation, or performance of a Valsalva maneuver

- **cricoarytenoid muscle, lateral** intrinsic laryngeal muscle that adducts the vocal folds through forward rocking and rotation of the arytenoids (paired)

- **cricoarytenoid muscle, posterior** intrinsic laryngeal muscle that is the primary abductor of the vocal folds (paired)

- **cricothyroid muscle** intrinsic laryngeal muscle that primarily controls pitch by making the vocal folds tense

- **extrinsic laryngeal muscles** strap muscles in the neck, responsible for adjusting laryngeal height and for stabilizing the larynx

- **infrahyoid muscle group** collection of extrinsic laryngeal muscles including the sternohyoid, sternothyroid, omohyoid, and thyroid muscles

- **intrinsic laryngeal muscles** muscles within the larynx responsible for abduction, adduction, and longitudinal tension of the vocal folds; controlling the area of the glottic aperture are the cricothyroid, lateral cricoarytenoid, transverse and oblique arytenoid, posterior cricoarytenoid, and thyroarytenoid muscles

- **muscle fasciculus** bundle of muscle fibers enclosed by a sheath of connective tissue

- **muscle fiber** long, thin cell; the basic muscle unit that is excited by innervation

- **respiratory muscles** any of the muscles for inhalation or exhalation, which include the diaphragm, muscles of the rib cage (parasternal, internal and external intercostals, and scalene), abdominal muscles (internal and external obliques, transversus abdominis, and rectus abdominis), and muscles of the upper airways, which are essential to maintain airway patency

- **skeletal muscle** striated, or voluntary, muscle

- **smooth muscle** muscle type found in viscera and the walls of the gastrointestinal tract; membrane ion channels provide for longer action potentials

- **stapedius muscle** inner ear muscle connecting neck of stapes bone with medial wall of middle ear; contraction pulls the stapes to slightly stiffen the ossicular chain

- **striated muscle** muscle whose contractile proteins are arranged into specific striated units; most skeletal muscles (those attached to the bones of the body) and also the pharynx, larynx, and esophagus contain striated muscles

- **suprahyoid muscle group** one of the two extrinsic laryngeal muscle groups; includes the stylohyoid muscle, anterior and posterior bellies of the digastric muscle, geniohyoid, hyoglossus, and mylohyoid muscles

- **thyroarytenoid muscle (also vocalis)** relaxes (decreases tension) of the vocal folds and lowers the pitch of the voice tone; runs from the inner surface of the thyroid cartilage to the muscular process and outer surface of the arytenoid

muscle tone degree of tension in a muscle at rest

muscular dystrophy, oculopharyngeal gradual dysarthria onset after beginning of facial weakness (from condition onset after age 20), with hypernasality following; also marked by pharyngeal muscle weakness

musculoskeletal tension disorder laryngeal hyperfunction in response to stress

mutation change producing new effects; hereditary physical biochemical change in the codons that make up genes; mutational process; strain or trait stemming from mutation

mutism inability or refusal to speak; lack of vocal or verbal expression

mutism, elective condition in which an individual chooses not to speak in certain circumstances; the lack of speech is situational and will not appear to reflect an inability to speak

mutual gaze shared eye contact with a partner to signal attention

myasthenia gravis autoimmune disease characterized by muscle weakness and progressive fatigue; may result from a malfunction of the myoneural junction, causing failure in inducing normal muscle contraction

myelencephalon portion of embryonic brain from which the medulla oblongata develops

myelin fatty, white tissue that surrounds large axons to provide an insulating coating; the so-called white matter of the brain takes its color from myelin

myelinated fiber differentiated from fiber without a myelin sheath; sensory and motor neurons with myelin conduct action potential much faster than unmyelinated neurons

myelo-, myel- prefix: pertaining to spinal cord or bone marrow

myelography radiography for identifying and studying traumatic or pathologic spinal lesions; visualization enabled by photography of contrast medium

myelomeningocele spina bifida type caused by vertebral column cleft resulting in paralysis of the legs, bladder, and bowel

myenteric plexus nerve cell network between circular and longitudinal muscles in the esophagus, stomach, and intestinal walls

myocardial infarction (MI) heart muscle necrosis from blood blockage (by arterial obstruction, arteriosclerosis, or thrombus); a type of heart attack

myoclonus movement disorder characterized by series of sudden jerks

myoelastic-aerodynamic theory of phonation currently accepted hypothesis on the mechanism of vocal fold physiology, with compressed air exerting pressure on the undersurface of the closed vocal folds to overcome adductory forces and cause the folds to open; elasticity of displaced tissue (along with the Bernoulli effect) causes the vocal folds to snap shut, resulting in sound

myofibril subdivision of a muscle fiber; composed of a number of myofilaments

myofilament microstructure of periodically arranged actin and myosin molecules; subdivision of myofibril

myogenic response generated by muscle contractions

myoglobin small protein molecule, analogous to hemoglobin, that stores oxygen and transports it from the muscle capillaries into muscle fibers, facilitating oxygen diffusion

myology study of muscles and their parts

myopathy disease or abnormal condition of the muscles, especially skeletal muscles

myosin protein molecule that reacts with actin to form actinomycin for contraction of a myofilament

myotonia lack of muscle or muscle group relaxation after contraction (tonic spasm); problem with muscle membrane ion channels

myotonic dystrophy has both early onset and late onset (adult) forms, with delayed speech and language in early onset type, along with severe articulatory impairment secondary to neuromuscular disease; late onset form leads to articulatory impairmeny secondary to malocclusion and progressing myotonia

myringitis inflammation of the tympanic membrane

myringotomy procedure to drain fluid from the middle ear through a hole in the tympanic membrane

myxo- prefix: pertaining to mucus

M

N

Neuron

basic unit of the nervous system consisting of a cell body, axon, and dendrites

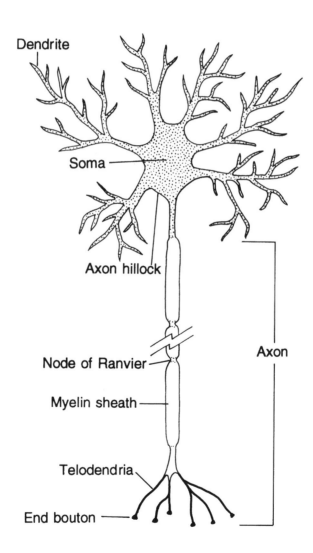

Dendrite

Soma

Axon hillock

Node of Ranvier

Myelin sheath

Telodendria

End bouton

Axon

Nager syndrome severe articulatory impairment, including compensatory articulation secondary to clefting and acute tongue backing secondary to prominent micrognathia; also marked by cleft or absent palate

naming to provide a name for; to state explicitly

- **caregiver naming** use of label to direct infant's attention to something

- **confrontation naming** naming a stimulus when asked to do so; a correct response to such questions as, *"What is this?"*

naris nostril (plural, nares)

narration a treatment technique involving the production of monologues along a story line

narrative representation of an event, idea, or story

- **chains, focused** narratives that organize a sequence of events around a character, but omit motivations for the character's actions

- **chains, unfocused** narratives based on elements linked together

- **complete narrative** story that includes all of the required elements of mature narratives

- **complex narrative** mature narratives that include subplots that are related to each other and overall plot

- **heaps** an early form of children's narrative in which unrelated elements are told in unorganized collections

- **metanarrative skill** ability to analyze and comprehend a story

- **narrative skill** ability to describe events in a sequential, chronologically correct, and logically consistent manner

- **primitive narrative (or centering)** narratives in which story elements are related in a conceptual way, but otherwise unorganized

- **protonarratives (or prenarratives)** the earliest forms of children's stories

- **topic-association narrative style** storytelling strategy in which several themes—some appearing tangentially related to one another—are linked to form a single story, with the speaker presuming shared knowledge with the listener

- **topic centered narrative style** storytelling strategy characterized by structured discourse on a single topic or a related group of topics, with elaboration of a main topic and little presupposition of shared knowledge between speaker and listener

narrow-band analysis an analysis in which the analyzing bandwidth is relatively narrow (such as 45 Hz in speech analysis); preferred when the interest is to increase frequency resolution, as in the analysis of harmonics for a voice

narrow transcription phonetic transcription in which sound modifications are marked, in addition to transcribing the phonemes in an utterance; usually involves the use of special symbols called diacritics or diacritic marks

nasal class of consonants made with a lowered velum. American English nasal consonants are [m], [n], and [ŋ]

nasalance an acoustic measure of nasal resonance, obtained with a Nasometer™

nasal assimilation substitution of a nasal consonant for a non-nasal (e.g., /n/ for /d/)

nasal formant the low-frequency resonance associated with the nasal tract. For men's speech, the nasal formant has a frequency of less than 500 Hz

nasality resonation of the vocal tone through the nasal cavities

nasal murmur the interval of nasal resonance associated with nasal sounds

nasal tract (nasal cavity) air cavity system of the nose

nasendoscope device used to examine internal organs illuminated by a fiberoptic tube inserted through the nose

naso- prefix: nose

nasogastric feeding feeding through a tube passed into the stomach via the nose

nasogastric tube (NG) tube a temporary, artificial means of providing nutrition and hydration via a tube inserted through the nose and into the aerodigestive tract

nasopharyngolaryngoscopy a direct visualization of the nares, nasopharynx, pharynx, and larynx employing a flexible fiberoptic scope with a light source. The positioning of the scope within the nares allows the patient to perform speech and nonspeech activities. A modification of this procedure is utilized during the fiberoptic evaluation of swallowing

nasopharynx the region of the pharynx posterior to the nasal cavity and superior to the velum

National Association of the Deaf (NAD) advocacy group for members of the Deaf Culture

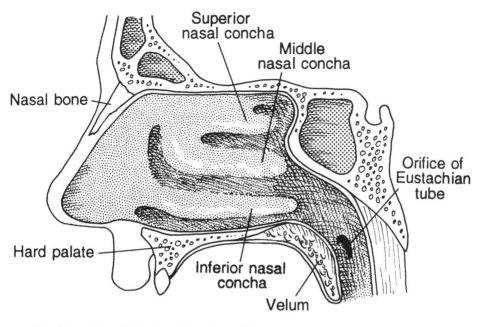

nasal tract (nasal cavity) air cavity system of the nose

native language magnet (NLM) theory a theory of the development of speech perception in the first year of life that accounts for the change from a language-general mode of speech perception to one that is language-specific

nativism the philosophical perspective that certain knowledge and abilities are innate

natural class a group of phonemes defined by a small number of features and related to important phonological regularities

natural settings nonclinical settings where most clients communicate; final treatment target; with infants and toddlers, treatment may be implemented in such settings; extending treatment to such settings is essential to promote response maintenance

nature-nurture evaluation of the relative contribution to a given ability, such as intelligence, of a person's genetic endowment as opposed to what the person acquires by interacting in the world

nebulizer equipment for introducing an extremely fine spray of medication deeply into lungs

neck constricted portion of a structure or vessel

neckloop a transducer worn around the neck as part of an FM assistive device system, consisting of a cord from a receiver; transmitting

signals via magnetic induction to a telecoil of a user's hearing aid

necro- prefix: pertaining to death

necrosis the death of living tissue

- **avascular necrosis** death of tissue due to deficient blood supply

- **central necrosis** damage to inner, deep areas of an organ or of tissue

- **ischemic necrosis** local blood supply stoppage causing hypoxia

negation is the use of words such as no, not, can't, all gone and the like to express the opposite of something that would otherwise be affirmed or true; denial, refusal, or rejection; in linguistics, denial can be expressed through syntactic or semantic means

negative major sentence type that expresses denial, rejection, or nonexistence

negative-pressure ventilation noninvasive mode of ventilatory support mode that employs negative pressure around the thorax to decrease intrathoracic pressure in relation to atmospheric pressure, causing inspiration. Expiration is passive. As a noninvasive mode, negative-pressure ventilation does not require an endotracheal tube or tracheostomy, but can be physically restricting to a patient

negative reinforcement procedure that increases the frequency of a behavior by removing an aversive stimulus contingent on each occurrence

neglect, hemispatial with a unilateral cerebral lesion, an inability to recognize or sense a stimulus presented to the side contralateral to the damage; unconscious perceptual omission

neo-, ne- prefix: new or strange

neologism novel word coined by an individual, but lacking shared meaning a with listener

neologistic jargon language use in aphasia marked by nonsensical, new words; words not found in the dictionary such as hayveness or appleholtent

neonatal period of the first 28 days after birth

neoplasia tumor formation process

neoplasm abnormal growth; tumor; may be benign or malignant

nerve bundle of fibers that connect the central nervous system (CNS) with other parts of the body; transmits afferent impulses from sensory receptors toward the brain and spinal cord and efferent impulses to effector organs

nerves, cranial 12 nerve pairs originating at the base of the brain that carry messages for such functions as hearing, vision, swallowing, phonation, tongue movement, smell, eye movement, pupil contraction, equilibrium, mastication, facial expression, glandular secretion, taste, head movement, and shoulder movement. Starting with the most anterior, cranial nerves (CN) are enumerated by Roman numerals: (CN I) olfactory, (CN II) optic, (CN III) oculomotor, (CN IV) trochlear, (CN V) trigeminal, (CN VI) abducens, (CN VII) facial, (CN VIII) acoustic (vestibulocochlear), (CN IX) glossopharyngeal, (CN X) vagal, (CN XI) accessory, (CN XII) hypoglossal. Several cranial nerves, especially CN V, CN VII, and CN VIII, include two or more separate functions, which are considered as independent nerves by some scientists. That classification would separate the masticatory nerve from the trigeminal (CN V), the glossopalatine from the facial (CN VII), and the equilibrium from the acoustic (CN VIII), making 15 pairs

nervous system vertebrate body system composed of the brain and spinal cord, nerves, ganglia, and receptor organ mechanisms; gathers and evaluates stimuli and sends impulses to effector organs; responsible for motion, sensation, thought, and control of various other bodily functions

- **autonomic nervous system** motor innervation system for cardiac muscle, smooth muscle, and gland systems, containing sympathetic and parasympathetic components

- **central nervous system (CNS)** brain and spinal cord, with tissue of gray and white matter; gray matter is composed of the cell bodies of neurons, with white matter made of the axons and dendrites of the neurons; white matter transmits inner-CNS impulses

- **parasympathetic nervous system** autonomic nervous system craniosacral aspect, with effects including bronchiole and pupil constriction, alimentary canal and smooth muscle contraction, heart rate moderation, and some glandular secretion

- **peripheral nervous system (PNS)** 12 pairs of cranial nerves and 31 pairs of spinal nerves, all outside the brain and spinal cord;. containing sensory and somatic motor fibers and the motor fibers of the autonomic nervous system

- **sympathetic nervous system** thoracolumbar autonomic nervous system portion, with effects including heart rate increase, bronchiole and pupil dilation, skin, viscera, and skeletal muscle vasodilation, peristalsis moderation, liver conversion of glycogen to glucose, and secretion of epinephrine and norephinephrine by the adrenal medulla. Sympathetic tends to prepare the body to deal with stress

Network of Educators of Children with Cochlear Implants (NECCI) professional organization of speech and hearing professionals and educators who are involved with children who receive and use cochlear implants

neural, neuro-, neur- prefix: pertaining to nerves or nervous system

neural anastomosis surgical or pathological linkage of two tubes; surgery connecting a branch of an undamaged nerve to a damaged nerve; treatment for some dysarthric clients; a branch of the intact XIIth cranial nerve may be connected to the damaged VIIth cranial nerve to restore function and appearance

neural folds the embryonic predecessor to the neural groove

neural groove the embryonic predecessor to the neural tube

neural spectrogram the transformation of an incoming speech signal to a neural signal by the auditory system; the transformation is thought to produce a neural version of the frequency-over-time information that can be seen in a speech spectrogram

neural tube the embryonic predecessor to the brain, spinal cord, and other central nervous system (CNS) tissue

neuraxis the axis of the central nervous system (CNS), unpaired CNS portion: spinal cord, rhombencephalon, and mesencephalon in comparison to the paired cerebral hemispheres and other dual structures

neurilemmoma tumor, synonymous with schwannoma

neuritic plaques tiny areas of degeneration of brain cortical and subcortical tissues; also senile plaques; one of the neuropathologies characteristic of Alzheimer disease

neuro- prefix: nerve

neurobiology life science covering neuroanatomy, neurophysiology, neurochemistry, and neuropharmacology

neurofibril filaments in nerve cell bodies, dendrites, axons, and synaptic endings

neurofibromatosis rare autosomal dominant disorder of neuromas developing on multiple cranial nerves as well as the alimentary tract, bladder, and endocrine glands

- **NF I: von Recklinghausen type** occasional mild dysarthria or dyspraxia; if cognitive impairment is present, speech and language can be delayed; marked by café au lait skin spots, cutaneous neurofibromas, macrencephaly

- **NF II: acoustic type** there may be speech development impairment, if CNS tumors develop; also marked by bilateral acoustic neuromas, café au lait skin spots, cutaneous neurofibromas, CNS tumors

- **NF III: mixed type** possible dysarthria and language impairment with brain involvement; also marked by CNS tumors, acoustic neuromas, and café au lait skin spots

- **NF IX: Noonan type** delayed or impaired speech and language in presence of cognitive disorder; is neurofibromatosis plus **Noonan syndrome**

neurolinguistics study of language processing by the brain

neurologist medical practitioner specializing in evaluating and treating disorders of the nervous system

neurology study of the nervous system and its disorders

neuroma, acoustic benign tumor of cranial nerve VIII often growing in the auditory canal. Signs and symptoms produced in cerebellum, lower cranial nerve, and brainstem. Can cause tinnitus, progressive hearing loss, headache, dizziness, and unsteady gait, with later stage symptoms of paresis and speaking/swallowing difficulty

neuromodulator a substance that modifies the function or effect of a neurotransmitter

neuromotor dysfunction dysfunction in motor ability arising from lesion or other problem within the nervous system or the neuromotor junction

neuromuscular junction the point of contact between a skeletal muscle fiber and the myelinated nerve innervating it

neuron basic unit of the nervous system consisting of a cell body, axon, and dendrites

- **bipolar neuron** a neuron that has axonic and dendritic processes extending from opposite poles of its cell body; typical sensory neuron of the special senses of hearing, smell, and sight

- **cholinergic neuron** neuron that secretes acetylcholine (ACh) at the terminals, including neurons within the central nervous system, including all of the alpha motor neurons that innervate skeletal muscle fibers, neurons within autonomic nervous system between pre- and postganglionic nerve fibers, and some postganglionic neurons that innervate cardiac and smooth muscle. Although ACh is released at all cholinergic synapses, the receptor on the postsynaptic membrane will differ for the type of synapse (i.e., muscaric or nicotinic)

- **interneuron neuron** with cell body and axon entirely in the central nervous system (CNS); interneurons relay initial sensory input throughout the CNS to motor neurons and other interneurons

- **internuncial neuron** between and connecting two other nerves

- **monopolar neuron** a neuron with a single bifurcating process arising from its cell body; typical neuron of general sensation

- **multipolar neuron** neuron with one axon and three or more dendrites; typical internuncial neuron and motor neuron

- **postganglionic neuron** the axons of the autonomic nervous system innervated by neurons from the CNS and that innervate visceral organs; postganglionic axons originate

N

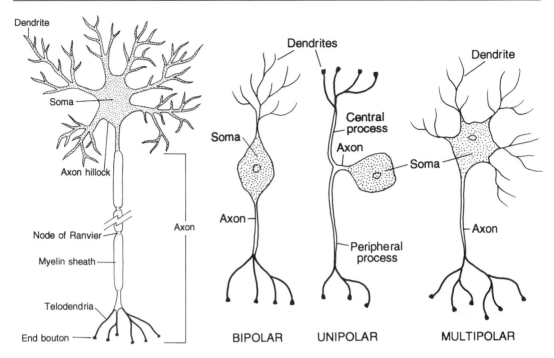

neuron basic unit of the nervous system consisting of a cell body, axon, and dendrites

from cell bodies within autonomic ganglionic tissues and terminate in such effector organs as smooth or cardiac muscle or glands

- **postsynaptic neuron** the neuron receiving input

- **preganglionic neuron** autonomic nervous system neuron that innervates ganglionic cells. The cell bodies of preganglionic neurons are situated within the central nervous system and send their axons to ganglia

- **sensory neuron (fiber)** transmits impulses from sensory sites toward the CNS; a neuron that consists of a long dendritic process that extends from the cell body to its target organ and an axon that synapses on an interneuron within the central nervous system. The cell body of the neuron usually resides within central nervous system locations like the dorsal horn of the spinal cord, the nucleus tractus solitarius, or the trigeminal sensory nuclei. The sensory fiber can end directly within the target organ or synapse and innervate a receptor organ (i.e., muscle spindle) within the tissue

neuron, motor activates skeletal musculature, with axons leaving the central nervous system and making functional contact with muscle (effector) tissue; also called postganglionic neuron

- **autonomic motor neurons** preganglionic motor neurons innervate glands or smooth muscle fibers via postganglionic (peripheral) neurons located in autonomic ganglions

- **final common pathway** the lowest motor neuron serving a muscle, muscle bundle, or gland

- **lower motor neuron** the final common neurological pathway leading to a skeletal muscle, including the anterior horn cell of spinal cord, nerve roots, and nerves

- **upper motor neuron** motor cortex neurons contributing to the pyramidal or corticospinal and corticobulbar tracts; termed motor neurons because stimulation leads to movement and upper motor neuron damage leads to movement disorders

neuropathology the study of the nervous system structure and function and the causes of brain or nervous system damage

neuropathy any functional disturbance or pathological change in the peripheral nervous system

- **ascending neuropathy** nervous system malfunction that begins in lower body portion and spreads upward

neuropeptides endogenous substance that influences neural sensitivity or action; polypeptides that serve hormonal transmission or other signaling functions in various tissues and are released by many nerves and by specialized (APUD [amine precursor uptake and decarboxylation]) cells within the mucosa of the gastrointestinal tract. Other important neuropeptides include gastrin, which stimulates gastric acid secretion after being released into the bloodstream and cholecystokinin which contracts the gallbladder after being released into the blood from duodenal cells. Others are vasoactive intestinal peptide (VIP), and substance P, which act as neurotransmitters or modulate the effects of other neurotransmitters in postganglionic autonomic synapses

neuropharmacology effects of drugs on the nervous system

neurotologist otolaryngologist specializing in disorders of the ear and ear-brain interface (including the skull base), particularly hearing loss, dizziness, tinnitus, and facial nerve dysfunction

neurotoxin poison that acts directly on central nervous system tissues

neurotransmitter chemical substance released by a stimulated presynaptic cell that crosses the synapse to inhibit or excite the postsynaptic cell; includes various amino acids, catecholamines, acetylcholine, certain peptides, and nitric oxide

neutrocclusion normal molar relationship between upper and lower dental arches

neutrophil granular—most common—white blood cell, essential for defense against bacteria and fungi that are short-lived with no capacity to divide that must be removed continuously from the bloodstream during ongoing infection; also tissue or cell that demonstrates no special attraction for basic or acid dyes

nevi small pigmented area in the skin (mole)

nicotinic associating with, approximating, causing, or moderating acetylcholine effects by autonomic ganglia and at the neuromuscular junctions of voluntary muscle

Nissen fundoplication surgical procedure used to treat gastroesophageal reflux; procedure involves wrapping of the fundus of the stomach around the gastroesophageal junction

nitric oxide free-radical, colorless gas serving as a neurotransmitter that is released from neurons of the CNS, enteric, and peripheral nervous systems; inhibits gastrointestinal motor function; in addition to neurotransmission, participates in vasodilation, macrophage cytotoxicity, lipid lowering therapy, and platelet aggregation inhibition

noci- prefix: to harm or injure

node a knot, knob, or swelling; in acoustics, a region of no vibration in a standing wave; in linguistics, a point in a tree diagram that connects the lines representing different constituents (see illustration, p. 160)

nodes the valleys (regions of no vibration) in a standing wave pattern

nodes of Ranvier regions of myelinated nerve fibers in which there is no myelin

nodose ganglion the inferior ganglion of the vagus nerve, containing cell bodies concerned with special visceral sensation and general visceral afferents from the viscera; also called inferior ganglion

nodule small atypical knot

- **vocal fold nodules** benign growths on the surface of the vocal folds; usually paired and fairly symmetric; generally caused by chronic, forceful vocal fold contact (voice abuse); form at the point of maximum vocal fold adduction

noise unwanted sound; a sound that interferes with perception of another sound

- **ambient noise** noise in a particular listening environment: usually a mix of near and distant sounds

- **background noise** extraneous noise that masks the acoustic signal of interest

- **impulse noise** a burst of sound, as produced by a gunshot or an explosion; has an instantaneous rise time and short duration

- **pink noise** a noise that has a spectrum shaped so that the energy is concentrated in certain regions, for example, to match the long-term average spectrum of speech

- **quantization noise** a signal distortion that results from an inadequate number of quantization levels in digitizing a signal

- **turbulence noise** source sound produced with a continuous spectrum. Turbulence noise sources result from the random variation of air pressure created when air particles pass through a narrow constriction at high velocity

- **white noise** noise having energy at all frequencies audible to the human ear; randomlike signal with a flat frequency spec-

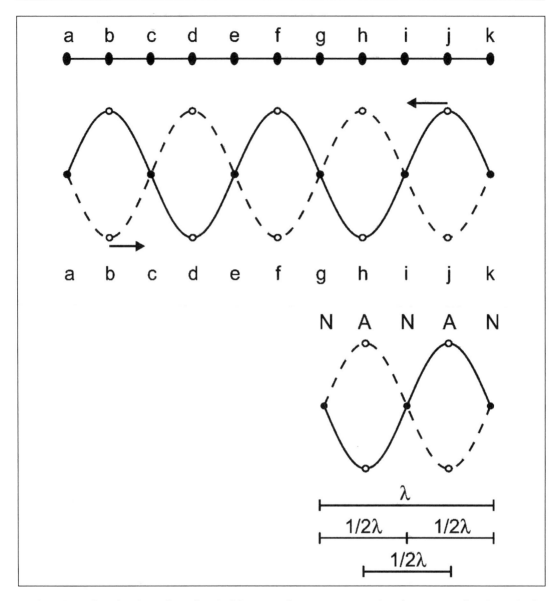

nodes the valleys (regions of no vibration) in a standing wave pattern (as shown on a vibrating string)

trum, in which each frequency has the same magnitude

- **wide-band noise** white noise

noise exposure level of noise and duration of exposure

noise-induced hearing loss (NIHL) sensorineural hearing loss resulting from excessive levels of sound; auditory trauma caused by loud sound and resulting in permanent hearing loss

noise-induced permanent threshold shift (NIPTS) permanent decrease in an individ-

ual's hearing thresholds as a result of exposure to excessive sound levels

noise-induced temporary threshold shift (NITTS) transient shift in an individual's hearing thresholds as a result of exposure to excessive sound levels; temporary threshold shift

noise reduction the difference in sound pressure level of a noise measured at two different locations

noise-to-harmonic ratio (NHR) a general evaluation of noise in a signal; includes jitter, shimmer, and turbulent noise

nomenclature a system of names or terms, particularly of a given science, discipline, or art

non- prefix: absence

nonexistence early reflexive relation in which a word indicates an object is not present where it would be expected

nonfluent aphasia a category of aphasia characterized by halting, broken, or absent speech; word retrieval deficits; and motor planning deficits caused by lesion(s) in the anterior language area and left premotor cortex (Broca's area); includes Broca aphasia, transcortical motor aphasia, and global aphasia

nonlinear amplification amplification system that does not provide a one-to-one correspondence between input and output at all input levels

nonlinear dynamics mathematical study of aperiodic, deterministic systems that are not random and cannot be described accurately by linear equations; study of nonlinear systems whose state changes with time

nonlinear system any system in which the output is disproportionate to the input

nonprototype members of categories that are poor as generalized examples of the category

nonpurulent nonsuppurative, does not form pus

nonrestrictive clause the information in the clause merely elaborates on the topic, as in "which is comfortable" in "the weather, which is comfortable, is just what you wanted"

nonverbal communication conveying attitudes or ideas through gesture and/or facial expression, without the use of words, whether spoken, written, or gestured

Noonan syndrome delayed or impaired speech and language in presence of cognitive impairment, with articulatory impairment secondary to malocclusion; also marked by small stature, webbed neck, vertebral anomalies, occasional cleft palate

Noonan type neurofibromatosis delayed or impaired speech and language in presence of cognitive disorder; is neurofibromatosis plus **Noonan syndrome**

norepinephrine a catecholamine hormone released as an adrenergic mediator at most sympathetic postganglionic endings; vasoconstrictor that can increase blood pressure; noradrenaline

norm standards derived from a sample of the population of interest thought to represent typical values of the characteristic under study or test

normalization a correction for variance

- **speaker normalization** the correction or scaling that reduces interspeaker variability in acoustic measures such as formant frequencies

- **time normalization** the correction or scaling that reduces variability in the durations of sound sequences

nosocomial infection infection acquired in a hospital at least 72 hours after admission; commonly caused by *Candida albicans*, *Escherichia coli*, herpes zoster virus, hepatitis virus, *Pseudomonas*, or *Staphylococcus*

nosocomial pneumonia pneumonia chiefly caused by gram-negative organisms acquired in a hospital, especially in association with endotracheal intubation and mechanical ventilation

notch an indentation

notch filter a filter that attenuates a given frequency band of the input signal

noun one of a class of words that can be the subject of a verb, be singular or plural, can be substituted by a pronoun, and that refers to a circumstance, activity, idea, or creature; word that names the subject of a discourse or sentence; any word except for a pronoun that has the grammatical functions of subject or object of a verb, object of a preposition, predicate after a copula, or a name of an absolute construction

- **common noun** labels any one of a group of beings or things and may be accompanied by limiting modifiers (as, a or an, some, every, and my)

- **count noun** names items that can be counted as individual units (e.g., pennies, forks); compare mass noun

- **mass noun** nouns that express items perceived as integral wholes that cannot be divided (e.g., milk, sand, water); compare count noun

- **proper noun** names an official title, name, or geographical division

noun phrase group of words without subject or predicate composed of a noun and its associated modifiers

noun-verb-noun strategy language development comprehension strategy that relies strictly on word order

N

noy unit for a subjective measure of perceived noisiness expressed in terms of loudness of a stimulus

nucleus the part of the cell that contains the genetic material; an aggregate of neuron cell bodies within the brain or spinal cord; the most prominent word in an utterance; the sonorant peak of a syllable

- **caudate nucleus** a major deep brain cell body of gray matter that is part of the basal ganglia (basal nuclei)

- **cochlear nucleus** initial brainstem nucleus of the auditory neural pathway found within the pons and subdivided into anteroventral, posteroventral and dorsal cochlear nuclei; primary origin of source of the lateral lemniscus, or central auditory pathway

- **dorsal nucleus** of vagus nerve a pool of preganglionic parasympathetic neurons that innervate several internal organs including the heart and those of the gastrointestinal tract. Some of its neurons innervate the smooth muscle of the esophagus sending their axons through the vagus nerve (CN X)

- **hypoglossal nucleus** one of the cranial motor nuclei with motor neurons that innervate the extrinsic and intrinsic muscles of the tongue. Only one muscle protrudes the tongue, with most motor neurons innervating muscles that retract the tongue or alter its shape

- **nucleus ambiguous** one of the cranial motor nuclei of the brainstem with motor neurons that innervate laryngeal, pharyngeal, and esophageal muscles

- **nucleus of solitary tract** one of the cranial sensory nuclei of the brainstem that receives sensory input from the oral, pharyngeal, and laryngeal regions. Some of the sensory input is involved with taste. Interneurons within discrete subdivisions of the nucleus serve multiple functions, including controlling blood pressure, respiratory regularity, swallowing, and taste

null in linguistics, an indicator that a particular position is not filled by a change in the form of a word in a particular context; symbolized by 0 (zero)

nutrition taking in nourishment, with nutrient assimilation for adequate body function and health maintenance

- **parenteral nutrition** nutrient administration other than through the alimentary canal, maintaining fluid and electrolyte balance, along with delivering glucose, saline solution, amino acids, vitamins, and medications

- **total parenteral nutrition (TPN)** nutritional needs provided exclusively through intravenous access and not the gastrointestinal tract; typically long-term, with nutrition administered through a catheter in the superior vena cava

Nyquist sampling theorem statement that a digital representation requires at least two sampling points for every periodic cycle in the signal of interest. Therefore, the sampling rate of digitization should be at least twice the highest frequency of interest in the signal to be analyzed. Unfortunately, the term "Nyquist frequency" is used inconsistently. Some use it to indicate the highest frequency of interest in an analysis; others employ it for twice the highest frequency of interest, that is, to the sampling rate needed to prevent aliasing (named for Harry Nyquist, 1889–1976)

nystagmus jerky sideways or vertical involuntary oscillation of the eyeballs; often indicative of a brain injury

otoscope

instrument for visual examination of the external ear and tympanic membrane

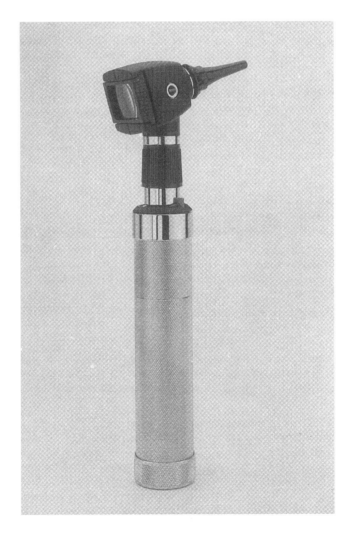

OAE (otoacoustic emission) sounds (usually echoes) from the hair cells of the inner ear that are only evidenced when the hearing organ is intact. There are four types of emissions: transient-evoked (TEOAE), distortion-product (POAE), spontaneous (SOAE), and stimulus-following. Only the first two are commonly used for clinical purposes; proposed as universal screening mechanism for infants at 3 months old as a fast, noninvasive, and inexpensive test of cochlear function

ob- prefix: against, in front of, toward

object in grammar, noun or pronoun that receives the action of the verb

indirect object grammatical object that is the secondary destination of the action of its verb (as dog in "I threw the ball to the dog")

objective physically measurable

object permanence (or **constancy)** awareness that an object has relative permanence even if it is removed from view

oblique diagonal

obstruction, acute upper airway occlusion of the route for passage of air into and out of the lungs, most commonly due to foreign bodies lodging in or around the larynx

obstructive lung disease airway disease classification in which airflow out of the lungs is impeded by narrowing of the small- or medium-sized airways due to spasm, inflammation, or scarring. Overinflation of the lung, prolongation of the expiration, air hunger, dyspnea, and respiratory insufficiency can result

obstruent a class of nonnasal speech sounds made with a radical obstruction of the vocal tract; the obstruents include oral stops, fricatives, and affricates

obturator a device that closes an aperture; for example, the obturator of a tracheostomy tube, which is placed in the outer cannula of the tracheostomy tube to extend past the blunted end, rounding it and easing insertion of the tube into the stoma site; for example, prosthetic device for bridging a cleft palate gap

occipital bone bowled bone at the back of the skull marked by the foramen magnum (opening for connection with the vertebral canal)

occipital lobe posterior lobe of each cerebral hemisphere; among other functions houses visual areas

occlusal surface the surfaces of teeth within opposing dental arches that make contact

occlusion state of being closed; in dentistry, the closing pattern of the masticatory surfaces of the upper and lower teeth (e.g., Angle's classification of occlusion)

occlusion effect hearing enhancement of the level of low-frequency sound in bone-conducted signals as a result of occlusion of the ear canal

occupational hearing loss noise-induced hearing loss incurred on the job

Occupational Safety and Health Act U.S. federal legislation passed to ensure safe and healthy work environments; resulted in the establishment of OSHA, NIOSH, and OSHRC

Occupational Safety and Health Administration (OSHA) Federal agency that regulates occupational health and safety hazards and establishes and enforces minimum standards for industrial hearing conservation programs

occupational therapy (OT) a rehab specialty that employs therapeutic work, self-care, and play activities to enhance independent function; can include adaptation of tasks or environment for achievement of maximum independence and to improve performance of activities of daily life (ADLs)

octave interval between two pitches with frequencies in the ratio of 2; musical duration of eight diatonic degrees; harmonic combination of two tones an octave apart

oculo- prefix: eye

oculo-auriculo-vertebral spectrum marked by misarticulation secondary to tongue motion asymmetry, malocclusion, and possible compensatory articulation secondary to clefting, with hypernasality common and hoarseness caused by unilateral vocal fold paresis; language is delayed and impaired in presence of cognitive impairment

oculo-dento-digital syndrome dysarthria commonly seen, with articulation impairment secondary to dental anomalies; also marked by microphthalmia, broad lower jaw, occasional cleft palate and neuropathy

oculopharyngeal muscular dystrophy gradual dysarthria onset after beginning of facial weakness (from condition onset after age 20), with hypernasality following; also marked by pharyngeal muscle weakness

odonto- prefix: pertaining to tooth or teeth

odynophagia pain on swallowing

ohm impedance measure; electrical resistance between two points of a conductor when a constant difference of potential of 1 volt, applied between these points, produces in this conductor a current of 1 ampere, the conductor not being the source of any electromotive force; from German scientist Georg Simon Ohm (1782–1854)

- **mho** unit of measure of admittance; as reciprocal of impedance, the word is ohm spelled backward

olfaction the sense of smell, mediated by the first cranial nerve (CN I)

oligo- prefix: a little, a few; too little, too few

oliva egg-shaped smooth prominence on the ventrolateral surface of the medulla oblongata, lateral to the pyramidal tract; also called inferior olive

olive, lateral superior nuclear aggregate of superior olivary complex involved in processing interaural intensity differences; also dorsal nucleus of trapezoid body; also called dorsal nucleus of trapezoid body

olive, medial superior nucleus in the lower brainstem where some second-order neurons synapse with third-order neurons of the ascending auditory pathways. Important region for comparing inputs from the two ears

olivocochlear bundle efferent auditory nerve fibers that originate from the periolivary nuclei, following the vestibular nerve to the cochlear nerve in the inner ear and eventually to the hair cells

- **crossed olivocochlear bundle** portion of efferent auditory pathway leading to the outer hair cells, apparently integral to the processing of a signal in noise

- **uncrossed olivocochlear bundle** originates in the olivary complex and courses to the inner hair cells

-oma suffix: neoplasm or tumor

omo- prefix: pertaining to shoulder

one-way (speaking) valve valve placed on the hub of a tracheostomy tube to allow air to enter on inspiration. On expiration, the valve is closed and air cannot escape the tracheostomy tube. Rather, the trapped air is redirected through the vocal folds and into the upper airway to use for speaking and swallowing

onomatopoeia words that mimic the sounds associated with the objects or events they represent, such as zip, buzz, or sizzle

onset the pitch height of the first full syllable in an utterance; beginning of phonation: consonant or consonant sequence that precedes the nucleus of a syllable

- **easy onsets** a treatment technique for producing speech by directing breath through relaxed vocal folds; initiating vocalization and then initiating articulatory movements

- **gentle phonatory onset** a stuttering treatment target; initiating voice in a gentle, soft, easy, relaxed manner; also a treatment target in treating hard glottal attack

ontogeny the development or course of development of an individual organism

opaqueness signs or symbols that do not reveal specific resemblance to their referents and are not readily guessable

open class a large set of morphemes to which new members are readily added; includes nouns, verbs, adjectives, and adverbs; contrasts with closed set

open quotient the ratio of the time the glottis is open to the length of the entire vibratory cycle

open-set testing or training task that does not provide a set of choices to the patient

open syllable syllable that ends with a vowel or diphthong (i.e., bay, toe); in phonological disorders, open syllables can result from omission of final consonants

operant a group of behaviors that operate on the environment and are affected by the consequences that follow their occurrence

operant behavior behavior that is influenced by the consequences it produces

operant (or instrumental) conditioning a learning model in which desired behavior or progressive steps toward it are prompted by a reward or other reinforcement

operant theory an explanation of learning that attributes behavior change to the occurrence of environmental consequences

operational stages of Piaget's cognitive development developmental psychological processes as identified by Jean Piaget (1896–1980), an early theorist of the constructivist theory of instruction and learning

- **concrete operational stage (elementary and early adolescence)** operational thinking (capability to reverse mental actions) develops, with intelligence seen in systematic and logical symbol manipulation of concrete concepts; egocentrism diminishes

- **formal operational stage (adolescence and adulthood)** intelligence becomes linked to logical use of abstract concept symbols
- **preoperational stage (toddler and early childhood)** intelligence seen in symbol use, growing language maturity, and development of memory and imagination; egocentrism dominates

operculum appearing as a lid, flap, or covering

ophthalmologist medical practitioner specializing in diagnosis and treatment of diseases of the eye

ophthalmoscope instrument used to examine structures in the interior of the eye

Opitz syndrome delayed speech and language onset, with impaired language development and possible compensatory articulation pattern secondary to clefting; also marked by hypertelorism, cognitive impairment, cleft palate and lip

opsonization biological process of making bacteria or other antigens more vulnerable to phagocytosis by macrophages such as leukocytes

optical pointer a device that focuses a beam of nonvisible light (e.g., infrared) or other energy (e.g., sonar) on the surface of a communication system

orad toward the oral cavity or mouth

oral approach educational philosophy for deaf children that emphasizes the use of amplification, speech reading, and auditory training to develop oral/aural skills to encourage a mainstream lifestyle

oral cavity the region extending from the orifice of the mouth in the anterior and bounded laterally by the dental arches and posteriorly by the fauces

oralism method of instruction for deaf children that emphasizes spoken language skills to the exclusion of manual communication

oral phase of swallowing early stage of swallowing, in which a bolus is formed and propelled toward the pharynx through repeated contractions of the tongue

oral preparatory phase of swallowing stage of swallowing in which the tongue gathers the food bolus and forms it into a centrally located globular mass ready to be propelled over the back of the tongue

oral secretions the mixture of saliva and organisms residing in the mouth

oral sounds speech sounds made exclusively with oral transmission of sound energy (lacking nasal quality or nasal transmission of sound energy)

orbicular circular or rounded

order of mention strategy language development comprehension strategy that assumes the first event mentioned occurred earlier than events in the remainder of a sentence

organelle specialized aspect of a cell, could be likened to an organ in a cell; includes Golgi complex, mitochondria, centriole, endoplasmic reticulum, ribosomes, and lysosomes

organic disorder disorder caused by structural malfunction, malformation, or injury, as opposed to psychogenic disorders

organic language disorder language disorder associated with physiological causes such as brain damage or hearing loss

organic voice disorder disorder for which a specific anatomic or physiologic cause can be identified, as opposed to psychogenic or functional voice disorders

organization cognitive process of structuring patterns of interaction to deal more effectively with the environment

organ of Corti the structure in the middle scala of the cochlea that contains the hair cells, supporting cells, nerve fibers, and membranes that turn mechanical displacement into neural codes for auditory centers in the brain to interpret as sound; sensory organ of hearing; named for Alfonso Corti (1822–1888)

organs tissue of the body performing a function

orientation awareness of oneself and one's surroundings, generally permanent course of belief or endeavor; in biology, position shift by organs, organelles, or organisms because of an external stimulus

origin proximal and less movable attachment of a muscle; point of attachment of a muscle with relatively little movement; also the beginning point of a muscle and related soft tissue and starting location of a spinal or cranial nerve

oro- combining form: mouth

oropharyngeal transit time the time taken between the beginning of swallowing and the time the bolus passes out of the oropharynx

oropharynx the region of the pharynx bounded posteriorly by the faucial pillars, superiorly by the velum, and inferiorly by the epiglottis

ortho- combining form: straight, normal, correct

orthodontics dental speciality diagnosing and treating malocclusion and other tooth irregularities; also known as dentofacial orthopedics

orthography writing and/or spelling based on rules and/or standard usage

oscillation variation with time of periodic direction; changing and rhythmic vibration of a feature of an audible sound, such as the sound pressure or an aspect of a vibrating solid object

- **forced oscillation** oscillation imposed on a system by an external source

- **natural oscillation** oscillation without imposed driving forces

oscillator in the larynx, the vibrators responsible for the sound source, specifically the vocal folds

-osis suffix: specified condition or process

oss- combining form: a hardened or bony part

osseus composed of bone

ossicular chain collective term for malleus, incus, and stapes, the three tiny middle ear bones that transmit energy from the tympanic membrane to the cochlea

ossification formation of, conversion into bone

osteo- prefix: bone

osteology study of the structure and function of bone

osteopenia reduced bone calcification or density; bone mass reduction from decreased osteoid synthesis

osteoporosis abnormal reduction in density of bones; it may be idiopathic or secondary to other diseases

ostium opening

otitis an inflammation or infection of the ear; most typically in early childhood

- **acute otitis media** intense inflammation of the middle ear, which can be accompanied by pain, fluid drainage, hearing loss, fever, headache, vomiting; often caused by *Haemophilus influenzae* or *Streptococcus pneumoniae*

- **chronic otitis media** generally caused by such gram-negative bacteria as *Proteus, Klebsiella,* or *Pseudomonas*

- **otitis media** an inflammation of the middle ear; repeated (chronic) infections can lead to language delay

- **otitis media with effusion** fluid in the middle ear unaccompanied by symptoms of acute infection; also nonsuppurative otitis media or serous otitis media

oto- combining form: the ear

otoacoustic emissions (OAE) subaudible sounds generated by the cochlea either spontaneously or evoked by sound stimulation; used for infant screening

- **distortion-product evoked otoacoustic emissions (DPOAE)** acoustic energy created by stimulating the cochlea with two pure tones (f1 and f2). As a result of cochlear nonlinear processes, energy is created at several frequencies that are combinations of the two stimulating frequencies. The most easily recorded is the 2f1–f2 distortion product (technically, the cubic distortion product)

- **evoked otoacoustic emissions (TEOAE)** faint sounds generated by nonlinear cochlear processes in response to acoustic stimulation. They can be detected by placing sensitive recording equipment within the ear canal

otolaryngologist physician who specializes in the diagnosis and treatment of diseases of the ear, nose, and throat

otologist otolaryngologist specializing in disorders of the ear

otology the medical specialty that deals with the ear

otorhinolaryngologist physician trained in diseases of the ear, nose, and throat

otorhinolaryngology the medical specialty that deals with the ear, nose, and throat

otosclerosis anomalous formation in the ear of spongy bone near the stapes and fenestra vestibuli leading to progressive hearing loss

otoscope instrument for visual examination of the external ear and tympanic membrane (see illustration, p. 168)

ototoxic harmful to the structures of the ear, particularly the hair cells in the cochlea and vestibular organs, in addition to cranial nerve VIII

outcome conclusion or effect, as of treatment

- **functional outcome** environmentally based results of therapy that can be readily integrated into a patient's natural settings

outer ear the pinna and ear canal leading to the eardrum (tympanic membrane)

output energy or information exiting a listening device; also information transferred from a

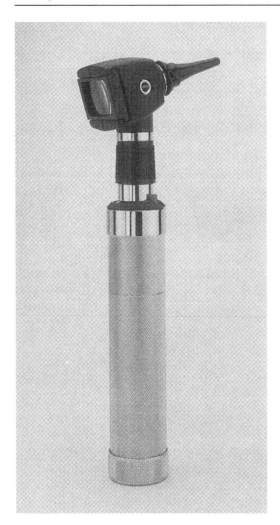

otoscope instrument for visual examination of the external ear and tympanic membrane

computer or AAC system to an external device, such as a display screen, disk drive, printer, or modem

output limiting limiting the output of a listening device by means of peak-clipping or compression

oval window the opening into the ear's scala vestibuli; where the footplate of the stapes transmits movements of the ossicular chain to the cochlea

overbite the vertical overlap of maxillary incisors over the mandibular incisors when molars are occluded; mostly measured on the perpendicular to the occlusal plane

overextension word that overgeneralizes to items that do not represent the conventional referents for the word

overjet horizontal overlap of upper teeth over lower teeth; typically measured parallel to the occlusal plane

overlap phenomenon the occurrence of the same speech disfluencies in normally speaking preschool children and children believed to show signs of early stuttering

overtone partial above the fundamental in a spectrum

oxidation process of combining with oxygen, with oxygen content increased

oximeter noninvasive electronic device for determining arterial oxygen saturation via a probe placed on a highly oxygenated area of the body

oxygen (O₂) colorless, tasteless, odorless gas needed for animal and plant life—essential for human respiration

P

Pharynx

throat; a respiratory and digestive passageway from the larynx to the oral and nasal cavities; the region above the larynx, below the velum, and posterior to the oral cavity. Composed of muscle and lined with mucous membrane; changes in pharyngeal shape allow formation of various vowel sounds

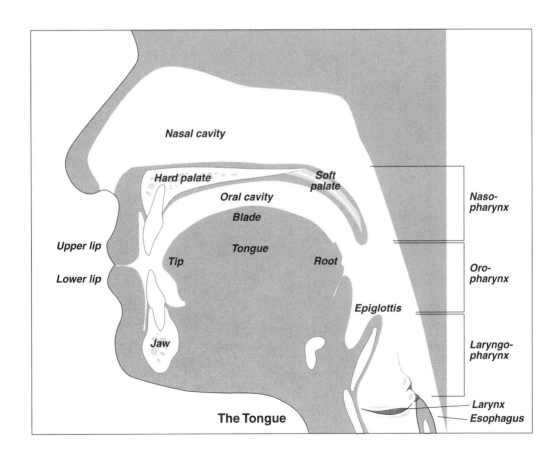

pachy- prefix: thick

pacing speech treatment technique that consists of using an external source to cue the rate of speaking

pacing board a wooden board that has a series of colored slots separated by ridges; used in reducing the speech rate of clients with motor speech disorders. The speaker touches one slot for each word spoken

PaCO$_2$ the partial pressure of carbon dioxide in the arterial blood; represents the amount of carbon dioxide dissolved in blood plasma. PaCO$_2$ is one of the values reflected in a arterial blood gas study

palatal lift prosthesis for mechanically elevating a soft palate that is functionally impaired; generally to correct velopharyngeal insufficiency (VPI) and resulting hypernasal speech

palate roof of mouth; partition between oral and nasal cavities

- **cleft palate** a congenital defect resulting from incomplete fusion of the horizontal palatal segments; fissure may be complete (extending into the nasal cavities from open hard and soft palates) or cleft may be incomplete or partial; often accompanies cleft lip; seen about once in every 2,500 live births, affecting more females than males

- **hard palate** the bony portion of the roof of the mouth, made up of the palatal processes of the maxillae and the horizontal plates of the palatine bones

- **soft palate** the muscular portion of the roof of the mouth (also called the velum); located posterior to the hard palate; forms the back portion of the roof of the mouth

palatine tonsils lymphoid tissue between the fauces, often considered "the" tonsils

palato- combining form: pertaining to the roof of the mouth

palatoplasty surgical repair of the palate

palilalia speech in which one's own words and phrases are repeated, often with increasingly rapid rates and decreasingly accurate articulation; typically in the middle and end of utterances; for example, "The man walked down the street the street the street the street"

palliative treatment medical therapy aimed at relieving or reducing intensity of symptoms, but not necessarily to cure

palmar pertaining to the palm of the hand

palpate to examine by means of touch and pressing with the palms of the hands and the fingers

palsy abnormal physical state distinguished by paralysis

pan- combining form: all

pancreatitis inflammation of the pancreas. Alcohol abuse is the most common cause of chronic pancreatitis and a principal cause of acute pancreatitis

- **hemorrhagic pancreatitis** pancreatitis with bleeding into pancreas; possible etiologies are gall stones or alcoholism

panic disorder a disorder characterized by sudden, unexpected, and persistent episodes of intense fear, accompanied by a sense of imminent danger and an urge to escape

pantomime a method of communication in which the speaker acts out a message by gestures and body movements; a target communication skill for some nonverbal or minimally verbal individuals who can use gestures and bodily movements; unlike other gestural systems, employs whole- as well as part-body movements; often more concrete and easier to understand than other gesture systems

papilloma small benign epithelial tumor that may appear randomly or in clusters on the vocal folds, larynx, and trachea and elsewhere in the body. Believed to be caused by various types of human papillomavirus (HPV), some of which are associated with malignancy

papillomatosis widespread papilloma development

- **florid oral papillomatosis** scattered evidence on lips and oral mucosa of benign squamous papilloma

- **juvenile papillomatosis** fibrocystic disease of the breast in young women

- **laryngeal papillomatosis** multiple laryngeal squamous papilloma seen most commonly in young children, which may be transmitted by HPV infection from the birth canal

para- prefix: beside; partial, disordered

paradigm internal map or world view that provides a broad conceptual framework for thought and action

paragrammatism use of semantically and morphologically intact sentences that, however, are semantically empty; use of inappropriate words and inflections; associated with fluent aphasias

paralinguistic codes speech production aspects such as intonation, loudness, rate, rhythm, and stress that accompany a spoken message to express attitude or emotion

parallel play instances in which children engage in similar play activity in proximity to one another, but do not actually interact

parallel talk a language-stimulation technique, wherein an adult matches language to an activity a child is performing

parallel teaching instruction of bilingual children from two teachers working as a team—each using a different language. The term specifically means a second-language teacher and the classroom teacher planning together, but teaching independently

parallel training method with a user introduced to a new set of complex skills at the same time as they are mastering an easier set of skills

paralysis loss or impairment of voluntary motor function or sensation or both from injury, disease, or toxic damage; type and degree of paralysis depends on whether the damage is to the central nervous system or the peripheral nervous system

- **acute ascending paralysis** successive flaccid paralysis in order of the legs, trunk, arms, and finally muscles of respiration

- **bilateral vocal fold paralysis** loss of the ability to move both vocal folds, caused by neurologic dysfunction

- **compression paralysis** paralysis from external pressure on a nerve

- **facial paralysis** facial muscle paresis—often unilateral—from peripheral facial paralysis (lesion of facial nerve peripheral to nucleus) or central facial paralysis of a lesion of the cerebrum or upper brainstem

- **progressive bulbar paralysis** incremental atrophy of the muscles of the tongue, lips, palate, pharynx, and larynx; often caused by motor neuron disease

- **pseudobulbar paralysis** atrophy of the tongue and lips, similar to progressive bulbar paralysis, but with bilateral lesions (supranuclear); marked by swallowing and speech problems, along with intermittent unemotional laughter or crying

- **unilateral vocal fold paralysis** immobility of one vocal fold, due to neurological dysfunction

paranoia fairly rare condition of abnormal suspicious delusions (popularly linked to term "per-secution complex"); paranoiac patterns often follow high-dose chronic stimulant use and may occur during withdrawal from sedative hypnotics

paraphasia unintentional substitution of words or sounds in words; verbal paraphasia is the substitution of one word for another, and literal paraphasia is the substitution of one sound in a word for another. Caused by feedback failures at the internal abstract level or at an internal self-monitoring stage

- **phonemic paraphasia** unwanted substitution of a phonemically similar word for an intended word

- **semantic paraphasia** unintended substitution of a semantically similar word for an intended word

paraplegia paralysis of both lower limbs, along with trunk; often caused by spinal cord injury or disease

parasite organism living in or on by taking nourishment from another organism

parasympathetic nervous system one of the two divisions of the autonomic nervous system. It is defined anatomically by postganglionic fibers that arise from ganglia close to the organ they innervate. Acetylcholine is the neurotransmitter released from parasympathetic neurons; effects include bronchiole and pupil constriction, alimentary canal and smooth muscle contraction, heart rate moderation, and some glandular secretion

parathyroid glands small paired endocrine glands usually embedded on posterior surface of the thyroid gland that secrete a hormone regulating calcium and phosphorus metabolism

parenchyma the functional substance of an organ, as differentiated from connective or supporting tissue; in the lungs, distal airspaces are parenchymal

parenteral nutrition nutrient administration other than through the alimentary canal, maintaining fluid and electrolyte balance, along with glucose, saline solution, amino acids, vitamins, and medications

- **total parenteral nutrition (TPN)** nutritional needs provided exclusively through intravenous access and not the gastrointestinal tract; typically long-term, with nutrition administered through a catheter in the superior vena cava

parentese (also motherese or child-directed speech) distinctive style of speech exhibited by caregivers with toddlers, characterized especially by exaggerated prosody

paresthesia abnormal burning, prickling, tickling, or tingling sensation

parietal forming or located on a wall

parietal bone one of the pair of bones forming the cranium sides

parietal pleura the outermost of two membranes surrounding the lungs; inner surface of thoracic cavity

Parkinson disease a neurologic disorder resulting from deficiency of dopamine, especially in the substantia nigra and usually resulting in the classic symptom triad of tremor, bradykinesia, and rigidity

parotid gland largest salivary gland, situated in front of, and below, the ears

parotitis inflammation of the parotid gland; infectious parotitis is commonly known as mumps

pars part of a structure or area

pars flaccida a flaccid portion of the tympanic membrane in the superior region

partial sound sinusoid that is part of a complex tone; in voiced sounds, the partials are harmonic, implying that the frequency of the nth partial equals n times the fundamental frequency

partial leak intentional leak maintained in a tracheostomy tube cuff to allow a patient access to airflow through the upper airway for the purposes of speaking, swallowing, and airway clearance

partial pressure pressure expended by one gas in a gaseous mixture or liquid, with the pressure directly connected to the concentration of that gas to the mixture's total pressure

- **partial pressure of carbon dioxide in arterial blood (PaCO$_2$)** portion of all blood gas pressure exerted by carbon dioxide, which decreases during heavy exercise, with uncontrolled diabetes, or with diseases of the kidneys or liver

- **partial pressure of oxygen in arterial blood (PaO$_2$)** part of total blood gas pressure expended by oxygen, which is lower than typical in persons with obstructive lung disease, asthma, and some blood diseases, as well as healthy persons during vigorous exercise

particle an elementary subatomic energy and/or matter units (as a molecule, atom, proton, electron, or photon); in English, a word

that combines with a verb to form an expression with idiomatic meaning

partner, frequent communication a particular person with whom another often converses; often a family member

pascal (Pa) international standard unit of pressure or stress; one newton (N) per meter squared (m^2); from French mathematician Blaise Pascal (1623–1662)

Pascal's law pressure is transmitted rapidly and uniformly throughout an enclosed fluid at rest; applies especially to hydraulics

passaggio in singing, the break between vocal registers

Passavant's ridge (or pad) a muscular bulge that projects from the posterior nasopharyngeal wall to assist velopharyngeal closure, formed by contraction of the pharyngeal superior constrictor during swallowing or other activities

pass band a band of frequencies minimally affected by a filter

passive grammatical construction in which action is done to a subject and not by the subject ("you will receive a grade" is passive and "I will give you a grade" is active); the words "am, is, are, to be," and so on should not be confused with the passive voice

patent open

patho-, -pathy prefix or suffix: disease

pattern playback machine invented in the 1950s that allowed investigators to create the first versions of artificial speech by painting formants on an acetate belt, which were then converted into sound

pause short interruption of the voice to indicate the boundaries and relations of and within sentences

- **filled pause** a pause or gap between utterances that is associated with a vocalization, such as a hesitation sound involving a prolonged vowel or nasal; for example,"I think that his name was . . . mmmmmmm . . . John"

- **interturn pause** gap in vocalizing that occurs at the end of a speaking turn when the speaker stops talking

- **intraturn pause** gap in vocalization that occurs within a single speaking turn

pauser response nerve response characterized by an initial on-response followed by silence and subsequent low-level rate throughout stimulation

pectoral pertaining to the chest or thorax

pedagogy profession, art, and science of teaching

pedi-, pedo- combining forms: pertaining to child; foot

peduncle stalklike connecting part

-penia suffix: deficiency

peptide substance of more than two amino acids, with the amino group of one member joined to a carboxyl group of another

per through; passing through; before

percentile figure on a scale of 100; percentile rank of 75 denotes that 25% of total scores were above and 75% scored below

perception process of attending to, identifying, and interpreting stimuli

perceptual magnet effect the finding that the best members of a category function as perceptual magnets for surrounding stimuli

perceptual map representation stored in memory that indicates the relationships among a variety of stimuli; specifically, the distances from one another

perceptual organization the ability to group sounds into categories

percussion in medicine, the use of mechanical stimulation on the chest wall, either manually or via various devices, to loosen secretions from the bronchi and possibly increase the ease of their removal during suctioning or coughing; also diagnostic procedure to estimate fluid amount in body cavity or evaluate size and condition of internal organs

percutaneous endoscopic gastrostomy (PEG) artificial means of providing nutrition and hydration via a tube placed through the esophagus into the stomach via endoscopy, with the tube connected to nutrition source though an opening in the stomach. This type of tube is generally more comfortable for a patient than a nasogastric tube. It appears to carry the same risk of aspiration, especially if aspiration precautions (i.e., elevation of the head during feeding) are not allowed; a similar procedure is percutaneous endoscopic jejunostomy

performance versus intensity (PI) function curve illustrating percentage correct score to speech intensity. Useful for all types of speech test materials. Ordinarily, performance increases monotonically with increasing intensity

performative a speech act in which the utterance itself performs the intended act, such as promising, teasing, and apologizing

perfusion migration of fluid through an organ or body area; flow of blood or other fluid per unit volume of tissue, as with ventilation/perfusion ratio; therapeutic introduction through bloodstream of drug to isolated body area

peri- prefix: around

pericardium fibroserous sac surrounding the heart and sources of the great vessels

perilingual hearing loss loss acquired during the stage of spoken language acquisition

perilymph clear fluid of the ear's scala vestibuli and scala tympani, separating the osseous labyrinth from the membraneous labyrinth

perimysium fibrous sheath surrounding primary muscle bundles

period in physics, the time interval between repeating events; shortest pattern repeated in a regular undulation; a graph showing the period is called waveform. In medicine, a stage of a disease; specified duration; colloquialism for menses

period doubling one form of bifurcation in which a system that originally had x period states takes on $2x$ periodic states, with a change having occurred in response to a change in parameter or initial condition; can precede a chaotic state

periodic having predictable repetition; recurring at regular times

periodic behavior repeating over and over again over a finite time interval. Periodic behavior is governed by an underlying deterministic process

periodontal pertaining to tissues that surround and protect the teeth

period time in physics, duration of a period

peripheral relative to the periphery; in biology, about the surface, outside, or surrounding area of a body structure or organ

peripheral device hardware that is physically separate from a computer. Examples include video monitors, disk drives, printers, alternative keyboards, and touch tablets

peripheral nervous system the major division of the nervous system that lies largely outside the bony protection of the skull and spinal column; 12 pairs of cranial nerves and 31 pairs of spinal nerves, all outside the brain and spinal cord, containing sensory and somatic motor fibers and the motor fibers of the autonomic nervous system

peristalsis a coordinated propulsive contraction of the esophagus that occludes the esophageal lumen to propel the bolus through the esophagus and into the stomach. When the contraction follows a pharyngeal swallow and begins at the cricopharyngeal level, it is a primary peristalsis. If the contraction is stimulated by residual bolus that has been left behind, or by distension (e.g., from reflux), it is called secondary peristalsis; also serial contraction of other smooth muscle to force bile through the bile duct and urine through the ureter

perlocutionary the component of a speech act consisting of the effect of a speech act on a listener

perlocutionary stage the stage of communication development from birth to approximately 6 months in which caregivers infer intentions by infants

permanence (or constancy), object awareness that an object has relative permanence even if it is removed from view

permeability property of allowing a substance (such as heat, gas, liquid) to pass through a structure, such as a membrane

perseveration involuntary continued use of a gesture, spoken word, or vocal utterance that is not appropriate but cannot be inhibited or stopped; a common consequence of brain injury following stroke

personal amplifier assistive listening device in which a remote microphone is hard-wired to a receiver/amplifier

personal FM system assistive listening device in which a remote microphone transmits to a receiver/amplifier via an FM radio wave

personality disorder general term for behavioral problems marked usually by lifelong maladaptive patterns of lifestyle and social adjustment, varies in quality from psychosis and neurosis

• **antisocial personality disorder** a pervasive pattern of disregard for and violation of the rights of others. The disorder is characterized in part by risk taking, criminality, and pathological lying

• **borderline personality disorder** a disorder beginning in early adulthood that features a pattern of unstable self-image, moods, and

interpersonal relationships; marked by viewing persons or situations as either all good or all bad

perturbation change from predicted behavior; disturbance of direction, equilibrium, or distribution; in chaos theory, a minor bump

• **amplitude perturbation quotient** a relative evaluation of short term (cycle-to-cycle) variation of peak-to-peak amplitude expressed in percentage

• **pitch period perturbation quotient** a relative evaluation of short-term (cycle-to-cycle) variation of the pitch periods expressed in percentage

• **relative average perturbation** relative evaluation of cycle-to-cycle variation of noise-to-harmonic ratio, and voice turbulence index

• **smoothed amplitude perturbation quotient** a relative evaluation of long-term variation of the peak-to-peak amplitude within the analyzed voice sample, expressed in percentage

• **smoothed pitch perturbation quotient** a relative evaluation of long-term variation of the pitch period within the analyzed voice sample expressed in percentage

perturbation measures indexes of irregularity or instability, especially in the laryngeal waveform. The common measure of perturbation include jitter, shimmer, and signal-to-noise ratio

pes a footlike structure

petechiae small bleeding points under the skin

petit mal seizure obsolete term for absence seizure, a brief loss of consciousness or slowing of thought processes sometimes accompanied by clonic movements

Pfeiffer syndrome articulatory distortions secondary to maxillary deficiency, malocclusion, and anterior skeletal open bite; also marked by craniosynostosis, hypertelorism

pH a value (abbreviation for potential hydrogen) on a scale representing the acidity or alkalinity of a substance (e.g., blood). pH levels express the hydrogen ion concentration of a solution, with neutral at 7.0, acid below 7.0, and alkaline above 7.0

-phage, -phagia suffix: eating

phagocyte cell that surrounds and destroys microorganisms and debris

phagocytosis envelopment and destruction of toxic matter by phagocytes as an important biological defense mechanism against infection

pharmacology sources, chemistry, actions, and uses of drugs

pharyngeal-esophageal (P-E) segment a part of the pharynx and the esophagus. Muscle fibers from the cricopharyngeus, esophagus, and inferior constrictor blend at this site to create a sphincter that can reduce the cross-sectional area of the esophagus

pharyngeal phase of swallowing bolus passage through the pharynx and into the esophagus in coordination with respiration to assure air supply continuation and aspiration prevention

pharyngeal tonsil the mass of lymphatic tissue within the nasopharynx; also called adenoids

pharyngoplasty reparative surgery on the pharynx for cleft palate and/or velopharyngeal insufficiency, as well as for snoring

pharynx throat; a respiratory and digestive passageway from the larynx to the oral and nasal cavities; the region above the larynx, below the velum, and posterior to the oral cavity. Composed of muscle and lined with mucous membrane; changes in pharyngeal shape allow formation of various vowel sounds

phase manner in which molecules are arranged in a material (gas, liquid, or solid); angular separation between two events on periodic waveforms

phase-locking the tendency of a neuron to respond to a particular phase of an acoustic signal

phase plane plot representation of a dynamic system in state space

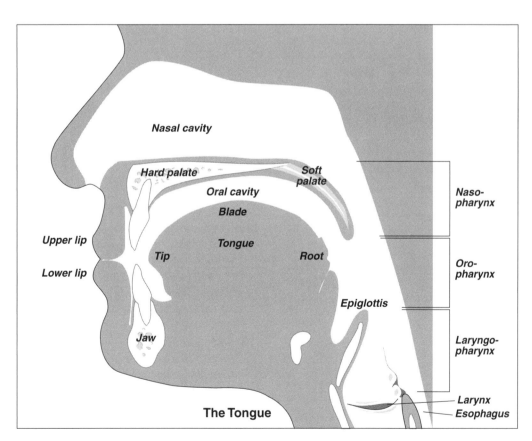

pharynx throat; a respiratory and digestive passageway from the larynx to the oral and nasal cavities; the region above the larynx, below the velum, and posterior to the oral cavity. Composed of muscle and lined with mucous membrane; changes in pharyngeal shape allow formation of various vowel sounds

phase space a space created by two or more independent dynamic variables, such as positions and velocities; utilized to plot the trajectory of a moving object

phase spectrum a display of the relative phases versus frequency of the components of a waveform

phase transition a qualitative change in the behavior of a system

phenotype expression of genetic characteristics of an individual; some phenotypical aspects, such as blood groups, are determined by heredity, with others capable of alteration by environmental factors

phenylketonuria (PKU) autosomal recessive inherited disorder in which infants have excessive phenylketones and other phenylalanine metabolites in the urine, which, if untreated, leads to mental retardation; treatment is a diet low in phenylalanine. Most states in U.S.A. require PKU screening for all neonates

-phobe suffix: person who fears a specific thing

phobia morbid irrational fear of a explicit thing that can lead to a panic state; manifested typically by fatigue, palpitations, faintness, nausea, tremor, and perspiration

phonation the production of vocal tone through the physiological process of setting the approximated vocal folds into vibration with exhaled air

- **inhalation phonation** a technique of voice therapy to evoke true vocal fold vibration in clients who are aphonic

- **maximum phonation time (or maximum phonation duration)** the duration in seconds that an individual is capable of sustaining phonation

- **myoelastic-aerodynamic theory of phonation** widely accepted theory on the mechanism of vocal fold physiology, which posits that compressed air exerts pressure on the undersurface of closed vocal folds, with the pressure overcoming adductory forces, causing the vocal folds to open; elasticity of the displaced tissued(along with the Bernoulli effect) causes the vocal folds to snap shut, resulting in sound

- **pressed phonation** type of phonation characterized by small airflow, high adductory force, and high subglottal pressure. Not an efficient form of voice production. Often associated with voice abuse and common in patients with lesions such as nodules

- **soft phonation index (SPI)** a measure of the ratio of lower frequency harmonic energy to higher frequency harmonic energy. If the SPI is low, then the spectral analysis will show well-defined higher formants

phonatory onset, gentle a stuttering treatment target; initiating voice in a gentle, soft, easy, relaxed manner; also a treatment target in treating hard glottal attack

phonatory system the system, including the laryngeal structures, through which phonation is achieved

phone an individual instance of a speech sound production notated within brackets (i.e., [ ])

phoneme the smallest unit of speech sounds used to distinguish words and morphemes in a language. Examples include m in man, or s in this. Different languages have different sets of phonemes. Notated within slashes (i.e., / /)

- **voiceless phoneme** phoneme produced without vibration of vocal folds

phonemic a phonetic change that is sufficient to change the meaning of a word in a particular language

phonemic synthesis blending of discrete phonemes into correctly sequenced, coarticulated sound patterns

phonetically balanced (PB) word lists sets of words that contain speech sounds with the same frequency of occurrence as in everyday conversation

phonetic boundary midpoint for identification by a given listener between two phonetic categories

phonetic categories all speech sounds belonging to a particular class, such as all sounds composed of a certain set of defining features, such as open or closed

phonetic features the smallest building blocks of speech; phonetic units are bundles of phonetic features

- **voiced-voiceless** a phonetic feature of speech distinguished in syllable-initial positions by voice onset time; an acoustic feature that describes the timing between two events in speech, the onset of laryngeal voicing and the onset of other acoustic events that mark the release of the sound; voiced sounds are produced when these two events occur nearly simultaneously, voiceless sounds when the release of the sound precedes voicing by more than 40 ms

phonetic form rules the underlying universal rules that generate the basic syntactic relationships in the deep structure of a sentence

phonetic prototypes stimuli from a phonetic category that are judged by native speakers to be exceptionally good instances of the category

phonetics study of speech sounds, including sound formation, acoustic properties, and perception

phonetogram recording of highest and lowest sound pressure level versus fundamental frequency that a voice can produce; phonetograms are often used for describing the status of voice function in patients; also called voice range profile

phoniatrics scientific study and treatment of voice problems

phonics method of teaching early reading based on recognizing the sounds of letters and combinations of letters, particularly syllables

phono-, phon- combining form: pertaining to sound, especially speech or voice

phonological awareness understanding of the sound structure of language, including the recognition that words are composed of syllables and phonemes and applying this knowledge

phonological delay, phonological disorder development of the phonological system that is slower than normal in accuracy or completeness or that follows an atypical pattern

phonological process a systematic error pattern that affects a class of speech sounds, wherein one type of sound is substituted for another or a class of sounds is deleted in certain word contexts

phonological processes multiple ways in which children simplify adult production of speech sounds; these include such categories of processes as deletion processes, substitution processes, and assimilation processes; persistent processes in children are targets of intervention; treatment is directed against eliminating a phonological process

- **final consonant deletion** an error pattern in which a child omits the consonant at the end of the word

- **gliding** an error pattern in which a child substitutes a glide /w/ or /j/ for /ʃ/ or /r/

- **stopping** substitution of a stop for a fricative or an affricate (e.g., /p/ for /f/)

- **substitution processes** a group of phonological processes in which one class of sounds is substituted for another; in phonological treatment, the target is to eliminate such processes

- **velar fronting** substitution of an alveolar for a velar (e.g., /t/ for /k/)

phonological processing the language-specific aspects of phonetic perception; listeners of different languages learn which phonetic units are contrastive in the language and the rules about how those units can be combined

phonological systems approach any treatment approach for remediating speech errors that is based on the phonological system as a whole. The process is designed to teach children new phonological rules so that systematic error patterns change and the child's phonological system becomes more adult-like

phonology, phonological system the speech sound system of a language, including all the elements and their rules for combination

photophobia extreme dislike and avoidance of light

photoreceptors sensory receptors for visual stimulation, such as a rod or a cone in the eye's retina

phrase groups of words that are structurally related and form a single grammatical unit, but lack either a subject or verb

phrase structure rules underlying universal rules that generate the basic syntactic relationships in the deep structure of a sentence

phrasing the use of prosodic cues to mark the beginning or the ending of phrases

phrenic nerve the nerve that controls the diaphragm and is responsible for inspiration. Composed primarily of fibers from the third, fourth, and fifth cervical nerves (largely the fourth)

phrenoesophageal ligament, or **membrane** an extension of the fascia of the diaphragm that anchors the gastroesophageal junction in the hiatus of the diaphragm. The membrane contains collagen and elastic fibers that allow the gastroesophageal junction to move up into the hiatus on swallowing and then move back down to its resting position. Degeneration and laxity of the membrane is a feature of hiatus hernias, with functioning also related to gastroesophageal reflux (GER)

physiatrist a medical doctor who specializes in physical medicine or the rehabilitation of body parts or functions compromised through physical impairment or disease

physical therapy (PT) a rehabilitation specialty who targets the restoration of optimal functioning following trauma; daily functions of standing, transferring, and walking are common goals, with methods being such physical means and agents as exercises, manipulation, massage, and cold and/or heat application

physics science that deals with the forces and composition of matter, particularly interaction between matter and energy

physiology the study of function of the body and its components

Piaget's stages of cognitive development developmental psychological processes as identified by Jean Piaget (1896–1980), an early theorist of the constructivist theory of instruction and learning

- **concrete operational stage (elementary and early adolescence)** operational thinking (capability to reverse mental actions) develops, with intelligence seen in systematic and logical symbol manipulation of concrete concepts; egocentrism diminishes

- **formal operational stage (adolescence and adulthood)** intelligence becomes linked to logical use of abstract concept symbols

- **preoperational stage (toddler and early childhood)** intelligence seen in symbol use, growing language maturity, and development of memory and imagination; egocentrism dominate

- **sensorimotor stage (infancy)** intelligence evidenced through motor activity without symbol use until very end of stage

pia mater delicate innermost of the three meninges covering the brain and the spinal cord; contains many blood vessels to nourish nervous tissue

pica craving to eat such nonfood items as dirt, clay glue, chalk, starch, or ice

pictographs symbol sets that are simple pictures representing actual things. Illustrative picture symbols representing drink, tree, and bus are examples of pictographs

picture communication symbols (PCS) pictorial representations developed by the Mayer-Johnson Company

picture exchange communication system (PECS) a training approach used to promote interactive symbolic communication. This technique teaches a child to initiate a communicative act in which he or she exchanges a picture symbol in order to receive a concrete outcome

picture symbol sequences an encoding system that uses picture sequences to retrieve pre-stored messages (e.g., I + spoon = I'm hungry)

pidgin language a simplified hybridization of two language systems, typically used for trading purposes or in conducting business

Pierre Robin syndrome now known as Robin sequence

pillar cells of Corti supportive cells of the organ of Corti

pineal shaped like a pine-cone

pinna auricle, visible portion of the outer ear

pit a depression or indentation, usually small

pitch sound property—especially a musical tone—determined by the frequency of the waves producing it; highness or lowness of sound; a standard frequency for tuning instruments; variation in the human voice and relative vibration frequency that adds to the total meaning of speech; definite relative pitch that is a significant speech phenomenon. In hearing mechanism, is coded by the periodicity of phase-locked action potentials for very low frequencies by both the periodicity of firing and which fibers are firing (place code) for low and middle frequencies and by place code alone for high frequencies (above about 5000 Hz).

- **concert pitch** also known as international concert pitch. The standard of tuning A4. reference pitch has changed substantially over the last 200–300 years

- **habitual pitch** the perceptual correlate of vocal fundamental frequency habitually used by an individual

- **intrinsic pitch of vowels** in normal speech, certain vowels tend to be produced with a significantly higher or lower pitch than other vowels, for example, high vowels have a higher pitch than low vowels

- **optimal pitch** the perceptual characteristic representing the ideal or most efficient frequency of vibration of the vocal folds

- **pitch declination** gradual fall in fundamental frequency over time

- **pitch direction** perceived pitch change

- **pitch height** average pitch level

- **pitch matching** experiment in which subjects are asked to produce the pitch of a reference tone

- **pitch range** the perceptual correlate of the range of fundamental frequency variation possible for an individual

- **pitch slide** a smooth movement from one pitch height to another

- **pitch slope** change in fundamental frequency over time

- **pitch variation** the range of pitch heights from lowest to highest

pitch determination algorithm (PDA) (also pitch extraction) a procedure used to extract the fundamental frequency of a speech signal. Although the term pitch strictly should be used to refer to a perceptual phenomenon, it is often used in speech analysis in reference to fundamental frequency

pitch period perturbation quotient a relative evaluation of short-term (cycle-to-cycle) variation of the pitch periods expressed in percentage

- **smoothed pitch perturbation quotient** a relative evaluation of long-term variation of the pitch period within the analyzed voice sample expressed in percentage

pivot grammar a description of children's early grammar that describing a limited number of words (pivots) occurring only in certain positions and a larger set of words (open) combined with them

pixel from *pic*ture *el*ement, the smallest visual information portion used to construct an image, as in a computer monitor

placenta uterine vascular tissue that allows diffusive metabolic exchange of respiratory and nutritive products between a mother and fetus

place of articulation a phonetic feature of speech sounds that specifies the location in the vocal tract where the point of major constriction occurred when the sound was produced; the place feature specifies whether a sound was produced with a bilabial closure, an alveolar closure, and so on

place theory of hearing theory of hearing that states frequency processing of the cochlea arises primarily through differential displacement of locations along the basilar membrane and, subsequently, stimulation of the hair cells of the stimulated regions

plane generally, a flat surface; in anatomy, a two-dimensional surface that either intersects the body or is tangential to it

plantar pertaining to the sole of the foot

plantar flexion bending the foot downward in the direction of the sole

plantar response reflex action of the toes when the outer surface sole of the foot is stimulated from heel to toe

plaques, neuritic tiny areas of degeneration of brain cortical and subcortical tissues; also called senile plaques

-plasia combining form: formation or development

plasma fluid aspect of circulating blood and lymph

plastic capable of being molded

plasticity in neurology, malleability of the central nervous system prior to stabilization of neural function; alteration of neurons to conform better to immediate environmental influences, often associated with a change in behavior; neural reorganization may be possible to some extent across the lifespan, as well as following injury (compensatory plasticity), and in response to learning

-plasty combining form: molding, forming

plate in anatomy, a thin, flat structure, especially a thin bony layer

platelets structures in the blood necessary for proper clotting

plausibility reasonable; the notion that information communicated is a likelihood

plausible event strategy language development comprehension strategy that relies on determining the most probable state of affairs

play audiometry behavioral method for testing the hearing thresholds of young children, in which correct identification of a stimulus presentation is rewarded by allowing the child to participate in a play-oriented activity

play, cooperative play behavior in which children interact for common advantage

play, parallel instances in which children engage in similar play activity in proximity to one another, but do not actually interact

play, solitary play behavior in which a child plays independent of others, even those in close proximity

play, symbolic play behavior in which one item is used to represent another

play, vocal infant sound productions exhibiting long strings of varied syllables

pleura serous membrane covering the lung (visceral pleura) and lining the inner chest wall (parietal pleura). Between these two layers a potential space (the pleural space) can become filled with fluid (pleural effusion) or pus (empyema)

pleural pertaining to the pleurae of the lungs

pleural space the fluid-filled space between the parietal and visceral pleura

pleurisy inflammation of the pleural linings of the lungs

plexus interjoining network of nerves and blood or lymphatic vessels

plosive consonant produced by creating complete blockage of airflow, followed by the buildup of air pressure, which is then suddenly released, producing a consonant sound

plot the central theme that provides the focus for story elements

Plummer-Vinson syndrome (also described as the Paterson-Kelly syndrome) dysphagia, iron-deficiency anemia, upper esophageal inflammation with web formation, angular stomatitis, and atrophic gastritis. Predominantly affects females between the ages of 40 and 70 years

pneumo- combining form: pertaining to air or to lungs

pneumomediastinum presence of air within the mediastinum; generally caused by emphysema or ruptured pulmonary bleb (blister) in infants at risk from respiratory distress syndrome or aspiration pneumonia and in older children by acute asthma, bronchitis, pertussis, or cystic fibrosis

pneumonia inflammation of the lung, usually of infectious (i.e., viral or bacterial) origin. Pneumonia can also be related to aspiration of either gastric contents with high acid levels or oropharyngeal contents containing bacteria

- **aspiration pneumonia** bronchopneumonia following aspiration into the bronchi of foreign material (vomit or food particles)

- **nosocomial pneumonia** chiefly caused by gram-negative organisms acquired in a hospital, can be associated with endotracheal intubation and mechanical ventilation

pneumonitis a disease distinguished by inflammation of the lungs

- **aspiration pneumonitis** inflammation (not necessarily due to infection) of the lung following aspiration

- **chemical pneumonitis** lung inflammation due to aspiration of irritating chemicals

pneumotachograph device used to instantaneously measure the volume rate of airflow

pneumothorax trapped air or gas in the pleural space of the thorax causing lung collapse; can be caused by open chest wound, severe coughing spasms, or have an unidentified etiology; can be induced for therapeutic reasons or for radiographic measurement techniques

pocket a saclike space

-poiesis combining form: production of or formation

Poincaré section a graphic depiction of a discernable pattern in a phase plane plot that does not have an apparent pattern, with the premise that the motion of a single variable of a complex system reflects the dynamics of the entire system; mathematician developer Jules-Henri Poincaré (1854–1912) is generally believed to be the first scientist to examine ideas that have become chaos theory

point vowels the three vowels (/i/, /a/, and /u/) at the articulatory and acoustic extremes in vowel space

poly- combining form: many

polyglot someone competent in several languages; or a mixture of languages

polymodally mapped information that is stored in the brain in a way that is not specific to any one sensory modality

polymorphous having various forms

polymyositis inflammatory disease of many muscles, especially skeletal muscle, characterized by swelling, pain, sweating, and tension

polyposis presence of several polyps

polyp, vocal small bulge of tissue on vocal fold mucosal surface; usually unilateral and benign

pons the more rostral region of the brainstem above the medulla oblongata, in which sensory and motor nuclei are surrounded by ascending and descending pathways and netlike arrangements of neurons defined as the reticular formation; the tegmentum of the pons (dorsal portion) contains the abducens nerve nucleus, facial nerve nucleus, trigeminal nerve motor and sensory nuclei, CN VIII cochlear division nucleus and vestibular division nuclei, and the superior olive

positive end expiratory pressure (PEEP) the maintenance of airway pressures above atmospheric throughout the expiratory phase of ventilation for improving oxygenation. PEEP can be set at differing levels according to patient need

- **auto-PEEP** amount of air left in the lungs after a maximum expiration; positive end expiratory pressure ensures that the lungs do not collapse after a maximum expiration. The placement of a one-way valve (Passy-Muir) in the ventilatory circuit may create additional auto-PEEP beyond what is supplied from ventilation

positive pressure ventilation mechanical ventilation that creates air pressure higher than atmospheric to push air into the lungs; can be invasive or noninvasive

positive reinforcement a stimulus that when presented contingent on a given response increases the likelihood of that response

positron emission tomography (PET) imaging of body (especially brain) sections by tracking positron-emitting radionuclides; depending on the radionuclides employed, researchers can measure regional cerebral blood flow, blood volume, oxygen uptake, and glucose transport and metabolism, in addition to locating neurotransmitter receptors

possessive grammatical case signaling that an entity is associated with, held, or owned by a possessor

post- prefix: after; behind

postconceptual age number of weeks following conception, approximately 2 weeks less than gestational age

posterior toward the back

postero- combining form: behind

postganglionic neuron cell body located in an autonomic ganglion, with an axon terminating in smooth or cardiac muscle or a gland

postlingual for hearing loss, deficit incurred after the acquisition of spoken language

postnatal after birth

postpolio syndrome progressive fatigue, weakness, and pain in patients with a remote history of acute paralytic poliomyelitis

postsynaptic inhibition an input to nerve or muscle cells that decreases the chance of their membrane channels opening and conducting action potentials through hyperpolarization

postsynaptic neuron the neuron receiving input

posttraumatic amnesia (PTA) memory loss accompanied by agitation and confusion following traumatic brain injury (TBI) from just after the injury or on awakening from coma

postural strategies in swallowing therapy, changing of a patient's head or body posture (to eliminate aspiration) that changes the position of the pharynx and the direction of food flow without increasing a patient's work or effort during a swallow

potassium pump in cells, energy-dependent pushing of the potassium ion (K^+) across the cell membrane employing the energy of K^+-activated adenosine triphosphatase; membrane potentials are determined by K^+

potential situation of tension in a source of electricity, enabling the source to function under specific conditions—potential is to electricity as temperature is to heat

- **action potential (AP)** sequential electrochemical polarization and depolarization associated with longitudinally propagated change of potential across a cell membrane, reflecting activation of excitable cells such as nerve or muscle

- **auditory evoked potential (AEP)** small electrical potential superimposed by auditory input on the steady-state electrical activity of the brain. Usually detectable only by signal averaging

- **endocochlear potential** constant positive potential of the ear's scala media

- **endogenous evoked potential** evoked potentials that are relatively invariant to changes in the eliciting physical stimulus, but are highly influenced by subject state and require an internal or mental activity (e.g., perceptual or cognitive process) to generate the potential

- **evoked potential** electrical activity in the brainstem or cerebral cortex elicited by a specific stimulus; a stimulus may affect the auditory, somatosensory, or visual pathway, each producing a characteristic brain wave pattern

- **hair cell intracellular resting potential** negative electrical potential difference between the ear's endolymph and the potential of the hair cells

- **membrane potential/resting potential/ standing potential** to some degree, each cell in the body pumps ions across cell membranes to keep an electrical potential difference across the membrane; ions travel in and out of a cell through channels in the membrane; passive channels allow free movement; chemically gated channels are selective, for example, with sodium-selective channels pumping sodium (and some calcium) out of cells and allowing potassium in; voltage gated channels are only open for some potentials

- **somatosensory evoked potential** cortical and subcortical response to repetitive stimulation of sensory fibers of the peripheral nerves that are averaged by computer

- **spike potential** brief electrical voltage changes that occur in certain smooth muscle and are related to such ionic channels as calcium

- **summating potential** sustained direct current (DC) shift in the endocochlear potential that occurs when the organ of Corti is stimulated by sound

power source, vocal the expiratory system including the muscles of the abdomen, back, thorax, and the lungs; responsible for producing a vector of force that results in efficient creation and control of subglottal pressure

Prader-Willi syndrome speech and language delayed, with articulatory impairment secondary to hypotonia; marked by hyperphagia obesity, cognitive deficiency

pragmatics study of speech acts and the contexts in which they are performed, along with the societal-dependent aspects of communicative interaction; exploration of the rules of social interaction such as turn taking and topic maintenance, as well as the accepted contexts for questioning and assigning titles to conversational partners

- **metapragmatics** conscious intentional awareness of ways to effectively use language in various contexts, as in knowing politeness and impoliteness

pre- prefix: before; in front of

prechaotic behavior predictable behavior prior to the onset of chaotic behavior, such as period doubling

precipitating factor aspect that results in the onset of a language or communication problem

predictability, word amount of fill-in-the-blank meaningfulness in a preceding spoken context. In predictability-high (PH) sentences, preceding semantic-contextual information is presented in the form of clue words; no such clue words are available in predictability-low (PL) sentences

prediction the scientific goal of identifying the variables that reliably precede a phenomenon; forecast based on information, examination, scientific evidence

predictive assessment AAC assessment process consisting of a focused evaluation that evaluates those skills necessary for developing an AAC prescription by matching the skills of a nonspeaking individual to the features of a given AAC system. Predictive assessment is sometimes referred to as the "feature-matching" process

predisposing factor aspect of or in an individual that increases likelihood of a language and/or communication skills impairment

preemphasis in speech analysis, a filtering that boosts high-frequency energy relative to low-frequency energy. Because speech normally contains its strongest energy in the low frequencies, these frequencies would dominate analysis results, if preemphasis were not performed

preganglionic neuron autonomic nervous system neuron that innervates ganglionic cells. The cell bodies of preganglionic neurons are situated within the central nervous system, with axons terminating in autonomic ganglia

prelingual hearing loss loss incurred before the acquisition of spoken language

prenatal before birth

preposition part of speech that delineates a relation between words in a sentence and includes such words as of, on, in, between

prepositional phrase most common aspect in which prepositions function, with the phrase beginning with a preposition and including modifier(s) followed by a noun (object of the preposition); prepositional phrases are modifiers, acting as adjectives or adverbs

presbycusis progressive loss in auditory function associated with the aging process

prescriptive grammar a collection of rules that purports to dictate correct grammatical structures to the speakers of a language

prescriptive hearing-aid fitting strategy for fitting hearing aids by using a formula to calculate the desired gain and frequency response; formula incorporates pure-tone audiometric thresholds and, usually, information about uncomfortable loudness levels

press of speech use of excessive content of speech, as if the speaker needs to press on

pressure derived measure representing force expended over an area; force of the interaction of gravity and the atmosphere

pressure support ventilation addition of preset positive pressure breaths to the inspiratory phase of ventilation; helps reduce the work of breathing. Can be used with cycled ventilatory modes or with CPAP

prevalence percentage of cases of a specific disease or disorder existing in a given population at a certain time; compare incidence

prevocalic voicing assimilation process substitution of a voiced sound for voiceless sound preceding a vowel (e.g., /b/ for /p/ in prevocalic positions)

prevoicing the onset of voicing before the appearance of a supraglottal articulatory event; for example, for stops, prevoicing means that voicing precedes the stop release; also called voicing lead

prima donna literally means "first lady"; soprano soloist, especially the lead singer in an opera

primitive/infantile reflexes automatic responses that produce change in muscle tone and movement of the limbs; typically present in newborns; examples include the asymmetrical and symmetrical tonic neck reflexes, including:

- **asymmetric tonic neck reflex (ATNR)** can be elicited by turning a supine infant's head laterally. Visible evidence includes extension of the extremities on the chin side or flexion on the occiput side. The ATNR is commonly persistent in children with severe motor deficits related to cerebral palsy

- **Moro reflex (startle reflex)** elicited with infant in supine position. The head is allowed to drop back suddenly from at least 3 cm off a padded surface. On extension of the neck, there is a quick symmetrical abduction and upward movement of the arms followed by opening of the hands. Adduction and flexion of the arms can then be noted

- **positive support reflex** can be elicited by suspending an infant around the trunk or axillae with the head in neutral or midline flexed position. The infant is bounced five times on the balls of the feet. The balls of the feet are then taken into contact with the table surface. Co-contraction of opposing muscle groups of the legs occurs, resulting in a position capable of supporting weight

- **tonic labyrinthine reflex** can be evaluated in supine or prone position. In supine, infant's head is extended 45° below the horizontal and then flexed 45° above the horizontal. While the neck is extended 45° the limbs extend. With the neck flexed 45°, the limbs flex

primitive streak a feature of the embryonic disk that generates the mesoderm

primo passaggio "first passage"; in music, the first register change perceived in a voice as pitch is raised from low to high

prion proteinaceous infectious particle believed to cause transmissible neurodegenerative diseases; does not trigger a typical immune response

pro- prefix: before; in front of

probability the ratio of the number of outcomes in a comprehensive grouping of equally credible outcomes that lead to the total number of likely outcomes of a given event

probe microphone microphone transducer that is inserted into the external ear canal for the purpose of measuring sound near the tympanic membrane

probes procedures used during speech therapy to assess generalized production of clinically established responses; administered every time a few exemplars are trained to assess generalized productions

problem solving generating a variety of potentially effective responses to a situation that needs a solution and then recognizing and implementing the most effective response

process a prominence of an anatomical structure

process instruction an emphasis on "doing" in the classroom rather than on creating a product. A focus on procedures and techniques rather than on learning outcomes; learning "how to" through inquiry rather than learning through the transmission and memorization of knowledge

process verb word that refers to unobservable activity or gradual changes

productions the expression or encoding of an idea in an utterance

prognathism atypical facial formation in which one or both jaws project forward

prognosis the projected outcome of injury, disease, or disorder; may pertain to the projected outcome of recovery with or without treatment

programmable hearing aid hearing aid in which several parameters of the instrument, such as gain, are under computer control

progressive advancing; occurring over time; in defining disease process, generally means unfavorable

P

progressive bulbar paralysis incremental atrophy of the muscles of the tongue, lips, palate, pharynx, and larynx; often caused by motor neuron disease

progressive systemic sclerosis (PSS) autoimmune connective tissue disorder leading to progressive fibrosis of the dermal layer of the skin, of smooth muscle, or of other visceral tissues

projection fibers neural tracts running to and from the cerebral cortex, connecting it with distant locations

prompt in treatment, supplementary cue added to an original stimulus to increase the likelihood of a correct response; in language development, caregiver involvement that stimulates responses from a child to encourage continuation of a verbal exchange; prompts may be verbal or nonverbal

pronate to place in the prone position

pronation a turning down or outward; for example, turning the palm of the hand downward; muscles used to perform this function are called pronators

prone body in horizontal position with face down

pronominalization process of replacing a noun or noun phrase with a pronoun form (or pronominal)

pronoun words that can replace a noun or noun phrase through anaphoric or cataphoric reference

- **relative pronoun** pronouns that introduce relative clauses, which act as adjectives for the noun they follow (e.g., The boy *who* came thanked me)

proprioception the awareness, often subconsciously, of weight, posture, movement, position in space in relationship to the body; based on sensory input from nerve terminals in joints and muscles in conjunction with vestibular information

prosencephalon in embryology, the forebrain, from which the telencephalon and diencephalon will arise

proso-, pros- prefix: forward or anterior

prosody production features of speech, such as intonation, stress, rate, and rhythm, that provide its melodic character; also, suprasegmental aspects of spoken language; the dynamic melody, timing, rhythm, and amplitude fluctuations of fluent speech

- **exaggeration** prosodic behavior overemphasis as a treatment technique

- **facilitator** the prosodic context that makes a task easier or simpler

- **phrasing** the use of prosodic cues to mark the beginning or the ending of phrases

prostaglandin one of a group of physiologically active unsaturated fatty acids causing such effects as vasoconstriction and vasodilation, stimulation of bronchial or intestinal smooth muscle, and antagonism to hormones that influence lipid metabolism

prosthesis fabricated replacement for a missing or dysfunctional body part

protein major foundation for muscle, blood, skin, hair, nails, and internal organs; one of a large group of naturally occurring complex nitrogenic organic compounds composed of amino acid compounds, with 22 noted as being vital for living cells; the body can synthesize 13 amino acids (called nonessential) and the 9 essential amino acids can only be obtained from dietary intake

protensity estimated duration of an experience is often termed its protensity and provides a psychological correlate for the physical concept of duration

proto-, prot- prefix: primitive; simple form

protoconversation early interaction between caregivers and infants that includes elements such as turn taking

protodeclaratives early infant vocal and gestural behaviors that suggest commanding or requesting action on the part of an infant

protoimperatives early infant vocal and gestural behaviors that suggest commanding or requesting action on the part of a infant

protonarratives (or prenarratives) earliest forms of children's stories

protoplasm living matter; the basic substance from which animal and plant cells are formed

prototype earliest design or model from which similar things are copied

protoword early infant vocalization that has wordlike function and may lead to words

protuberance a bulge or prominence above a structure's surface

proverb brief statement of societal truth or principle, often in metaphorical form

proxemics the study of personal space in social interactions, including interpersonal communication

proximal situated nearest to the center of the body; opposite of distal, with the shoulder proximal and the hand distal

pseudo- combining form: false

pseudobulbar paralysis lips and tongue paralysis characterized by dysphagia, dysphonia, and/or dysarthria, along with spasmodic cheerless laughter or nonanguished crying; etiology is supranuclear lesions and upper motor neuron bilateral involvement

pseudophrase early approximation of multiword utterances through production of conventional two-word phrases (e.g., *allgone, nomore*) in which the individual elements do not occur elsewhere independently

psychiatrist a physician specializing in mental disorders

psychoacoustician researcher studying the psychological correlate of auditory stimulus parameters

psychogenic caused by psychological factors rather than physical dysfunction; can result in physical dysfunction or structural injury

psycholinguistic encoding processes (speech programming) mental actions by which words are retrieved from memory and assembled into a code that can direct the movements of speech structures

psycholinguistics the branch of linguistics concerned with studying the mental operations that are related to and undergird the speaking and understanding of language

psychological dependence a condition resulting from repeated use of a drug (or other enabling mechanism) in which an individual must continue the dependence to satisfy a strong emotional need; the need for something that results from the continuous or periodic use of what is depended on. This need may be characterized by mental and/or physical changes in users that make it difficult for a dependent person to change or stop a dependent habit

psychologist professional licensed to evaluate and treat behavioral/emotional disorders

psychosis psychiatric diagnosis of a major disorder causing gross distortion or disorganization of mental capacity, communication, affective response, and capacity to determine reality that limits or prohibits a person's ability to handle everyday life. Typically psychoses are divided into organic brain syndromes (i.e., Korsakoff syndrome) and those also having some functional aspects (schizophrenia, bipolar disorder)

- **acute psychosis** a disturbance in thinking that is often accompanied by delusions and visual or auditory hallucinations. An acute psychosis may be caused by alcohol or other drug withdrawal, drug toxicity (most commonly in conjunction with abuse or cocaine, methamphetamine, or psychedelic agents), or schizophrenia

ptosis drooping (usually from paralysis) of upper eyelid(s); prolapse or sag of any organ or organ part

puberty the period of development in which sexual maturation and rapid growth occur

Public Law (P.L.) 94-142 the Education for All Handicapped Children Act of 1975, which mandated a free and appropriate education (FAPE) for every child with disabilities between the age of 3 and 18 years (extended to ages 3 to 21 in 1980), ensured rights of due process, and mandated individualized education plans (IEPs) and a least restrictive environment (LRE)

Public Law (P.L.) 99-457 the Education of the Handicapped Act Amendments of 1986 mandated preschool services for youngsters with disabilities and set up Part H to help states develop a multidisciplinary, comprehensive system of infant early intervention services

Public Law (P.L.) 101-336 Americans with Disabilities Act (ADA) of 1990 prohibits employment discrimination and exclusion from public services and accommodations, requires telecommunication relay services for those with hearing impairment and/or speech impairment, and established an Architectural and Transportation Barriers Compliance Board

Public Law (P.L.) 101-431 Television Decoder Circuitry Act of 1990 required television sets of 13-inch and larger screens to be manuctured with closed-captioning capacity

Public Law (P.L.) 101-476 the 1990 Education of the Handicapped Act Amendments, retitled the legislation to Individuals with Disabilities Education Act (IDEA); reauthorized P.L. 94-142 and expanded accepted handicapping conditions that qualify for services, transition services for youths 16 years and older, and made provision for the use of assistive technology

Public Law (P.L.) 103-218 the Technology-Related Assistance for Individuals with Disabilities Act Amendments of 1994, known as the Tech Act, provided states with a means to establish projects focused on systems change and to increase consumer access to assistive technology devices and services

Public Law (P.L.) 105-17 the Individuals with Disabilities Act Amendments of 1997, which seeks to enhance parental involvement; calls for attention to racial, ethnic, and linguistic diversity to prevent inappropriate identification and labeling; promotes a safe school environment; and establishes a mediation process for parents and providers

pulmonary compliance expandability measure of the lungs

pulmonary dysmaturity syndrome disorder of preterm infants characterized by hypoxia, with lungs having thickened alveolar walls and blebs

pulmonary edema swelling of alveoli in the lung from fluid leaking from the capillaries; can lead to significant respiratory distress

pulmonary fibrosis, interstitial scarring and abnormal deposition of collagen within alveolar walls, leading to increased stiffness of lungs and impaired oxygenation; may be caused by autoimmunity, drug hypersensitivity, infection, irradiation, or occupational exposures

pulmonary function test one of variety of assessment techniques that can provide both diagnostic and therapeutic information based on the lungs' capacity to exchange oxygen and carbon dioxide; tests include measuring the amount of air a person can maximally exhale after a maximum inspiration and the time required for that expiration; and by determining the ability of the alveolar capillary membrane to transport oxygen into the blood and carbon dioxide from the blood into the expired air

pulmonary system the breathing apparatus, including the lungs and related airways

pulse arterial rhythmical dilation from increased blood volume caused by each pump of a heart contraction

pulse register glottal fry; the vocal register characterized by low fundamental frequency, with syncopated vibration of vocal folds; characterized by a pattern of short glottal waves alternating with larger and longer ones and with a long closed phase

pulse sequence in MRI, a series of electromagnetic pulses used to excite the spins of body protons and generate the signal used to construct a magnetic resonance image

punishment the contingent presentation of an aversive stimulus that results in a decrease in the probability of a response

- **type I punishment** delivering a stimulus contingent on a behavior that results in its decrease
- **type II punishment** removing a stimulus contingent on a behavior that results in its decrease

pure tone sinusoid; simplest tone; produced electronically; in nature, even pure-sounding tones like bird songs are complex

pure-tone audiometry test to check an individual's capability of discriminating frequencies, including comparison of air conduction and bone conduction tests

pure-tone average (PTA) average of hearing thresholds at 500 Hz, 1000 Hz, and 2000 Hz

purulent referring to pus, which is a liquid formed in certain infections that contains fluid composed of tissue cells mixed with bacteria

pushing voice treatment technique that involves the speaker pressing against an immovable object while vocalizing

Pygmalion effect a self-fulfilling prophecy, in which a student and/or client's outcome is based on expectations of others in the person's environment; based on a legend about a benefactor bringing a statue to "life" to meet the expectations of the benefactor; can be positive or negative

pyloric stenosis narrowing of the sphincter at the lower end of the stomach, blocking food from entering the small intestine; can be congenital or secondary to a sphincter ulcer or fibrosis

pyramidal tract (corticobulbar and corticospinal) white matter through which motor impulses travel; descending fibers dealing with voluntary and reflex muscle activity

pyridoxine water-soluble vitamin of the B group

pyriform pear-shaped

pyriform sinus pouch or cavity constituting the lower end of the nasopharynx located to the side and partially to the back of the larynx; typically there are paired sinuses

pyrosis heartburn; burning painful feeling in the esophagus; generally caused by reflux of gastric contents (GER)

Q in the manual alphabet

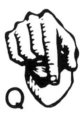

quad-cane broad-based cane with four legs that provides increased stability for standing or walking

quadra-, quadri prefix: four

quadrangular membrane elastic, mucosa-covered membrane extending from the sides of the epiglottic cartilage to the corniculate and arytenoid cartilages; forms the aryepiglottic fold and the wall between the pyriform sinus and larynx

quadriplegia paralysis of all four limbs and body trunk from below the level of a spinal cord injury, notably in the fifth to the seventh vertebrae

quality the psychological correlate of spectrum

quality control actions; measures put into place by organization, department, or other workplace to help assure successful production; for those with ADD, ability of an individual to self-verify personal actions

quantization the assignment of discrete values to the amplitude dimension of an analog signal; process by which a continuous variation in amplitude is represented as a sequence of discrete values; necessary to represent the signal in a digital computer

quantization noise a signal distortion resulting from an inadequate number of quantization levels in digitizing a signal

quasiperiodic a behavior that has at least two frequencies in which the phases are related by an irrational number; a form of motion that is recurrent, but never exactly repeating

quefrency the time axis in a cepstrum; transliteration of frequency

question interrogative presentation, such as the form employed for testing information acquisition; interrogative clause or sentence

- **intonation question** question that is signaled by change in intonation rather than by change in syntax

- **tag question** question added to the end of a statement

- **wh-question** interrogative sentence beginning with a wh-word, such as who, what, where, when, how, and why

- **yes/no question** interrogative sentence associated with a rising intonation or inversion of subject and auxiliary (e.g., You can come? or Can you come?)

questioning, neutral questions asked from a nonjudgmental position of curiosity, with the intent of understanding clients' concerns, exploring interactive patterns, and identifying resources to facilitate change

questionnaire speech assessment procedure for conversational fluency and communication handicap, in which respondents provide subjective information about their listening and communication difficulties by answering questions on a form designed to elicit diagnostic information

quotient, abduction the ratio of the glottal half-width at the vocal processes to the amplitude of vibration of the vocal fold

quotient, amplitude perturbation a relative evaluation of short term (cycle-to-cycle) variation of peak-to-peak amplitude expressed in percentage

quotient, open the ratio of the time the glottis is open to the length of the entire vibratory cycle

QWERTY standard keyboard arrangement, from the six leftmost letters in the second row from the top of a keyboard

R

Reflex

preprogrammed neuromuscular response to stimuli; involuntary motor act

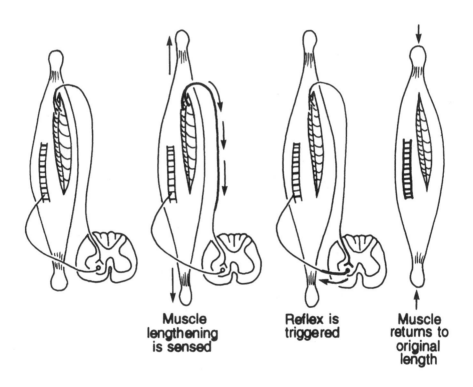

Muscle
lengthening
is sensed

Reflex is
triggered

Muscle
returns to
original
length

racism a system of privilege and penalty based on race; based on a belief in the inherent superiority of one race over others and acceptance of economic, social, political, and educational differences based on such supposed superiority

radian the angular measure obtained when the arc along the circumference of the circle is equal to the radius length

- **radian frequency** the number of radians per second covered in circular or sinusoidal motion

radiation absorbed dose (rad) unit of absorbed dose of ionizing radiation, with 1 rad equal to 100 ergs of ionizing radiation per gram of tissue or other absorbing material; a measure of the radiation dose a patient receives with X rays or radionuclides

radiation characteristic in source-filter theory of speech production, radiation of sound from the lips to the atmosphere; typically expressed as a 6-dB per octave increase in sound energy (hence, a high-pass filter)

radiation, ionizing high-energy electromagnetic waves (such as X rays, gamma rays) and particulate rays (i.e., electrons, neutrons, alpha particles, beta rays, heavy nuclei) that dissociate material in their paths into ions; directly affects living organisms by retarding development or destroying cells, also leading to gene mutations and chromosome breaks; animal tissues with high atomic weights, such as calcium, soak up higher doses from a given radiating source than does soft tissue

radioallergosorbent test (RAST) radioimmunoassay technique to identify IgE that has been combined with known allergens to determine antigen-antibody reaction

radiographic swallowing study/modified barium swallow a moving X ray of oropharyngeal swallow on designated bolus consistencies; barium is a radiopaque substance used to enhance X-ray contrast

radiolabel a compound that has a radionuclide attached to it and can be imaged with a gamma camera after ingestion or injection of the compound into the body

radionuclide isotope (or nuclide) of an element with unstable nuclei that emit radiation at a known rate of decay

radiopharmaceutical medication labeled with a radionuclide for diagnosis (tracing) or therapy

radiotherapy treatment employing gamma or Xrays to impede malignant cells through radiation damage

radius shorter and lateral bone of the forearm; the line that connects the center of a circle with any point on the circumference

ramus major branch or division of a blood vessel or nerve; part of the mandible

random behavior action that never repeats itself and is inherently unpredictable

range, dynamic the difference in decibels between an individual's threshold of hearing sensitivity for a sound and the level at which the sound becomes uncomfortably loud; in electroacoustics, the difference between the least and most intense signals in an analysis or display

range of motion (ROM) the extent of movement possible in a particular joint measured in degrees of a circle; also, a set of physical exercises designed to preserve or promote such movement

Ranvier, nodes of regions of myelinated nerve fibers in which there is no myelin

raphe biological seam or ridge formed at the line of union of two symmetrical halves of a structure

- **palatine raphe** elevation in hard palate midline extending the length of the hard palate mucosa

- **pharyngeal raphe** central posterior line of the pharynx where muscular fibers connect and partly interlace

- **raphe linguae** median tongue groove

rapid eye movement (REM) the rapid, jerky movements of the eyes which occur during certain stages of the sleep cycle when dreams occur

Rapp-Hodgkin syndrome compensatory articulation pattern secondary to clefting and hypernasality and articulatory placement problems secondary to clefting and maxillary deficiency; hoarseness secondary to hypohidrosis and dry vocal folds; maked also by ectodermal dysplasia

rapport harmonious connection based on mutual respect and trust

rarefaction a decrease in density; minimum pressure area in a medium crossed by waves that can be compressed (as sound waves)

rate variability when speech is produced at different rates, the physical characteristics of individual phonetic units vary and the phonetic boundary between two categories is shifted, making it impossible to specify an absolute physical value for a phonetic unit

re- prefix: back or again; curved back

Compression

Rarefaction

rarefaction a decrease in density; minimum pressure area in a medium crossed by waves that can be compressed (as sound waves)

reactance portion of impedance of an alternating-current circuit caused by capacitance or inductance or both and that is expressed in ohms; symbol is X

- **elastic reactance** the rejection of low-frequency vibrations as a result of the stiffness of the vibrating object. Elastic reactance goes up drastically as the frequency of the attempted motion decreases

- **mass reactance** the loss of energy that occurs when a mass is moved back and forth at a high frequency. The greater the mass, the more difficulty one encounters trying to move it back and forth at rapid rates. Moving a mass back and forth at low frequencies is considerably easier

real-ear gain gain of a hearing aid measured with a probe microphone at the tympanic membrane; the difference between the SPL in the external ear canal and the SPL at the field reference point for a specified sound field

real time an operation that takes no more time than the incoming signal itself

real-time captioning captioning of a person's speech in real time

real-time speech the transitory, ephemeral nature of an ongoing speech signal; when speech is presented in a real-time manner, listeners must quickly recognize phonemes, syllables, and words based on preceding linguistic-contextual cues and ongoing acoustic-phonetic information

real-time ultrasound sonographic process that provides multiple, rapid images of anatomical structure in motion

reasoning evaluation of arguments, drawing of inferences and conclusions, and generation and testing of hypotheses

rebus depiction of words or syllables by pictures of objects or by symbols that resemble the intended words or syllables in sound

received pronunciation (RP) the dialect of British English spoken by those attending public schools (the equivalent of private schools in the United States) and universities such as Oxford and Cambridge

receiver component that converts electrical energy into acoustic energy, as in a hearing aid; or component of an FM system worn by a listener that receives FM signals from a transmitter; or individual who receives a message from a sender

reception classes/centers programs for students newly arrived from another country

receptive aphasia a neurogenic language disorder in which comprehension of written and spoken language is impaired and linked to effortless communication of malformed and substituted words; also called sensory aphasia, Wernicke aphasia

receptive field the region of the body that, when receiving a particular stimulus, will excite a sensory fiber to discharge action potentials toward the cell body

receptive language ability an individual's skill in understanding language

receptor sensory nerve ending that reacts to stimulation; cell portion that mixes with a drug, hormone, or chemical intermediary to change the cell function

- **baroreceptors** pressure sensors; pressure-sensitive nerve endings in various cardiac or airway walls that provide for physiologic adaptation to blood or air pressure changes; homeostasis depends on baroreception

- **chemoreceptor** sensory organ that is sensitive to properties of specific chemicals, especially taste and smell; also, specialized cells (i.e., neural receptors) in the central nervous system that respond to gas levels in the blood, especially levels of CO_2, for activating the muscles of inspiration

- **exteroreceptor** skin or mucous membrane peripheral end organ that responds to external agent stimulation

- **interoceptor** sensory receptor responsive to stimuli originating inside the body

- **mechanoreceptor** sensory receptor sensitive to mechanical stimulation such as pressure on or distortion of the skin or other membrane

- **photoreceptor** sensory receptor for visual stimulation, such as a rod or a cone in the eye's retina

- **proprioceptor** sensory receptor that responds to stimuli concerning body position or orientation

- **stretch receptors** specialized neural cells in the walls of the lung and thorax that during inspiration respond to lung and thorax movement by sending impulses to the respiratory center to cease movement of the inspiratory muscles; sensory receptors that monitor stretch in a muscle

- **taste receptor** specialized chemoreceptor that responds to substances dissolved in oral fluids; various different substances activate different types of membrane channels or transmembrane

- **telereceptor** sensory receptor responsive to stimuli originating outside of the body

- **thermoreceptor** sensor responsive to temperature

recess small cavity

recessive gene one of a gene pair lacking the ability to be evidenced if its more dominant allele is present; only evident in homozygous state

reciprocal marked by mutual agreement and/or interchange

reciprocal teaching alternating roles between a client and clinician, allowing the client to assume the role of teacher as well as learner

recognition the perceptual process of identifying a stimulus as having been previously known or experienced; the ability of individuals to attend to and identify a particular item's or individual's presence

- **speaker recognition** the determination that a particular speaker produced a given speech signal; also called voice recognition

recoil pressure, elastic the alveolar pressure derived from extended (strained) tissue in the lungs, ribcage, and the entire thorax after inspiration (measured in pascals)

recombination language developmental process of combining two shorter language constructions into a longer construction; in genetics, formation of new gene arrangements within a chromosome

recording setting down permanently in writing or through instruments

- **differential recording** the electrophysiologic technique based on the recording of action potentials from a limited spatial region by use of bipolar electrodes connected to a differential amplifier

- **electrophysiological recording** any recording of electrical activity generated by physiological processes; technique of using micropipettes or metal to record inside or outside of neurons and muscle cells. Micropipettes placed in these two types of cells can record action potentials in millivolts. Micropipettes and metal electrodes placed outside this tissue records extracellular signals that are much smaller—in the microvolt range

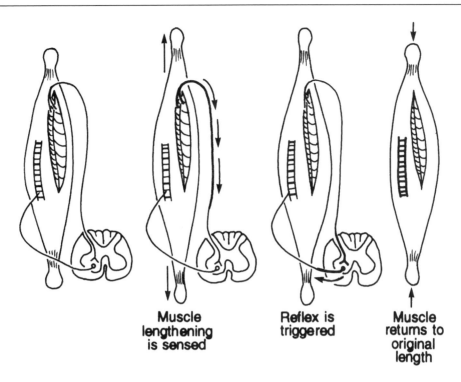

Muscle lengthening is sensed   **Reflex is triggered**   **Muscle returns to original length**

reflex   preprogrammed neuromuscular response to stimuli; involuntary motor act

recounts narrative type that relates a series of events

recovery, spontaneous unassisted resolution of deficits created by a disease or injury such as stroke

recreational therapy (RT) a rehabilitation specialty that targets the use of leisure or recreational activities as part of the therapeutic process

recurrent laryngeal nerve (RLN) branch of the vagus nerve (cranial nerve X) that serves cardiac, tracheal, and esophageal branches

- **recurrent laryngeal nerve resection** treatment procedure for adductor spasmodic dysphonia, with RLN unilaterally resectioned to paralyze one of the vocal folds to prevent hyperadduction

reductionism a style of thinking that studies complex phenomena by breaking them down into small and simple parts

reduplication in language development, an early approximation of a multiword utterance by repeating a conventional word with an identical phonetic shape or intonational contour; also any repeated syllable in babbling

reduplication assimilation process repetition of a syllable, resulting in substitution of one for another (e.g., wawa for water)

reference something pointing to another or a synonymous source of information

- **joint reference** establishing an object as the shared topic of communication

referential identifying a stimulus as the topic for communication

referential learning a language-learning strategy based primarily on the acquisition of words that refer to objects

referential words early words whose primary purpose is to refer to objects

reflecting a technique in which a therapist, from a position of unconditional positive regard, restates the feelings and content that a person is expressing

reflex preprogrammed neuromuscular response to stimuli; involuntary motor act

- **acoustic reflex** a bilateral reflex of the stapedius muscle in the middle ear; it is activated by sounds of high intensity and reduces the transmission of energy into the inner ear, providing protection from loud noise

- **asymmetrical tonic neck reflex (ATNR)** a postural reflex commonly observed in typically developing infants younger than 6 months and often seen in children with cerebral palsy. When the head is rotated, the ATNR causes an extension in the arm and leg on the side to which the face is turned, while the opposite side increases in flexion; can be elicited by turning an infant's head laterally in a supine position. Visible evidence includes extension of the extremities on the chin side or flexion on the occiput side. The ATNR is commonly persistent in children with severe motor deficits

- **gag reflex** normal neural reflex activated through touch of the posterior pharynx or soft palate; employed to check the integrity of the vagus and glossopharyngeal nerves

- **infantile/primitive reflexes** automatic responses that produce change in muscle tone and movement of the limbs. These reflexes are typically present in newborns; however, they can persist in individuals with brain damage through lifespan; include the asymmetrical tonic neck reflex and Moro (startle) reflex

- **Moro reflex** a primitive reflex elicited with infant in supine position. The head is allowed to drop back suddenly from at least 3 cm off a padded surface. On extension of the neck, there is a quick symmetrical abduction and upward movement of the arms followed by opening of the hands. Adduction and flexion of the arms can then be noted. Typically disappears by about 6 months of life but may persist in neurological damage

- **positive support reflex** can be elicited by suspending an infant around the trunk or axillae with the head in neutral or midline flexed position. The infant is bounced 5 times on the balls of the feet. The balls of the feet are then brought into contact with the table surface. Co-contraction of opposing muscle groups of the legs occur, resulting in a position capable of supporting weight

- **reflexive cry** infant cry behavior in response to physiologic stimuli

- **reflexive smile** infant smile behavior that is in apparent response to internal physiologic stimuli

- **specific activity reflex** a reflex that affects an individual body part

- **symmetrical tonic neck reflex (STNR)** a postural reflex often seen in children with cerebral palsy. When the neck is extended, the arms extend and the hips flex. When the neck is flexed, the arms flex and the hips extend

- **tonic labyrinthine reflex** an early reflex that can be evaluated in supine or prone position. In supine, infant's head is extended 45° below the horizontal and then flexed 45° above the horizontal; with the neck extended 45°, the limbs extend; with the neck flexed 45°, the limbs flex

- **uncrossed acoustic reflex** stapedius muscle contraction recorded with sound stimulus and immittance recording probe in the same ear

reflexive relations ways in which objects relate to themselves, including existence, nonexistence, disappearance, and recurrence

reflux a flowing back, as in the case of fluids in the body

reflux esophagitis inflammation of the esophageal mucosa, resulting from reflux of gastric contents into the esophagus; a condition that can present clinically as heartburn, chest pain, or dysphagia. Endoscopically, the mucosal appearance can range from normal to a single or few erosions in the distal esophagus to extensive ulcerative tissues. Histologically, it shows changes in the architecture of the epithelium and infiltration by inflammatory cells. Chronic reflux can be complicated by the development of stricture of Barrett's esophagus

reflux laryngitis inflammation of the larynx due to irritation from gastric juice

refractive eye surgery surgery to correct lack of visual acuity

refractory period, absolute period following depolarization of a cell membrane during which stimulation will not result in further depolarization

refractory period, relative also known as refactory state or phase, which is from about −60 mV during the action potential phase 3, when a strong stimulus can produce a depressed response

reframing a review of a situation that results in a change in meaning or value attributed to the situation even though the facts remain the same. This change in thinking is expected to result in subsequent changes in behavior related to the situation

- **cognitive reframing** a relapse prevention skill training strategy that helps a patient who has been drug-dependent find new responses to high-risk factors

Refsum syndrome probably late speech deterioration with ataxia onset in adult years, which can lead to dysphonia; also marked by retinitis pigmentosa, peripheral sensory and motor neuropathy

register vocal qualities; often register refers to a series of adjacent tones on the scale that sound similar and seem to be generated by the same type of vocal fold vibrations and vocal tract adjustments (such as vocal fry, modal, and falsetto); any of the varieties of a language employed in a particular social context

- **falsetto register** a very high-pitched register, sometimes restricted to male voices
- **modal register** the vocal register used during normal conversation (i.e., vocal register used most frequently)
- **pulse register** glottal fry; the vocal register characterized by low fundamental frequency, with syncopated vibration of vocal folds; characterized by a pattern of short glottal waves alternating with larger and longer ones, and with a long closed phase
- **whistle register** the highest of all registers (in pitch). It is observed only in females, extending the pitch range beyond F6

rehabilitation the restoration of physical, mental, communicative, social, or vocational skills following a disabling injury or disease

- **audiologic rehabilitation** often used synonymously with aural rehabilitation or aural habilitation; sometimes may entail greater emphasis on the provision and follow up of listening devices and less emphasis on communication strategies training and speech perception training
- **aural rehabilitation** intervention aimed at minimizing or alleviating the communication difficulties associated with hearing loss; may include diagnosis of hearing loss and communication handicap, amplification, counseling, communication strategies training, speech perception training, family instruction, speech-language therapy, and educational management

rehearsal, covert treatment technique of practicing targeted behaviors when alone; a rehearsal of a skill or act that is not visible to outside observers, for example, subvocal rehearsal in language tasks

reinforcement stimulus that strengthens by added material assistance or support

- **negative reinforcement** procedure that increases the frequency of a behavior by re-

moving an aversive stimulus contingent on each occurrence

- **positive reinforcement** stimulus that when presented contingent on a response increases the likelihood of that response

reinforcer any stimulus presented contingently that increases the frequency or strength of a response

- **automatic reinforcer** sensory consequence of responses that reinforce those responses (e.g., the sensation a child with autism derives from banging his or her head)
- **conditioned reinforcer** stimulus that takes on reinforcing properties as a result of association with a known reinforcer
- **generalized conditioned reinforcer** stimulus that obtains reinforcing potential from association with a variety of other reinforcing stimuli
- **primary reinforcer** stimulus that has reinforcing potential because of the mechanism's survival value
- **secondary reinforcer** stimulus that gains reinforcing potential through association with primary reinforcers
- **social reinforcer** a variety of conditioned reinforcers frequently used in treatment sessions; these include verbal praise, attention, touch, eye contact, and facial expressions; resistant to satiation effect; may not work with nonverbal clients

Reinke's edema swelling of Reinke's space from chronic smoking or hypothyroidism

Reinke's space loose connective superficial layer of the lamina propria in the vocal fold

Reissner's membrane in the ear, membranous separation between scala vestibuli and scala media

relapse recurrence, especially of a disease; reversion to use of any mind-altering chemical following a period of abstinence

relational concepts knowledge about how objects and events relate to each other

relational words words that refer to abstract relationships between objects

relative average perturbation a relative evaluation of short-term (cycle-to-cycle) variation of the pitch periods expressed in percentage

relative pronoun pronouns that introduce relative clauses, which act as adjectives for the noun they follow (e.g., The boy *who* came thanked me)

R

relay system system employed by persons with significant hearing loss who have access to telephone communication; the individual contacts a relay operator who transmits messages between caller and person called by means of teletype and/or voice

reliability extent to which a test yields similar results with repeated administration

- **alternative form reliability** evaluating the reliability of a test by having the subject take two different forms of the same test and comparing the performances

- **split-half reliability** measure of consistency between the halves of a test or other procedure (one way of assessing possible practice effects)

- **test-retest reliability** measure of test consistency from one presentation to the next

remediation process of achieving a remedy

remote control hand-held device that permits adjustments in the volume or changes in the program of a programmable electronic device, including a hearing aid

renal relating to the kidneys

reorganization, intersystemic speech treatment strategy that pairs speaking with a rhythmic activity such as pushing a button or squeezing a ball

repair strategies tactics implemented by a participant in a conversation to rectify breakdowns in communication

- **conversational repairs** devices used by individuals to clarify messages within a conversation

- **specific repair strategy** repair strategy used to rectify a communication breakdown that provides explicit instruction to the communication partner about what to do next

- **stacked repair sequences** successive attempts to clarify an utterance in which additional elements are included in each subsequent attempt

requests, clarification one communicative partner signals to the other that there has been a communicative breakdown

research design, cross-sectional research design in which groups of subjects are assessed at a given point in time, as in comparing subjects at different ages

research design, longitudinal research design that follows the continuous development of its subjects

research design, single-subject research design in which an individual subject serves as his or her own control

reserpine antihypertensive medication

residential care facility caregiving institution providing custodial nurturence to individuals incapable of independent living

residual error error in speech left over from earlier development; usually referring to a small number of errors that were once developmentally typical

residual hearing the hearing remaining in a person who has hearing loss

residual volume amount of gas remaining in the lungs after maximal voluntary expiration. This volume, which does not contribute to effective gas exchange, is increased in patients with obstructive lung diseases

residue material left in the oral, pharyngeal, or laryngeal cavity after the swallow

resistance quantity or property of opposition to electron movement (current) through a conductor (unit: ohm), which is equal to the voltage drop across an element divided by the current through the element; in general, a passive force opposing another active force

- **airway resistance** impeded flow of gases during ventilation because of turbulent flow or obstruction in the upper and/or lower airways

- **drug resistance** ability of pathogens to survive drugs that were previously toxic to the disease-causing agents; happens through spontaneous mutation or selective pressure after use of the specific drug

- **expiratory resistance** resistance to flow of expiratory phase of respiratory cycle

- **glottal resistance** resistance to flow at the glottis

- **nasal resistance** resistance to flow at the velopharyngeal aperture

resonance peak occurring at certain frequencies (resonance frequencies) in the vibration amplitude in a system that possesses compliance, inertia, and reflection; resonance occurs when the input and the reflected energy vibrate in phase; the resonances in the vocal tract are called formants

resonant frequencies frequency of stimulation to which a resonant system responds most vigorously

resonation modification of the vocal tone produced through changing the shape and size of the spaces in the vocal tract; clinically, the oral/nasal balance in voice quality

resonator for the voice, primarily the supraglottic vocal tract, which is responsible for timbre and projection

resonatory system the portion of the vocal tract through which the acoustical product of vocal fold vibration resonates; usually the oral, pharyngeal, and nasal cavities combined; sometimes only the nasal cavities and nasopharynx

resorb to absorb again

respiration the process of exchange of gas between an organism and its environment; also, the physiologic process of ventilating the body to inhale fresh air and exhale used air

- **abdominal respiration** breathing with the diaphragm providing the primary action

- **Cheyne-Stokes respiration** pattern with gradual depth and rate increase followed by a decrease leading to apnea

- **cycle of respiration** completion of both inspiration and expiration phases of respiration

- **respiration rate** number of cycles of respiration per minute

- **thoracic respiration** respiration powered mainly by muscles that raise the ribs, causing expansion of the chest

respiratory control center the part of the central nervous system that coordinates the control of respiration; the reticular formation in the brainstem mediates the automatic control of breathing, responding to specialized chemoreceptors

respiratory muscles any of the muscles involved in inhalation or exhalation, which include the diaphragm, the muscles of the rib cage (parasternal, internal and external intercostals, and scalene); the abdominal muscles (internal and external obliques, transversus abdominis, and rectus abdominis), and muscles of the upper airways, all of which are essential to maintain airway patency

- **auxiliary respiratory muscles** accessory muscles of breathing that assist in the expansion or compression of the rib cage by fixing, elevating, or depressing the ribs. They include muscles of the thoracic cavity, abdominal wall, and back. Contraction may allow for deep inhalation, forced exhalation, or performance of a Valsalva maneuver

respiratory physiology the study of function in respiration

respiratory tract the physical system involved in respiration, including the lungs, bronchial passageway, trachea, larynx, pharynx, and oral and nasal cavities

- **lower respirator tract** the portion of the respiratory tract that consists of the trachea and lungs

- **upper respiratory tract** the part of the respiratory tract that consists of the nasal and oral cavities, pharynx, and larynx

respirometer instrument for determining extent of respiratory movements and/or for detailing oxygen consumption or carbon dioxide production

respite care short-term care for home-based patients who typically are cared for by family, provided to allow family caregivers relief from constant patient care

response a reaction to a stimulus

- **auditory brainstem response (ABR)** also called BAER (brainstem auditory evoked response); an electrophysiologic record of the synchronous discharge of auditory nerve fibers in response to a click or brief tone burst. It is the most commonly available procedure for assisting in the diagnosis of hearing impairment in infants and young children. It can also be used to uncover hidden damage to the auditory nervous system

- **conditioned response** response reinforced though repeated connection to its natural stimulus

- **evoked response** change in the electrical activity in a nervous system area when an incoming sensory stimulus passes; can be somatosensory, auditory, or visual

- **frequency response** a function or functions that specify the relation between amplitude response and frequency characteristics, showing the manner in which the gain and phase of a system vary with the frequency of a stimulus

- **galvanic skin response (GSR)** emotional arousal change measure from electrodes attached to the skin that record real-time changes in perspiration and related autonomic nervous system activity

- **immune response** reaction to an antigen, such as antibody production, which can lead to evoked sensitivity

- **mode of response** manner or method of a response; includes imitation, oral reading, and conversational speech

R

- **off-response** a contraction that occurs with a latency period following the end of a stimulus. The off-contraction of esophageal smooth muscle, for example, is associated with depolarization of the muscle cells and the generation of spike potentials; also called off-contraction
- **pauser response** nerve response characterized by an initial on-response followed by silence, and subsequent low-level rate throughout stimulation
- **plantar response** reflex action of the toes when the sole of the foot is stimulated

response, neural

- **build-up response** neural responses characterized by slow increase in firing rate during the initial stages of firing
- **chopper response** neural responses characterized by periodic, chopped temporal pattern that is present throughout stimulation
- **onset response** neural response in which there is an initial burst of activity related to the onset of a stimulus, followed by silence
- **primary-like response** neural response patterns of brainstem fibers that have characteristics similar to those of the auditory nerve

resting lung volume the volume of air remaining within the lungs after quiet tidal expiration; also called expiratory reserve volume

resting membrane potential cells have membranes selective for the movement of charged particles across them and that separate charged particles and chemicals. The membranes have channels to selectively move some of these charged particles and to prevent the movement of other charged chemicals. The separation of potassium and sodium across a resting cell, such as a neuron or muscle cell, leads to voltage across the membrane labeled the resting membrane potential

resting potential voltage potential differences that can be measured from cells at rest

restoring force a force that returns an object to stable equilibrium

restrictive clause descriptive clause that is integral for the concrete meaning of the word it qualifies, as in: "that you wanted" in "the weather that you wanted is not in the cards"

restrictive ventilatory defect classification of respiratory pathology in which the patient's ability to fully inflate the lungs is diminished. May be due to neuromuscular diseases (causing respiratory muscle weakness), to defects in the thoracic spine, ribs, or pleura (causing a mechanical obstruction to lung inflation), or to fibrosis or surgical removal of the lungs

resuscitation restoration from potential or apparent death

- **cardiopulmonary resuscitation (CPR)** reestablishment of cardiac action and pulmonary ventilation by means of artificial respiration, along with closed-chest compression or open-chest heart massage
- **manual bagging** the process of supplying breaths by a manual resuscitation bag, often used to oxygenate a patient before attempting intubation or when a patient is temporarily disconnected from mechanical ventilation
- **mouth-to-mouth resuscitation** artificial ventilation of an overlap of patient's mouth (plus nose for infants and small children) with the mouth of the person doing the resuscitation blowing to inflate the patient's lungs in tandem with an unassisted expiratory phase; repeated 12 to 16 times a minute

reticulo-, reticul- combining form: netlike

reticular formation thick neuron cluster inside the brainstem, including the medulla that controls consciousness level, among other critical functions; areas in the formation constantly monitor body state for functioning of swallowing, stomach fluids, and facial movements, as well as tongue and eye action

retina the structure at the back of the eye of filmy nervous tissue membrane that is continuous with the optic nerve, receiving images of external material and transmitting visual impulses to the brain

retract to draw back, shorten

retro- prefix: backward, toward the rear

retroflex in phonetics, a backward turning or pointing of the tongue tip, as may occur in producing /r/

retrograde the direction of movement of an electrical signal (i.e., action potential) or chemicals in the reverse direction from the normal conduction of action potentials of the neuron. For a biological motor fiber, retrograde conduction would be movement of an action potential or chemical toward the cell body

retrograde amnesia a loss of memory (amnesia) for events that occurred before the brain injury or the neurologic disorder; contrasts with anterograde amnesia

return map similar to phase plane plot, but analyzed data must be digital. This graphic technique represents the relationship between a point and any subsequent point in a time series

reverberation persistence or prolongation of sound in an enclosed space, resulting from multiple reflections (echoes) of sound waves off hard surfaces after the source of the sound has ceased. Reverberation time (RT 60) is the time required for a steady-state sound to decay 60 dB from its initial peak amplitude offset

reversibility possibility that the subject and object phrase nouns could logically change places

Reynold's number (R) ratio of viscous and inertial forces in a fluid defined by the formula R=rVD/μ, where: r = density of fluid, μ = viscosity in centipoise (CP), V = velocity, and D=- inside diameter of pipe; nondimensional index of the development of turbulence; after Osborne Reynolds (1842–1912), English scientist

rheumatism one of many inflammatory conditions of the bursae, joints, ligaments, or muscles marked by pain, movement limitation, and degeneration

rheumatoid factor (RF) antiglobulin antibodies often found in the serum of sufferers from some kinds of rheumatism or arthritis or rheumatoid arthritis; also found in conjunction with such diseases as tuberculosis, leukemia, and connective tissue disorders

rhino-, rhin- combining form: pertaining to or resembling the nose

rhinoanemometer instrument that measures nasal airflow and nasal resistance to airflow

rhinorrhea liquid discharge from the nasal mucous membrane

rhinoscopy nasal cavity inspection

- **anterior rhinoscopy** with or without nasal speculum use, examination of the nasal cavity anterior portion

- **median rhinoscopy** looking at the roof of the nasal cavity and ethmoid and sinus openings employing a nasopharyngoscope or nasal speculum

- **posterior rhinoscopy** checking the nasopharynx with a rhinoscope or nasopharyngoscope

rhinosinusitis inflammation of the lining membrane of a paranasal sinus

rhinovirus large group of individual small ribonucleic acid viruses that cause more than one-third of acute respiratory illnesses

rhombencephalon embryonic division of the brain from which the pons, cerebellum, and medulla oblongata ultimately arise

rhythm the temporal or stress pattern of speech; intermittent replacement of strong and weak elements in the flow of speech

rich interpretation method analyzing children's utterances considering the linguistic and nonlinguistic context

right hemisphere impairment (RHI) a constellation of linguistic and extralinguistic deficits created by damage to the right cerebral hemisphere. May include impaired perception, visual field neglect, alterations in certain emotions, and reduced ability at tasks that require synthesis or inference

rima vestibuli space between the false (ventricular) vocal folds

Robin sequence disorder with association of a small lower jaw (micrognathia), wide U-shaped cleft palate, and upper airway obstruction; previously known as Pierre Robin syndrome

- **Robin deformation sequence** during gestation, the mandible is prevented from growing forward by some type of mechanical force

- **Robin malformation sequence** intrinsic to a developing baby, such malformation might be any that causes the mandible to be small or cause the tongue to interfere with palatal shelf growth

role playing treatment technique involving a form of dramatics in which an individual adopts the character of a real or imagined person to practice a desired behavior or to analyze a hypothetical situation

roll off characteristics of filters that specify their ability to shut off frequencies outside the pass band; for example, if a low pass filter is set to 2 kHz and has a roll off of 24 dB/octave, it will attenuate a 4 kHz tone by 24 dB and a 8 kHz tone by 48 dB

rollover effect paradoxic decrease in the performance-intensity function at high sound levels. A characteristic of retrocochlear hearing disorder

root lowest part of an organ that is within other tissues; in linguistic tree diagrams, a high-level node; a base form or point of origin

rostral beak-shaped

rostrum a beaked or hooked structure

rotation gyration of a bone around its center axis

- **external rotation** movement of an anterior surface turning outward; for example, when the long access of a bone (leg or arm) turns outward

- **internal rotation** movement of an anterior surface turning inward; for example, when the long access of a bone (leg or arm) turns inward

rotator muscle rotating a structure around its axis

rounding an articulatory description referring to the rounding (or protrusion) of the lips; applied to vowels, rounding is associated with a lowering of the frequencies of all formants

round window in the ear, the opening between the scala tympani of the inner ear and the middle ear space

-rrhea suffix: a flowing

ruga, rugae fold or crease of tissue

S

Sinus

cavity or passageway

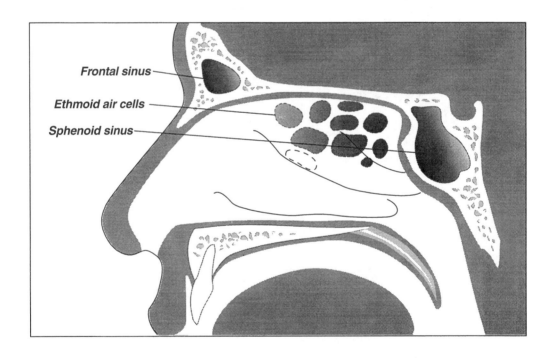

Frontal sinus

Ethmoid air cells

Sphenoid sinus

saccule sac or small bag

sacculus in the ear, smaller of the vestibular sensory mechanisms housed within the vestibule of the inner ear

sagittal an anatomic plane that divides the body into left and right sides

saliva fluid secreted within the mouth to lubricate the bolus for swallowing and to maintain moisture within the oral cavity; typically clear, slightly alkaline, and somewhat viscous

- **artificial saliva** an artificial, manufactured preparation of saliva containing glycoproteins and mucin

salivagram radionuclide study in which a small amount of saline with a high concentration radionuclide is placed on a child's tongue followed by scanning of the lungs with a gamma camera to look for radionuclide activity suggestive of aspiration

salivary flow normal flow of saliva from the parotid gland. Normal salivary flow is about 0.3–0.5 ml/min

sampling the process of making a series of measurements from a continuous (analog) signal

sampling rate the rate at which a signal or process is sampled; in digital processing of speech, the sampling rate specifies the intervals at which the analog waveform is converted to digital form

sampling theorem states that an analog signal waveform may be uniquely reconstructed without error from samples taken at equal time intervals. The sampling rate must be equal to, or greater than, twice the highest frequency component in the analog signal; also called Nyquist sampling theorum (for Harry Nyquist, 1889–1976)

saturation state of satiety; level at which an amplifier no longer provides an increase in output compared to input

saturation sound pressure level (SSPL) measure of the maximum hearing aid output—the point beyond which a hearing aid cannot amply

scaffolding approach teaching or coaching building on a student's repertoire of knowledge and understanding

scala media (cochlear duct) middle space of the cochlea created by the membranous labyrinth and containing the organ of Corti, bordered at the top by Reissner's membrane and at the bottom by the basilar membrane.

The major space in the scala media is filled with a fluid called endolymph, but the cells in the organ of Corti are protected from that fluid by a tight network called the reticular lamina. The cells of the organ of Corti are probably surrounded by perilymphatic fluid from the scala tympani

scalar real number and not a vector; quantity, such as mass or time, with a magnitude describable by a real number and no direction; also capable of being represented by a point on a scale

scala tympani division of the cochlear spiral canal situated on the basal side of the spiral lamina

scala vestibuli peripheral cavity of the cochlea that communicates with the middle ear via the vestibule and the oval window

scanning examining systematically and/or by point-to-point observation

- **AAC auditory scanning** whereby an AAC user activates his or her switch when he or she hears the desired item spoken

- **AAC circular scanning** the sequential presentation of symbol choices in a circular pattern

- **AAC directed scanning** a type of scanning in which an indicator moves for the length of time that a switch is pressed or activated

- **AAC group item scanning** scanning in which a cursor is moved to highlight groups of symbols, then single items in the selected groups. Row column scanning is an example of group item scanning—indicator stops at the selected item. Also called inverse scanning

- **AAC linear scanning** the sequential presentation of symbol choices, with a cursor highlighting one item or a set of items at a time in a line-by-line pattern

- **AAC multiple switch scanning** scanning using two or more switches

- **AAC predictive scanning** checking only potential symbol choices. On some devices, blank keys are not scanned. More sophisticated versions will only scan to symbols that are predicted based on previous selections

- **AAC row column scanning** this scanning method is commonly used with AAC systems. Quickly moves the cursor by first highlighting an entire row of symbols, then single symbols in the selected row

- **AAC scanning** an indirect method of AAC or computer access. The user makes choices through step-by-step switch activation. Usually employs a symbol array, a keyboard emulator, and one or more switches

- **AAC scanning patterns** the visual layout of pictures, symbols, or text and the manner in which the cursor indicator moves across patterns. Scanning patterns include linear, circular, and group item scanning

- **AAC scanning techniques** the methods by which an individual uses his or her switch to select a communication symbol. Scanning techniques include step scanning, automatic scanning, and directed scanning

- **AAC step linear scanning** a manual method of moving a cursor through a symbol array and selecting items. A user presses a switch to bring up the array. The user then presses and releases a switch to move the cursor across the array item-by-item. This process is repeated until the cursor reaches the desired item

- **AAC step scanning** technique in which an indicator moves to one item at a time each time a switch is activated

- **computed tomography (CT) scanning** specialized X-ray scan that produces thin (usually 10-mm thick) cross-sectional reconstructions of the body using computer back-projection techniques; also computerized axial tomography (CAT), a term that is mostly obsolete

- **functional magnetic resonance imaging (fMRI)** image of function is created from signals generated by the hemodynamics within the structure of interest, allowing observation of which body structures are active in specific functions; high-resolution images of neural activity are achieved through depictions of oxygen level and flow

- **helical computed tomography (CT)** scans produced by moving a patient at a constant rate through the bore of a CT scanner while the scanning tube is rotated around the patient. This produces a true volumetric dataset and allows standard transverse views, as well as images in any plane desired; also called spiral CT

- **magnetic resonance image (MRI) scanning** a highly sophisticated computerized X-ray imaging process that provides vivid pictorial details of internal hard and soft body tissues; a procedure used when attempting to specify the precise region, nature, and extent of an injury, anomaly, or anatomical feature

- **milk scanning** a radionuclide test for aspiration and gastroesophageal reflux (GER), with a small amount of radionuclide-labeled milk ingested by an infant being monitored

- **single-photon emission computed tomography (SPECT)** metabolic and physiological tissue function imaged by computer synthesis of single-energy photons emitted by radionuclides administered to the patient

- **spiral CT** synonymous with helical computed tomography scanning; scans produced by moving a patient at a constant rate through the bore of a CT scanner while the scanning tube is rotated around the patient. This produces a true volumetric dataset and allows standard transverse views, as well as images in any plane desired

- **trispiral tomography** allows a very thin and uniform focal plan, especially for inner ear visualization

- **ultrafast computed tomography** synonymous with fast CT scanning. A technique of CT scanning in which the X ray rapidly scans the patient in several planes; fast enough to freeze rapid motions such as occur in the oropharynx during swallowing

- **ultrafast magnetic resonance imaging (MRI)** scanning technique allowing rapid magnetic resonance imaging scans to be performed, with swallowing studies, among others, benefiting

scanning speech a speech pattern in which successive syllables tend to be separated in time and nearly equally stressed

scaphoid fossa in the ear, the region between the helix and antihelix, constituting a small elliptical depression above the pterygoid fossa on the pterygoid process of the sphenoid bone and providing attachment for the tensor veli palatini muscle origin

Schatzki's ring incomplete mucosal ring at the lower third of the esophagus, usually at the squamocolumnar junction. The upper surface of the ring is lined by squamous, esophageal epithelium, with the lower surface lined by columnar gastric epithelium. Typically accompanies chronic gastroesophageal reflux (GER) and may be associated with a hiatal hernia; also known as B ring

schema structured cluster of concepts and expectations; an abstract and generic knowledge structure stored in memory that preserves the relations among constituent concepts and generalized knowledge about a text, event, message, situation, or object

scheme   204   secondo passaggio

- **content or contextual schema** provides a generalized interpretation of the content of experience; organizes the facts and establishes a framework that imposes certain structures on events, precepts, situations, and objects, as well as facilitating interpretation

- **formal schema** linguistic form that organizes, integrates, and predicts relationships across propositions (e.g., additives [and, furthermore], adversative [although, nevertheless, however], causal [because, therefore, accordingly], disjunctive [but, instead, on the contrary], and temporal connectives [before, after, subsequently], as well as patterns of parallelism and correlative pairs [not only/but also; neither/nor])

scheme organized patterns of responding to stimuli

Schwann cells neural crest cells that make up a continuous wrapping (myelin) around peripheral nerve fibers

schwannoma, acoustic benign tumor of cranial nerve VIII that often grows in the auditory canal. Signs and symptoms produced in cerebellum, lower cranial nerve, and brainstem. Can cause tinnitus, progressive hearing loss, headache, dizziness, and unsteady gait, with later stage symptoms of paresis and speaking/swallowing difficulty; also know as as acoustic neuroma, acoustic fibroma, cerebellopontine angle tumor

Schwartz-Jampel syndrome tonic contractions of facial muscles, with progressive myotonia, skeletal dysplasia, and limited joint mobility; marked by later difficulty with articulation related to limited mouth movement and opening, accompanied by high-pitched voice and nasal resonance disorder secondary to progressive muscle contractions

science systematically organized and/or studied knowledge detailing collective truths or the functioning of general laws, particularly as gathered and tested through scientific method

scientific explanation identification and verification of the variables believed to cause an event to occur

scintigraphy images produced by a gamma camera recording the emissions of radionuclide energy from a patient; a radionuclide with an attraction to an organ to be studied is administered and the resulting radiation is recorded

- **gastroesophageal scintigraphy** radionuclide test for aspiration and gastroesophageal reflux (GER), with a small amount of radionuclide-labeled milk ingested by an infant being monitored; also called milkscan

scirrho-, sclero prefix: hard

scleroderma chronic thickening and hardening of the skin from collagen formation; part of a spectrum of connective tissue disorders that causes progressive fibrosis of the dermal layer of the skin, particularly of the face, hands, and feet

- **progressive systemic sclerosis (PSS)** autoimmune connective tissue disorder leading to progressive fibrosis of the dermal layer of the skin, of smooth muscle, or of other visceral tissues

-sclerosis combining form: hardening

sclerotherapy, variceal injections of sclerosing agents (hardeners) into dilated veins (varices) in the esophagus to stop or prevent bleeding

scolio- combining form: curved or twisted

scoliosis sideways twist to the spine

screening the use of tests that are quick and easy to administer to a large group to identify individuals who require further diagnostic testing

script a presumed mental representation of repeatedly occurring, sequenced events, episodes, or personal experiences; used in teaching advanced language skills including narrative skills; a description of baking cookies, or plan for running a hot dog stand is each a script; there needs to be a beginning and an end; actions people take or roles people play

sebaceous gland gland type found all over the body producing sebum that supplies the skin with oil

secondary reinforcer stimulus that gains reinforcing potential through association with primary reinforcers

second language extension an option in a secondary school, with the second language allotted extra time on the curriculum. Other students choose different subject options or more time on their first language

second language learning learning of a second language (L2) by an adult who was previously exposed only to a single language (L1)

secondo passaggio in music, "second passage"; the second register change perceived in a voice

secretin digestive polypeptide that functions as a hormone secreted by the duodenum to affect the pancreas and as a neurotransmitter in many regions of the CNS and enteric nervous system

sedative-hypnotic drug that depresses the central nervous system (CNS); includes barbiturates and benzodiazepines

seeing essential English (SEE) manual communication system that incorporates some signs of American Sign Language and some English syntax

segment an identifiable sound within a sequence of sounds that form a word; a phonetic or phonemic unit

segmental divided into segments; referring to the spinal cord; referring to phonetic elements of speech

segmentals speech sounds; as opposed to suprasegmental aspects of speech

segmentation the delineation of successive sound segments in a speech signal. Typically, segmentation yields units such as phonemes, allophones, or some other phonetic segment. Also, parsing spoken language into its constituent and successive segments; parsing sentences, words, or syllables into their constituent phonetic units

seizure sudden episode of uncontrolled electrical activity in the brain. If the abnormal electrical activity spreads throughout the brain, the result may be a loss of consciousness. One symptom of a seizure is convulsion, or twitching and jerking of the limbs. Seizures may occur as the result of head injury, infection, cerebrovascular accidents, withdrawal from sedative-hypnotic drugs, or high doses of stimulants (note grand mal, petit mal, and so on are being phased out)

- **absence seizure** brief loss of consciousness or slowing of thought processes sometimes accompanied by clonic movements; once termed petit mal seizure; an obsolete term

- **generalized tonic-clonic seizure** sudden onset of muscle contraction, often with cry or moan and a fall to the ground, giving way to clonic convulsive movements; contemporary nomenclature for the obsolete grand mal seizure label

selection restrictions constraints on words that can occur together because of the semantic features carried by each

selective enhancement relative benefit of auditory signal arising from resonance of the auditory mechanism

selective (focused) attention ability to focus on relevant stimuli while ignoring simultaneously presented, but irrelevant stimuli (i.e., distractors)

Self Help for Hard of Hearing People (SHHH) national organization for adults who have hearing loss

self-help groups general term for community-based organizations in which patients and caregivers share coping skills and mutual support for a variety of conditions

self-talk language-stimulation technique in which an adult describes what he or she is doing

semantics study of meanings: pertaining to both the surface and the underlying meaning of a language

- **convergent semantic production** ability to identify a topic based on inferences from associated words

- **divergent semantic production** ability to produce a diverse collection of words based on their association with a topic

- **lexical-semantic processes** language processes that deal with storage and use of word meanings

- **semantic complexity** measures the complexity of a linguistic structure by gauging the number of semantic relationships that must be discriminated to use the structure correctly

- **semantic features** perceptual features such as size, shape, color, and so on that define a conceptual class

- **semantic memory** individual's understanding of a word's meaning, including the words and concepts the person associates with that word

- **semantic network** pattern of associated words and concepts that evolve out of knowing a word. Also, a construct representing a mental system of nodes and links connecting lexical units; vocabulary building in such a network involves adding new nodes and links, as well as changing activation values of the links between nodes (e.g., building synonyms by strengthening the relationships between nodes)

- **semantic-syntactic rules** describes children's early grammar, emphasizing that expressing meaning provides the motivation for attempting to learn correct forms

s

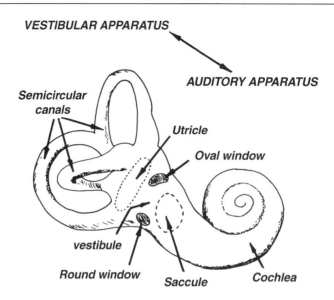

VESTIBULAR APPARATUS

AUDITORY APPARATUS

Semicircular canals

Utricle

Oval window

vestibule

Round window   *Saccule*   *Cochlea*

semicircular canals canals of the vestibular system, responsible for sensation of movement of the head in space. Also, three fluid-filled bony loops in the inner ear that contain fluid and contribute to maintaining balance

---

semi- prefix: half

semicircular canals canals of the vestibular system, responsible for sensation of movement of the head in space. Also, three fluid-filled bony loops in the inner ear that contain fluid and contribute to maintaining balance

- **lamina of semicircular duct** connective tissue between the ear's semicircular duct and the bony semicircular canal, enclosing the perilymph

- **lateral semicircular canal** the more horizontally placed semicircular canal that senses movement in the transverse plane of the body

sender individual who delivers a message, as opposed to a receiver

senile characteristic of old age

sensation the initial stage of perception, in which sense organs are affected by a physical stimulus; conversion effects of a stimulus exciting a sense organ into consciousness

sensation level (SL) the intensity level of a sound in dB expressed in relationship to an individual's threshold for the sound

sensitivity ability to feel through at least one sense; proportion of individuals screened with a positive test result for a disease a particular test is intended to search out

sensorimotor stage, Piaget's stages of cognitive development the earliest of Piaget's cognitive stages from birth to 2 years of age during which the child progresses from reflexive to voluntary behavior; intelligence is evidenced through motor activity without symbol use until very end of stage

sensorineural deafness, hearing loss deafness from disorders of the cochlear division of CN VIII, the cochlea, or the retrocochlear nerve tracts; loss that can be identified as mild, moderate, severe, or profound; measured in decibels

sensory having to do with the feeling or detection of other nonmotor input. For example, nerves responsible for touch, proprioception (position in space), hearing, and so on

sensory association area the cortical areas that assist in interpreting sensations

sensory neuron (fiber) a neuron that consists of a long dendritic process that extends from the cell body to its target organ and an axon that synapses on an interneuron within the central nervous system. The cell body of the neuron usually resides within central nervous system locations such as the dorsal horn of the spinal cord, the nucleus tractus solitarius, or the trigeminal sensory nuclei. The sensory fiber can end directly within the target organ or synapse and innervate a receptor organ (i.e., muscle spindle) within the tissue

sensory strip the postcentral gyrus of the parietal lobe, associated with somatosensory function (Brodmann areas 1, 2, and 3)

sentence a group of words that includes a subject and a predicate and is syntactically complete that is an assertion, question, command, wish, or exclamation that in writing usually begins with an uppercase letter and ends with appropriate closing punctuation and that in speaking is characterized by distinguishing patterns of stress, pitch, and pauses

- **complex sentence** a sentence composed of a main clause and an embedded subordinate clause

- **hierarchical sentence structure** the levels of constituent structures that relate the words and phrases of a sentence to its underlying structure

- **matrix sentence** a form of a sentence before embedding or after embedded aspects have been removed

- **passive sentence** a major sentence type in which the grammatical subject of the sentence is the passive recipient of the action in the verb

- **surface structure** the actualized production of a sentence by a speaker

sepsis infection spread from first site and into the bloodstream; initial infection is commonly from bacteria, but sepsis also occurs with fungal, parasitic, and mycobacterial infections, particularly in patients with compromised immune systems

septectomy surgical correction of a deviated nasal septum

septum a divider, partition, or wall

sequence term for constellation of developmental/health anomalies, in which each is derived sequentially from another anomaly or structural disorder; a single malformation, deformation, or disruption can secondarily cause other anomalies

- **Robin sequence** disorder with association of a small lower jaw (micrognathia), wide U-shaped cleft palate, and upper airway obstruction

sequence pattern syntactic device associated with text grammar that signals the description of a sequence of events or steps

sequences (or chaining) early narratives that relate heaps of elements that are related to a central topic

serotonin biogenic amine neurotransmitter that is a naturally occurring tryptophan derivative and that acts as a vasoconstrictor that stimulates smooth muscle and inhibits gastric secretion. Somewhat highly concentrated in the CNS basal ganglia and hypothalamus

set a number of similar things that are used together or that belong with one another

- **closed set** a stimulus or response set that contains a fixed number of items that are known to a patient

- **limited set** the response items in a stimulus or response set are limited by situational or contextual cues, for example, words related to summer

- **open set** a stimulus or response set that has no prior restrictions on its members

setting narrative characters, location, and circumstances

setting events the collection of stimuli present in a setting that are capable of influencing behavior

sex chromosome single pair of chromosomes responsible for sex determination. Females have two identical X chromosomes, whereas males have an X and Y chromosome (the Y chromosome's purpose is to reproduce the male phenotype)

shadowing treatment technique in which a speaker repeats the verbalizations of a model one or two syllables behind the model; a training experience in which a novice accompanies and observes a specialist

shaken baby syndrome child abuse characterized by whiplash-type intracranial injuries and long bone fractures; physical features often are not readily visible so that syndrome can be difficult to detect. A syndrome of child abuse characterized by intracranial injuries and long bone fractures; physical features often are not readily visible so that syndrome can be difficult to detect; parent-infant traumatic stress syndrome.

shaping gradual modification of a behavior, with variations progressively approximating a goal

shearing action in hearing, the bending action of the ear's hair cells arising from the relative movement of the basilar membrane and tectorial membrane during auditory stimulation

sheltered English content classrooms that provide support for English language development. The teacher uses English that is comprehensible by students (likely ESL), with course content at typical grade-level

S

shimmer index of instability in the laryngeal waveform, usually measured as variation in the amplitude of successive glottal cycles

shimmer percentage is the same as shimmer dB, but expressed in percentage instead of decibels. Both are relative evaluations of the same type of amplitude perturbation

short-bowel syndrome loss or resection of portions of small intestine resulting in malabsorption

short syndrome small stature, deficient subcutaneous fat, delayed dental eruption; speech onset can be delayed, with abnormal dental eruption pattern leading to articulation distortion, and an expressive language delay

short vowels vowels with an inherently short duration; [ɪ], [o], [ʊ]

Shprintzen-Goldberg syndrome craniosynostosis, micrognathia, contractures, cognitive impairment, hypertrophy of palate, airway obstruction; cognitive impairment can lead to severely delayed speech, with misarticulations secondary to malocclusion and hypertrophic soft tissue of the hard palate; cognitive impairment can also lead to severe expressive language delay and impairment

Shprintzen syndrome cleft palate, heart anomalies, learning disabilities, and ADHD; usually accompanied by delayed speech production onset, with global glottal stop substitutions in conjunction with clefts or VPI

shunt a diverter or bypass (generally tube) to collect fluid unwanted in one anatomical area and direct it to another area

sialometry salivary secretion function measurement

sicca syndrome, Sjögren syndrome dryness of the mucous membranes in head and neck from atrophy of the lacrimal and salivary glands. Tongue may be sore, coated, and fissured. Inability to produce tears leads to conjunctivitis, inability to produce saliva leads to inability to swallow dry food. Sjögren syndrome includes gland atrophy caused by autoimmune disease, including rheumatoid arthritis and lupus. Gland destruction or malfunction also occurs from radiation, excision, dehydration, and drugs

sickle cell anemia severe chronic autosomal recessive disorder most frequently seen in African American and Mediterranean populations that produces a form of hemoglobin that does not bind well with oxygen; red blood cells have a sickle; a leading cause of childhood stroke

signal, analog continuous variations in amplitude. The radiated sound-pressure waveform of speech is an analog signal, because its amplitude varies continuously in time

signal, common mode a signal or signal component presented to both inputs in a bipolar EMG electrode array, or to both inputs of a differential amplifier

signal duration perceptual correlate of signal length

signal length the length of a signal is determined by a physical measurement of the span of time occupied by the signal

signal processing manipulation of various parameters of a signal

signal-to-noise ratio (S/N) a measure of the ratio between signal energy and noise energy. In speech analysis, S/N usually is the periodic energy relative to noise energy. It is also the relationship between the sound levels of the signal and the noise at a listener's ear, commonly reported as the difference in decibels between the intensity of the signal and the intensity of the background noise (e.g., if the speech signal is measured at 70 dB and the noise is 64 dB, the signal-to-noise ratio is +6 dB)

signed English manual communication system that utilizes English word order and syntax

signing language for deaf people using hand movements

signing exact English (SEE2) a simplified version of Seeing Essential English

sign language system of manual communication in which hand configurations, positions, and movements are used to express concepts and linguistic information

silent period the temporary cessation of ongoing bioelectric (most often EMG) activity; for example, as a reflex inhibitory effect

silica gel agent that absorbs moisture, often used to store hearing aids

simian crease a single transverse palmar crease (as opposed to the more typical pattern of two incomplete palmar creases); seen especially in Down syndrome as a minor dysmorphology, but also occurs in some individuals without known disabilities or disorders

simile figurative language that directly states an analogous comparison of two unlike items, often joined by "like" or "as" (e.g., He's as clumsy as an ox!)

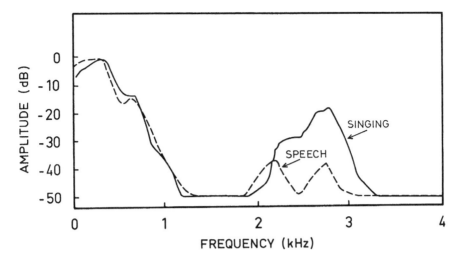

singer's formant   a high spectrum peak occurring between about 2.3 and 3.5 kHz in voiced sounds in Western opera and concert singing. This acoustic phenomenon is associated with "ring" in a voice and with a voice's capacity to project over background sound, such as a choir or an orchestra; a similar phenomenon of speaking voice, especially in actors, is the speaker's formant

Simpson-Golabi-Behmel syndrome cleft palate, cognitive deficiency, macrencephaly; delayed speech production onset secondary to cognitive impairment and misarticulation from poor oral motor coordination, along with possible compensatory articulation secondary to cleft palate; language can be delayed and impaired from cognitive deficiency

simultaneous communication educational approach used with individuals with severe and profound hearing loss that integrates aural/oral communication and manual communication; total communication

singer's formant a high spectrum peak occurring between about 2.3 and 3.5 kHz in voiced sounds in Western opera and concert singing. This acoustic phenomenon is associated with "ring" in a voice and with a voice's capacity to project over background sound, such as a choir or an orchestra; a similar phenomenon of speaking voice, especially in actors, is the speaker's formant

singing teacher professional who teaches singing technique (as opposed to voice coach)

singing voice specialist a singing teacher with additional training, and specialization in working with injured voices, in conjunction with a medical voice team

single-photon emission computed tomography (SPECT) metabolic and physio-logical tissue function imaged by computer synthesis of single-energy photons emitted by radionuclides administered to the patient

single-subject experimental design research design in which an individual subject serves as his or her own control

sinistro- combining form: left or left side

sinus a cavity or passageway

- **ethmoidal sinuses** air cells of the mucous membrane of the superior and middle meatuses of the nasal cavity sinuses

- **frontal sinus** air cell in the frontal bone of the cranium

- **paranasal sinuses** sets of dual air-filled passages in facial bones lined with mucous membrane and connected to the nasal cavity; frontal, sphenoidal, maxillary, and ethmoidal sinuses

- **pyriform sinus** pouch or cavity constituting the lower end of the nasopharynx located to the side and partially to the back of the larynx; typically there are paired sinuses

- **sinus of Morgagni** often confused with ventricle of Morgagni. Actually, the sinus of Morgagni is not in the larynx. It is formed by the superior fibers of the superior pharyngeal constrictor as they curve below the levator veli palatini and the eustachian tube. The space between the upper border of the mus-

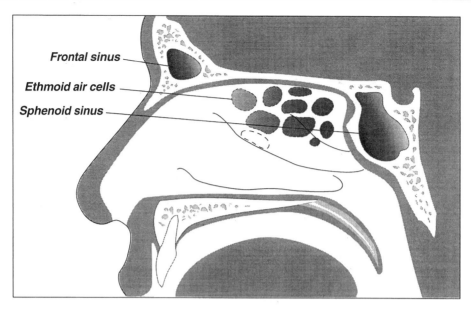

sinus   a cavity or passageway

cle and the base of the skull is known as the sinus of Morgagni and is closed by the pharyngeal aponeurosis

- **sphenoid sinus** air cell in the sphenoid bone

sinusitis infection of the mucous membrane of a sinus, especially the paranasal sinus cavities

sinusoid a graph representing the sine or cosine of a constantly increasing angle; in mechanics, the smoothest and simplest back-and-forth movement, characterized by a single frequency, an amplitude, and a phase; tone arising from sinusoidal sound pressure variations

sinusoidal motion the projection of circular motion (in a plane) at constant speed onto one axis in the plane; also called simple harmonic motion

situation-specific knowledge information gained by repeating experiences, which helps one predict what is likely to happen next in an ongoing situation and this, in turn, aids perception

situs invertus viscerum transposition of the viscera, as in the heart developing on the right side of the body or the liver on the left side

Sjögren-Larsson syndrome severe skin dryness and scaling, cognitive deficiency, spasticity; marked by delayed speech and language onset, along with dysarthria

skeleton bony structure of vertebrate body

skill behavior sequence learned through motor and sensory system coordination

skilled nursing facility/care long-term institutionalized care that provides continuous nursing and medical personnel; often for those with chronic injury or disability who need moderate to maximal assistance

skin protective membranous covering of the body

skull all bones of the head, especially the bony casing that houses the brain

sleep apnea a periodic cessation of breathing during sleep, often related to airway collapse from weakness of pharyngeal muscles. Symptoms include irregular breathing and loud snoring during sleep and excessive daytime sleepiness

small for gestational age (SGA) low birth weight of less than 2500 grams and weight below the 10th percentile for gestational age

social behavior behavior in relation to other persons that influences their behavior

social-cognitive theory learning theory that attributes behavior change to the meaning a person gives to situations, with behavior and learning linked to the meaning of circumstances and individuals having the ability to modify meanings through cognition; among social-cognitive learning variables are encoding strategies, personal constructs, expectancies, and self-regulatory systems and planning

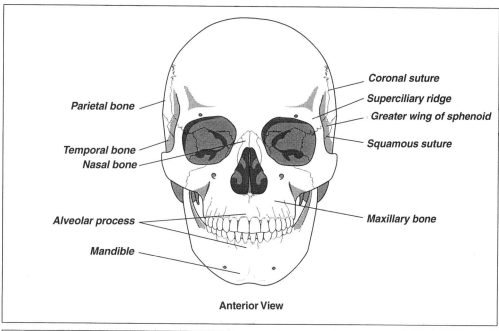

Anterior View

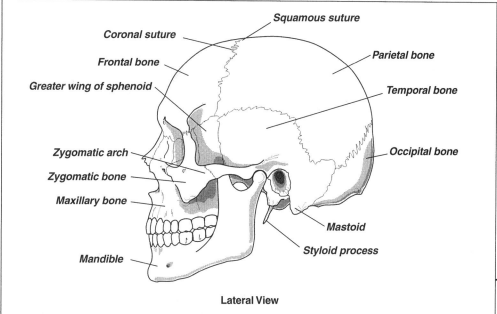

Lateral View

skull   all bones of the head, especially the bony casing that houses the brain

social context the nature of a setting and the status, roles, and agendas of the speakers in that setting

social interaction interchanges between at least two persons in which the behavior of one affects the other

social reinforcers a variety of conditioned reinforcers frequently used in treatment sessions, including verbal praise, attention, touch, eye contact, and facial expressions; such reinforcers are resistant to satiation effect; may not work with nonverbal clients

social smile a smile in response to another person's presence or behavior

sociolinguistics linguistics branch that studies the comparative interrelationship of language and society by examining language in everyday life; based on premise that language use symbolically reflects basic dimensions of social behavior and human interaction

sodium pump mechanism for transfer of sodium ions across cell membranes; current of positive ions moving into a cell leads to an action potential across the cell membrane; sometimes called sodium-potassium pump to recognize movement of both types of ion

soft glottal attack gentle glottal approximation, often obtained using an imaginary /h/

software programs that run on computers. Software (computer instructions specified by a programmer) is opposed to hardware (the electronic components of a computer). A related term is firmware, which denotes programs that are not intended to be changed

solid without an internal cavity; not liquid or gaseous

soma cell body; human body as differentiated from psyche or mind

somatic, -somatia-, somato- pertaining to the body

somatodyspraxia impediment in capability to plan nonhabitual skilled motor movements; awkwardness with new tasks

somatosensory evoked potential (SEP) evoked potential invoked by periodic stimulation of the touch and pain systems; employed during surgery to monitor neurologic function

somatosensory system nervous system aspects that accept and evaluate sensory information from the joints, ligaments, muscles, and skin

somesthetic pertaining to awareness of body sensation

somnolence sleepiness, drowsiness

sonorant consonant a consonant produced with a narrowing of the vocal tract, but with no pressure build-up behind the narrowing

sonority a concept that grades speech sounds according to their loudness, energy, or openness of the vocal tract

soprano uppermost (highest) singing voice

- **dramatic soprano** soprano with powerful, rich voice suitable for dramatic, heavily orchestrated operatic roles. Sings at least to C^6

- **lyric soprano** soprano with flexible, light vocal quality, but one who does not sing as high as a coloratura soprano

- **mezzo soprano** half soprano; common female range, higher than contralto but lower than soprano

- **soprano acuto** high soprano

- **soprano assoluto** a soprano who is able to sing all soprano roles and classifications

Sotos syndrome large stature, cognitive impairment, hypotonia, behavioral disturbances; marked by delayed speech onset secondary to hypotonia and developmental delay and articulation distortion from abnormal dental spacing

sound energy transmitted by longitudinal pressure waves in an elastic medium (such as air); although often considered to be what is heard by the hearing sense, sound exists without being heard: A tree falling in an unpopulated forest makes a sound

- **adventitious sound** may accompany typical breathing sounds, but not easily heard, such as wheezes, crackles, and gurgles

- **complex sound** a combination of sinusoidal waveforms superimposed on each other. May be complex periodic sound (such as musical instruments) or complex aperiodic sound (such as random street noise)

- **sound level** logarithmic, comparative measure of the intensity of a signal; the unit is dB

- **sound source** the generation of sound energy somewhere within the vocal tract, usually by narrowing of the airway; the larynx as source of voiced sound

- **sound spectrum** a graphic display, with frequency on the horizontal axis and amplitude on the vertical axis

- **sound wave** the acoustical manifestation of physical disturbance in a medium

sound field a free-field environment where sound waves are propagated

sound field testing determination of hearing sensitivity or speech recognition ability with stimuli presented through loudspeakers; often used in pediatric testing or hearing-aid evaluations

sound level meter an instrument designed to measure the intensity of sound in dB according to an accepted standard

sound pressure level (SPL) measure of the intensity of a sound, ordinarily in dB relative to 0.0002 microbar (millionths of 1 atmosphere pressure)

- **saturation sound pressure level 90** SSPL90; electroacoustic assessment of a hearing aid's maximum level of output signal, ex-

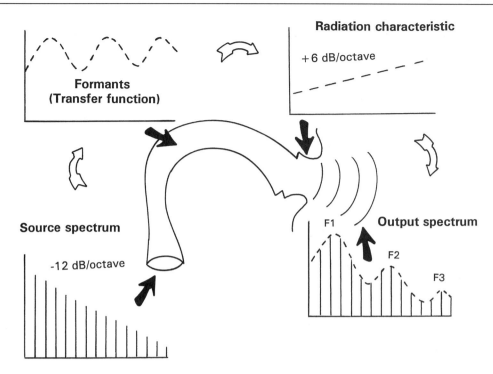

source-filter theory a theory of the acoustic production of speech that states that the energy from a sound source is modified by a filter or set of filters. For example, for vowels, the vibrating vocal folds usually are the source of sound energy and the vocal tract resonances (formants) are the filters

pressed as a frequency response curve to a 90-dB signal, with the hearing aid volume control set to full-on

soundproof impenetrable by acoustic energy

source-filter theory a theory of the acoustic production of speech that states that the energy from a sound source is modified by a filter or set of filters. For example, for vowels, the vibrating vocal folds usually are the source of sound energy and the vocal tract resonances (formants) are the filters

- **radiation characteristic** in source-filter theory, radiation of sound from the lips to the atmosphere; typically expressed as a 6-dB per octave increase in sound energy (hence, a high-pass filter)

source spectrum spectrum of the voice source

spasm a sudden, involuntary contraction of a muscle, muscle fibers, or a hollow organ (such as esophagus, colon, or artery); often associated with pain and dysfunction

- **bronchospasm** reflex constriction of the airways in response to a variety of stimuli, often associated with cough, wheezing, and mucus production

- **esophageal spasm** sudden dysphagia (inability to swallow), often in conjunction with a sense of chest constriction. It is characterized by intense dyspnea and occurs in croup, laryngeal ulceration, whooping cough, and laryngeal crises of locomotor ataxia; can also be caused by lodging of foreign bodies in the larynx and when aneurysms or mediastinal tumors press and irritate the recurrent laryngeal nerve

- **laryngospasm** involuntary muscular contraction of the larynx. This usually includes tight closure of the glottis and may occur during a procedure such as a fiberoptic examination of the larynx if the scope touches the false vocal folds, arytenoid cartilages, or true vocal folds

- **vasospasm** a brief abnormal constriction of a blood vessel

spastic dysarthria a type of motor speech disorder resulting from bilateral damage to the upper motor neuron (direct and indirect motor pathways) resulting in weakness, spastic paralysis, limited range of movement, and slowness of movement; may affect all aspects of speech and usually is not confined to only one aspect. Major

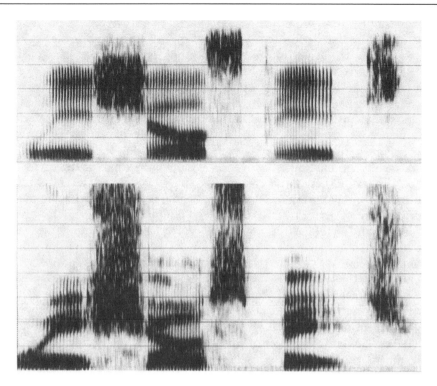

spectrogram   pattern for sound analysis containing information on intensity, frequency, and time; typically provides a three-dimensional display of time on the horizontal axis, frequency on the vertical axis, and intensity on the gray scale

speech problems include strained-strangled-harsh voice, hypernasality, slow rate, consonant imprecision, monopitch; and monoloudness

spasticity   condition usually associated with stroke or spinal cord disease in which stretch reflexes are exaggerated and may even occur spontaneously, producing involuntary muscle contractions

spatiotopic   the physical array of many of the regions of the cerebral cortex that defines the specific region of the body represented (e.g., the pre- and postcentral gyri)

speaking valve, one-way   a one-way valve placed on the hub of a tracheostomy tube to allow air to enter on inspiration. On expiration, the valve closes and air cannot escape the tracheostomy tube. Rather, the trapped air is redirected through the vocal folds and into the upper airway to be used for speaking and swallowing

specificity   the fraction of subjects without a condition that test negative for that condition; also known as the true negative rate; TN/(TN+FP), where TN is the number of true negatives and FP is the number of false positives

specific language impairment (SLI)   inability to use language to meet the requirements of most communication environments that often has no known cause, with common known causes including hearing impairment, traumatic brain injury, mental retardation, and other neurological or cognitive functioning impairment

spectral analysis   analysis of an acoustic signal to determine the relative magnitude of individual frequency components

spectrogram   pattern for sound analysis containing information on intensity, frequency, and time; typically provides a three-dimensional display of time on the horizontal axis, frequency on the vertical axis, and intensity on the gray scale

- **neural spectrogram**   the transformation of an incoming speech signal to a neural signal by the auditory system; the transformation is thought to produce a neural version of the frequency-over-time information that can be seen in a speech spectrogram

spectrograph   a machine used to create a frequency-over-time analysis of speech

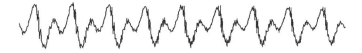

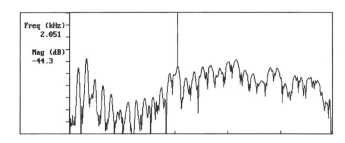

spectrum a graph showing the distribution of signal energy as a function of frequency; a plot of intensity by frequency; also known as Fourier spectrum or LPC spectrum depending on method of analysis

---

spectrographic analysis frequency-over-time analysis of the information in speech which is provided by a sound spectrograph

spectrum a graph showing the distribution of signal energy as a function of frequency; a plot of intensity by frequency; also known as Fourier spectrum or LPC spectrum depending on method of analysis

spectrum analysis analysis of a signal showing its partials

speculum retractor used to separate sides of a cavity to examine orifices and canals

speech dynamic production of voice sounds for communication through the processes of respiration, phonation, resonation, and articulation

- **altered speech** human speech that is recorded and then altered in some manner

- **buccal speech** produced from air trapped inside cheeks that can be called "Donald Duck speech." Can be used to produce words and short phrases following tracheostomy

- **caretaker speech** a simplified language used by parents to children to ensure understanding

- **child directed speech (CDS) (also motherese, parentese, or babytalk)** characteristic speech directed to toddlers and preschoolers by caregivers

- **choral/unison speech** a treatment technique consisting of the client speaking simultaneously with one (unison) or more (choral) speakers

- **clear speech** speech in which the speaker makes an effort to be easily understood; compared to ordinary conversational speech, it is often slower (with longer pauses between words and lengthening of some speech sounds), more apt to avoid modified or reduced forms of consonant and vowel segments, and characterized by a greater intensity of obstruent sounds, particularly stop consonants

- **compressed speech** speech that has had segments removed and then compressed and yet maintains intact frequency composition

- **cued speech** a system for making all the sounds of speech visible. In English it utilizes eight handshapes, placed in four different locations around the face, to remove any ambiguity about what is seen and heard by the person with a hearing impairment. Invented by physicist R. Orin Cornett, Ph.D., of Gallaudet College, it requires only cues to ensure one-time communication. Two of its special strengths are, first, that it allows virtually everything to be discussed as it happens around a child with hearing impairment and thus allows the child to learn much more language than is formally taught. Second, it supports a high likelihood that a child who uses it will be a fluent reader. It has been adapted for use in 53 languages and major dialects

- **digitized speech** storage of a real person's actual words and sentences in the form of digitized sounds that are recorded by a peripheral device that converts sound input from a stereo system, an instrument, or a microphone into a form that a computer can process, store, and play back as speech synthesis

- **esophageal speech** for persons following laryngectomy and vocal fold excision, speech is produced by taking air in through the mouth, trapping it in the throat, and suddenly releasing the air; upper parts of the throat/esophagus vibrate and produce sound in the air release; sound is shaped with lips, tongue, teeth, and other mouth parts in a manner similar to the presurgical method

- **expanded speech** recorded speech altered by duplicating small segments of the signal so that the speech sounds as if it were produced with a slow speaking rate; no additional spectral information is introduced

- **filtered speech** speech that has been passed through filter banks to remove or amplify frequency bands in the signal

- **fluent speech** characterized by the continuity or blending of words within phrases and a rapid rate that in adults is about 15 sounds per second

- **low-pass filtered speech** speech that has been passed through filter banks, leaving the lower, but not the higher, frequencies

- **rate variability** when speech is produced at different rates, the physical characteristics of individual phonetic units vary and the phonetic boundary between two categories is shifted, making it impossible to specify an absolute physical value for a phonetic unit present in the signal regardless of the rate of speech

- **real-time speech** the transitory, ephemeral nature of an ongoing speech signal; when speech is presented in a real-time manner, listeners must quickly recognize phonemes, syllables, and words based on preceding linguistic-contextual cues and ongoing acoustic-phonetic information

- **slurred speech** a sign of depressant intoxication; sometimes used to describe dysarthria

- **socialized speech** speech that is addressed to others and acknowledges their needs and interests

- **tracheoesophageal speech** speech facilitated by voice prostheses, which are devices employed following laryngectomy and vocal fold excision to enable speech production; most commonly, a surgical passage called a tracheoesophageal puncture (TEP) is created inside the stoma from the back wall of the trachea into the esophagus, with a valved tube enabling tracheoesophageal speech

speech act the concept of a unit of communication involving a speaker's intention, the linguistic form of the message conveying the intention, and the listener's interpretation of the message

- **direct speech act** a speech act in which the intention is expressed directly in the grammatical form of the utterance

- **illocutionary speech act** the component of a speech act that includes the outcome or effect intended by a speaker

- **indirect speech act** a speech act in which the speaker's intention is implied rather than expressed

- **performative speech act** speech act in which the utterance, itself, performs the intended act, such as promising, teasing, and apologizing

- **perlocutionary speech act** the component of a speech act consisting of the effect of the act on a listener

- **primitive speech acts** Dore's classification of intentions expressed by infants and toddlers through characteristic gestures and vocalizations

speech areas, motor cerebral hemisphere regions associated with motor control of speech

speech audiometry measurement of speech listening skills, including speech awareness and speech recognition

speech community collection of individuals who learn, share, and employ a particular set of linguistic codes that represent the universe of meanings characteristic of their particular culture

speech discrimination ability to distinguish meaningful differences between speech sounds

speech-language pathologist (SLP) professionals educated in the study of human communication, its development, and its disorders. By evaluating the speech, language, cognitive-communication, and swallowing skills of children and adults, the speech-language pathologist determines what communication or swallowing problems exist and the best way to treat them (source American Speech-Language Hearing Association, 1999, http://www.asha.org)

speech-language pathology specialty and academic discipline devoted to the study of the development, disorders, and differences of human communication

speech mode concept that speech is perceived in a special mode, unlike means employed to perceive nonspeech signals

speech perception the process by which a listener uses auditory (and sometimes visual) information to reach decisions about the phonetic structure and lexical composition of an utterance. Theories of speech perception vary in their assumptions about the size of the decision unit, basic strategy of analysis, and reliance on higher order linguistic information.

- **basic unit of speech perception** aspect of speech perception selected for analysis—can be either the phonetic feature, the phoneme, the syllable, or the word
- **categorical perception** the observation that listeners hear classes of similar sounds within a continuous range of sounds
- **cohort** a set of words that have a common initial sound sequence; the entire set presumably is activated until one word is selected
- **cross-modal speech perception** the perception of speech through two modalities, such as audition and vision, as in lipreading
- **cycling** in speech perception training, returning to a training objective that has been achieved with some success to provide reinforcement and additional skill
- **discrimination** ability to distinguish one stimulus from another
- **logogen** in speech perception, a theoretical passive sensing device associated with each word in a mental lexicon. Activation of a logogen is the means to recognition of a particular word
- **native language magnet (NLM) theory** theory of the development of speech perception in the first year of life that accounts for the change from a language-general mode of speech perception to one that is language-specific

speechreading speech recognition using auditory and visual cues

- **speechreading enhancement** the difference or ratio between speech recognition performance in an audition-only condition and an audition-plus-vision condition

speech recognition the ability to perceive and identify speech units

- **automatic speech recognition** (also called machine speech recognition) the recognition of speech by machine
- **equivalent lists** in speech recognition testing, test lists that contain items that are presumed to be equally difficult to recognize
- **error rate** in automatic speech recognition, the accuracy of speech recognition, typically expressed as the percentage of words correctly identified
- **live-voice testing** stimuli in a test of speech recognition are presented by a talker in real time
- **machine speech recognition** (also called automatic speech recognition) the recognition of speech by a machine, especially a computer. Most of these systems attempt to determine the phonetic sequences or words of an input signal
- **sound field testing** determination of hearing sensitivity or speech recognition ability with the stimuli presented through loudspeakers, often used in pediatric testing or hearing aid evaluations
- **speechreading** speech recognition using auditory and visual cues
- **speech reception threshold (SRT)** speech recognition threshold level, which is the lowest recognition level for spondee words at which 50% can be identified correctly
- **verbal auditory closure** the ability to use spoken contextual information to facilitate speech recognition

speech segmentation the separation of speech into units (such as phonemes, syllables, or words) that can be analyzed perceptually or instrumentally

speech synthesis the production of speech by artificial means; especially the generation of speech by computers or computer-controlled devices

speech variability individual units of speech (phonemes, words) are produced differently by different individuals, differently when produced in different phonetic contexts, and differently when produced at various rates of speech; each of these factors is responsible for the extreme acoustic variability observed in speech; acoustic variance for phonetic segments

speed the rate of change of distance with time; magnitude of velocity without regard for direction

spheroid shaped like a sphere

sphincter muscle band encircling a body passage or opening that, with constriction, tightens or closes an orifice, duct, or tube

- **lower esophageal sphincter (LES)** specialized muscle that closes the gastroesophageal junction and prevents gastroesophageal reflex by its tonic contraction; relaxes in response to swallowing
- **transient lower esophageal sphincter relaxation (TLESR)** relaxation of the lower

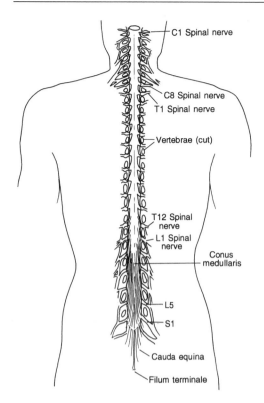

- C1 Spinal nerve
- C8 Spinal nerve
- T1 Spinal nerve
- Vertebrae (cut)
- T12 Spinal nerve
- L1 Spinal nerve
- Conus medullaris
- L5
- S1
- Cauda equina
- Filum terminale

spinal cord   the part of the central nervous sysem that extends as a continuation of the medulla oblongata and is housed in the vertebral column and gives rise to the spinal nerves

esophageal sphincter independent of associated swallowing activity; accounts for 60%–80% of gastroesophageal reflux activity

- **upper esophageal sphincter (UES)** formed by the cricopharyngeus muscle, which by its tonic contraction closes the lumen between the pharynx and the esophagus. Swallowing shortly thereafter relaxes the cricopharyngeus. Opening of the UES segment is enhanced by the pull from hyoid ascent and pressure exerted by the luminal bolus

spike potential   change in potential resulting from cell membrane stimulation

spike rate   rate of discharge of a neuron

spillage   material that has spilled into the pharynx before the pharyngeal swallow response has begun

spinal cord   the part of the central nervous sysem that extends as a continuation of the medulla oblongata and is housed in the vertebral column and gives rise to the spinal nerves

spinal cord injury   trauma to the spinal cord that causes paralysis of certain parts of the body and corresponding loss of sensation in that area for varying degrees of paraplegia and quadriplegia

spinal nerves   31 pairs of nerves connected to the spinal cord and numbered by the vertebral column level of their emergence; there are 8 cervical (C1–C8), 12 thoracic (T1–T2), 5 lumbar (L1–L5), 5 sacral (S1–S5), and 1 coccygeal pair; posterior nerve roots supply much of the body's muscle and skin function and some autonomic functions as well as sensory neurons; motor neuron axons are in the ventral roots, with the great sciatic nerve source in the sacral plexus

spinto   in music, pushed or thrust. Usually applies to tenors or sopranos with lighter voice than dramatic singers, but with aspects of particular dramatic excitement in their vocal quality. Enrico Caruso was an exemplar

spiral computed tomography (spiral CT)   synonymous with helical computed tomography scanning; scans produced by moving a patient at a constant rate through the bore of a CT scanner while the scanning tube is rotated around the patient. This produces a true volumetric dataset and allows standard transverse views, as well as images in any plane desired

spiral ligament of cochlea   thick lining of the bony cochlea that forms the cochlear duct outer wall serving as an attachment site for the basal lamina

spiral limbus   region of scala media from which the tectorial membrane arises

spirometer   device used to measure volume of inhaled and expired gasses in assessing pulmonary function; also called wet spirometer

spirometry   procedure for measuring the capacity of the lungs with a spirometer; incentive spirometry is a technique to encourage maximal deep breathing

spoiler   an obstacle in the path of airflow. In the production of fricative sounds, the upper and lower teeth can serve as spoilers to shape the noise spectrum

spondee   two-syllable word with equal stress on each syllable

spondee threshold (ST)   intensity level at which a listener correctly repeats 50% of spondee words

spontaneous recovery   unassisted resolution of deficits created by a disease or injury such as a stroke

sprechgesang   a treatment technique involving verbalizing using an exaggerated rhythm and stress but a normal intonation. This is often

stapedius muscle inner ear muscle connecting neck of stapes bone with medial wall of middle ear; in response to potentially injurious loud sounds, the muscle contracts to pull the stapes out of the oval window

---

a component of melodic intonation therapy (MIT)

squeeze pressure (also called contact pressure) in swallowing, pressure exerted on a sensor as the lumen is cleared of contents and obliterated. During peristalsis of the pharynx and the esophagus, squeeze pressures typically follow and exceed bolus pressure

S-structure abstract surface structure portion of government-binding linguistic theory

staccato abrupt authoritative musical instrument playing or singing of tones or chords; an explosive pattern of speech, as sometimes used to describe ataxic dysarthria

standard deviation (SD) statistical measure of the degree of variation (dispersion) from the mean; square root of the variance

stapedius muscle inner ear muscle connecting neck of stapes bone with medial wall of middle ear; in response to potentially injurious loud sounds, the muscle contracts to pull the stapes out of the oval window

stapes the smallest and innermost ossicle in the middle ear; resembles a small stirrup; its contact with the oval window transmits movements to the cochlea

Staphylococcus bacteria genus that is gram-positive and nonmotile; some species are found normally in skin and throat, with others causing severe purulent infections that can lead to nausea, vomiting, and diarrhea

• **Staphylococcus aureus** species often leading to abscesses, boils, endocarditis, osteomyelitis, and pneumonia

state relation condition expressed in early two-word utterances that express the status of objects, such as possession and attribution

state space in abstract mathematics, measurable space into which a random variable from a probability space is a measurable function

state verb word that links a subject to a stable or unchanging condition or attribute; the verb can often be considered synonymous with an equal sign

status post (s.p.) refers to a previous condition (disease or surgery) that may be pertinent to current considerations; for example, s.p. palatoplasty means that the individual had corrective palatal surgery

Steinert syndrome has both early onset and late onset (adult) forms, with delayed speech and language in early onset type, along with severe articulatory impairment secondary to neuromuscular disease; late onset form leads to articulatory impairment secondary to malocclusion and progressing myotonia

stem morpheme to which prefixes or suffixes can be combined to form new words; also called base

steno- combining form: narrow, short

stenosis narrowing of an anatomical area; laryngeal or tracheal stenosis may occur from injuries related to airway management procedures

- **subglottic stenosis** narrowing in the trachea below the level of the glottis that may result in airway obstruction and interfere with feeding

stent a device used for shape, support, and maintenance of patency of a lumen during surgery or after injury; device used in anchoring skin grafts

step scanning AAC scanning technique in which an indicator moves across one item at a time each time a switch is activated

stereocilia tiny cilia on the surface of inner ear hair cells

stereognosis ability to recognize objects through tactile sensation

sterno- combining form: pertaining to the sternum

steroid one of a large group of substances related to sterols, including sterols, D vitamins, bile acids, certain hormones, saponins, and glucosides of digitalis

- **anabolic steroid** derived from synthetic male hormones or testosterone to increase muscle mass and counteract effect of endogenous estrogen and may cause irreversible deepening or hoarseness of the voice

- **corticosteroid** potent substances produced by the adrenal cortex (excluding sex hormones of adrenal origin) in response to the release of adrenocorticoticotropic hormone from the pituitary gland, or related substances. Glucocorticoids influence carbohydrate, fat, and protein metabolism. Mineralocorticoids help regular electrolyte and water balance. Some corticosteroids have both effects to varying degrees. Corticosteroids may also be given as medications to alleviate various conditions, including inflammation, malignancy, suppressed immune system, and suppressed ACTH (adrenocorticotropic) secretion, as well as for hormone replacement therapy

Stickler syndrome micrognathia, maxillary deficiency, cleft palate, Robin sequence; marked by articulatory distortion secondary to malocclusion, with possible compensatory articulation secondary to clefting and VPI

stimulant any chemical that increases the activity of the body, usually resulting in sharpened reflexes, increased alertness and energy levels; classified according to system influences, such as cardiac, respiratory, gastric, hepatic, cerebral, spinal, and so on

stimulation, electrical the membranes of muscle and neurons have ionic channels that are sensitive to changes in electrical voltage. A transient change in voltage across a membrane of these two types of cells results in a progressive and transient change in ionic channels across the cells. Electrical stimulation is an experimental method to depolarize neurons and muscle cells using these ionic channels

stimulus something that can evoke or elicit a response

- **discriminative stimulus (Sd)** a stimulus that has been often present when a response has been reinforced and comes to influence the likelihood of that response occurring

- **functional stimulus** a stimulus that is causally related to the occurrence of a behavior

stochastic pertaining to a random variable

stoma-, stomato- combining forms: pertaining to mouth or opening

stoma, laryngeal opening made into the trachea between the thyroid glands to allow for breathing in patients with laryngectomy

stop speech sound characterized by a complete obstruction of the vocal tract; usually followed by an abrupt release of air that produces a burst noise

stop band band of frequencies rejected by a filter; the low region in a filter spectrum

stop consonant a consonant sound produced as a result of a complete closure formed by an articulator in the vocal tract

stop gap the acoustic interval corresponding to articulatory closure for a stop or affricate consonant; it is identified on a spectrogram as an interval of relatively low energy, conspicuously lacking in formant pattern or noise

stored knowledge information acquired during development that includes both linguistic (the mental lexicon, word meaning, the rules of grammar) as well as cognitive (information about the world, information about specific situations) sources of knowledge

story account of episode or happening; fictional narrative

story grammar the structure of narratives that may be treatment targets for children with language disorders

strain ratio of a change in length to an initial unstressed reference length; disfigurement of a material through application of force

strain gauge sensor whose resistance is a function of applied force

strepto- combining form: twisted

stress in speech, the product of a relative increase in fundamental frequency, vocal intensity, and duration to give prominence or emphasis to a word or syllable

- **contrastive stress drills** treatment method used to promote both articulatory proficiency and natural prosody, especially the stress and rhythm aspects of spoken language; used in treating apraxia of speech (AOS) in adults; varying phrases and sentences are used to teach placing stress on different words; stressed words or terms may be used to promote articulatory proficiency or simply to vary prosodic features of speech

- **emphatic stress** forceful expression manner often used to contradict the expectations of a listener

- **lexical stress** pattern of the stressed and unstressed syllables at the word level

- **stressed syllable** most prominent or noticeable syllable in a word or utterance

- **stress sequence** occurrence of stressed syllables at regularly perceived intervals

- **unstressed syllable** any syllable in a word or utterance that is not the most prominent syllable

stretch receptors specialized neural cells in the walls of the lung and thorax that during inspiration respond to lung and thorax movement by sending impulses to the respiratory center to cease movement of the inspiratory muscles; receptors that respond to the stretch in a muscle

stria line or streak

striated striped

striated muscle muscle whose contractile proteins are arranged into specific striated units; most skeletal muscles (those attached to the bones of the body) and also the pharynx, larynx, and esophagus contain striated muscles

stria vascularis vascularized tissue arising from the spiral ligament of the scala media

strident fricative with an intense noise energy; also called a sibilant; /s/ and /ʃ/ are examples. The nonstrident fricatives (/f/, /v/, /θ/, /ð/) have less energy

stridor upper airway high-pitched noise that indicates turbulent flow through a narrow airway, usually on inspiration, but can be on expi-

ration. Stridor is not a diagnosis itself but rather an indication of airway abnormality

stroboscopy means of capturing vibratory mode of the vocal folds for recording on video or computer disk; stroboscopic (short, intense bursts of focused light) illumination provides sampling of vocal fold position at different intervals in the vibratory cycle (phonation), which produces sequential still frames or slow motion images for research and diagnosis (see illustration, p. 222)

strobovideolaryngoscopy video recording with stroboscopy employing rigid instruments or flexible nasopharyngoscope for detailed evaluation of vocal fold motion in searching for small vocal fold lesions from scar, hemorrhage, or cyst

strohbass (German) glottal fry; also called pulse register

stroke injury to the brain secondary to some form of interruption in the blood supply; synonymous with a brain attack or cerebrovascular accident (CVA)

structuralism linguistic/philosophical perspective that language structure and organization is the inherent nature of the mind

Sturge-Weber syndrome cognitive impairment, seizures, intracranial calcification, malocclusion; speech delayed and language delayed and impaired secondary to cognitive impairment, with articulation impairment secondary to malocclusion caused by unilateral maxillary hyperplasia

stuttering articulatory or phonatory problem that typically presents in childhood and is characterized by anxiety about the efficacy of spoken communication, along with forced, involuntary hesitation, duplication, and protraction of sounds and syllables

- **accessory features** distinctive audible and visible characteristics of stutter events that result from excessive effort and tensing

- **core features of stuttering** part-word or sound repetitions and prolongations that mark the occurrence of stutter events; may exist without accessory features

- **episodic stuttering** the tendency for earliest signs of stuttering to be intermittent during the preschool years

- **stutter event** occurrence during speech that is interpreted to consist of a fluency interruption as perceived by the speaker, as well as the speaker's coping reactions

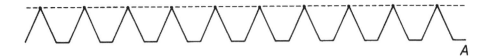

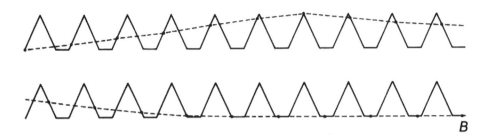

stroboscopy means of capturing vibratory mode of the vocal folds for recording on video or computer disk; stroboscopic (short, intense bursts of focused light) illumination provides sampling of vocal fold position at different intervals in the vibratory cycle (phonation), which produces sequential still frames or slow motion images for research and diagnosis

- **stuttering, adaptation, spontaneous recovery, and consistency** the tendency for stutter events to a decline in frequency by about 50% from the first to the fifth consecutive oral reading of a passage, return to their original frequency within several hours following adaptation, and occur on the same words when a passage is re-read aloud

- **stuttering disorder** characterized by the chronic occurrence of stutter events and their potentially handicapping effects on the speaker

style shifting modifications in style speakers make in response to social contexts or the status of their listeners

stylet a rigid probe used to assist in the insertion of a flexible tube, such as an endotracheal tube, into the body

stylo-, styl- combining forms: pertaining to the styloid process of the temporal bone

sub- prefix: under

subglottic beneath the glottis

subglottic pressure air pressure generated by the respiratory system beneath the level of the vocal folds; the unit most commonly used is centimeters of water and is the distance in centimeters that a given pressure would raise a column of water in a tube

subglottic stenosis narrowing in the trachea below the level of the glottis that may result in airway obstruction and interfere with feeding

subharmonic a frequency obtained by dividing a fundamental frequency by an integer greater than zero

subluxation partial separation or dislocation of a body part

submersion schooling in one language chosen by an educational administration

subordinate category subgroup of objects defined by a greater number of specific features than those defining the overall or superordinate category

subordinate clause an embedded clause that supplements the main clause in a complex sentence

subordinating conjunction a conjunction that introduces a clause serving as an adverb to describe time, location, cause, or conditions related to the main clause

substantive words classification of early words that occur in response to objects and classes of objects

substitution processes a group of phonological processes in which one class of sounds is substituted for another; in phonological treatment, the target is to eliminate such processes; major substitution processes include:

- **denasalization** substitution of an oral consonant for a nasal consonant (e.g., /d/ for /n/)

- **gliding** substitution of a glide for a liquid (e.g., /w/ for /r/)

- **stopping** substitution of a stop for a fricative or an affricate (e.g., /p/ for /f/)

- **velar fronting** substitution of an alveolar for a velar (e.g., /t/ for /k/)

successive single-word utterance utterance composed of two words spoken separately, where both words are related to the same context; taken by some as evidence of successive approximation of grammar

sucking/suckling in sucking, the body of the tongue is moved up and down by the activity of its muscles; suckling is a form of sucking present in the first few months of life in which backward movements of the tongue are pronounced

- **high-amplitude sucking (HAS)** a technique used to test infants' discrimination of speech sounds between the ages of birth and 4 months. Infants suck on a pacifier and the strength of each sucking response is measured using a pressure transducer

sulcus (pl., sulci) shallow depression or groove on an organ surface, generally those that occur on the convoluted cortical surface of the brain; also infoldings on the cerebral surface separating gyri

sulcus vocalis longitudinal groove, usually on the medial surface of the vocal fold

summating potential sustained direct current (DC) shift in the endocochlear potential that occurs when the organ of Corti is stimulated by sound

summation grouping of similar neural impulses or stimuli

sup- prefix: under; moderately

super- prefix: above; excessively

superficial near to the surface

superior the upper point; nearer the head

superior laryngeal nerve (SLN) one of the branches of the vagus nerve that innervates the laryngeal (cricothyroid) and the hypopharyngeal region; composed predominantly of sensory fibers, with a small component of motor fibers supplying the cricothyroid and upper esophageal striated muscle

superlative adjective form that expresses relative degree of an attribute when comparing more than two items (e.g., big versus bigger versus biggest)

superordinate category the highest conceptual level in a hierarchical classification of meanings, which includes all of the subgroups or subordinate categories in a given class

supination a turning upward; for example, turning the palm upward. The muscles that perform this function are called supinators

supine horizontal positioning of the body with head facing up

support commonly used in reference to the power source of the voice. It includes the mechanism responsible for creating a vector force that results in efficient subglottic pressure, along with the muscles of the abdomen and back, as well as the thorax and lungs; primarily in connection with the expiratory system

supra- prefix: above, over

supracricoid laryngectomy resection of the entire laryngeal cartilage, true and false vocal folds, preepiglottic fat, and the paraglottic space bilaterally; a portion of the epiglotttis may or may not be preserved

supraglottic above the level of the vocal fold; including the resonance system of the vocal tract, consisting of the pharynx, oral cavity, nose, and related structures

supraglottic laryngectomy resection of laryngeal structures above the level of the true vocal folds, including the superior portion of the laryngeal cartilage, the false vocal folds, the epiglottis, aryepiglottic folds, and preepiglottic space

suprahyoid muscle group external laryngeal muscles attached to the hyoid bone upper portion: the stylohyoid muscle, anterior and posterior bellies of the digastric muscle, geniohyoid, hyoglossus, and mylohyoid muscles

suprasegmental devices speech production effects, including intonation, stress, and rhythm, superimposed across the linguistic segments (i.e., words and phrases) to modify their meaning

surface structure the actualized production of a sentence by a speaker

surface wave a wave that moves along a surface; the vertical-phase difference observed on the vocal fold during vibration

surfactant chemical agent that reduces surface tension; lipoprotein surfactant secreted by pul-

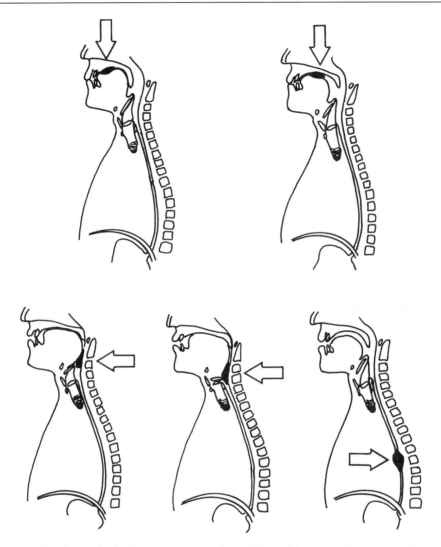

swallowing   deglutition; movement of nourishment from mouth to stomach; consists of sequential phases, which are subject to a variety of labeling schemes, depending on professional specialty. Arrow points to bolus

monary tissue allows gas exchange and enhances pulmonary tissue elasticity

suture   border or joint as between cranium bones; to stitch tissue together

swallowing   deglutition; movement of nourishment from mouth to stomach; consists of sequential phases, which are subject to a variety of labeling schemes, depending on professional specialty

- **esophageal phase of swallowing** bolus transport down esophagus and into stomach through coordinated contraction of smooth and striated esophageal muscles

- **oral preparatory phase of swallowing** stage of swallowing in which the tongue

gathers the food bolus and forms it into a centrally located globular mass ready to be propelled over the back of the tongue

- **oropharyngeal transit time** the time taken between the beginning of swallowing and the time of the bolus passaged out of the oropharynx

- **pharyngeal phase of swallowing** bolus passage through the pharynx and into the esophagus in coordination with respiration to assure air supply continuation and prevention of aspiration

- **preparatory phase** initial stage of bolus mastication and saliva amalgamation in anticipation of food transport from the mouth and through the pharynx and esophagus

- **squeeze pressure (also contact pressure)** pressure exerted during swallowing on a sensor as the lumen is cleared of contents and obliterated. During peristalsis of the pharynx and the esophagus, squeeze pressures typically follow and exceed bolus pressure

- **swallow apnea** the normal interruption of the respiratory cycle during expiration induced by a swallow

swallowing therapy regimen designed to help an individual swallow safely

- **direct therapy** patients practice swallow techniques with small amounts of food or liquid

- **indirect therapy** swallowing exercise programs or swallows of saliva during which no food or liquid is given

- **swallowing compensation** lessening of a swallowing problem by learned behavior, increased use of alternative mechanisms, or the inherent plasticity of the nervous system and of swallowing functions. Compensation may occur through use of postures that change pharyngeal dimensions and redirect bolus flow; through adaptations in bolus volume, delivery, or consistency; or through the use of sensory reinforcements or prostheses

- **swallowing treatment strategies/interventions** during the diagnostic radiographic study, management strategies to improve the swallow should be introduced, beginning with postural techniques, followed by introduction of techniques to increase oral sensation (when appropriate), and finally, diet (food consistency, viscosity) changes, if warranted

- **swallow maneuver** designed to place specific aspects of swallow physiology under voluntary control. Four swallow maneuvers have been developed to date: the supraglottic swallow; the super-supraglottic swallow; the effortful swallow, and the Mendelsohn maneuver

switch AAC hardware device that either opens or closes an electronic circuit, controlling the flow of electricity to an electronic device much like a light switch in the home turns the lights on (closed circuit) or off (open circuit)

- **switch latch timer** automated equipment that allows the user to use a switch to turn a device on and off, or to turn on a device for a specific length of time

- **switch mounting systems** custom-made or commercial adaptations designed to hold single switches in place

- **switch toys** battery- or radio-controlled toys that have been adapted for use with a single switch

syllable speech unit of either a single vowel (or a syllabic consonant) or a vowel and one or more consonants associated with it; often used to describe patterns of stress and timing in speech

- **disyllable** two syllables

- **heavy syllables** syllables that contain full vowels, such as /ɪ/, /e/ or diphthongized vowels such as /aɪ/, /au/, /ɔɪ/

- **light syllables** syllables that contain reduced vowels such as the schwa (/ə/), the r-colored schwa (/ɚ/), and the barred i (/ɨ/)

- **nonsense syllable** single syllable of speech that has no meaning

- **stressed syllable** the most prominent or noticeable syllable in a word or utterance

- **unstressed syllable** any syllable in a word or utterance that is not the most prominent syllable

sym- prefix: with or together

symbol representation that stands for or connotes another thing through kinship, alliance, custom, or incidental similarity; particularly a visible sign of abstraction, as the owl is a symbol of wisdom

- **presymbolic language** communication stage preceding uses of gestures, words, and actions to denote specific language concepts or words

- **tangible symbol** permanent, three-dimensional symbol that can be tactually discriminated and physically manipulated by an AAC communicator

symbolic function the cognitive process of using symbols to represent actual objects or events

symbolization the perceptual ability to identify the symbolic representation of objects or events with words

symbol systems personal sets of symbols assembled to form an ACC communication system, including means of representing abstract language, with mechanisms including pictographs, ideographs, and written language

symmetrical tonic neck reflex (STNR) a postural reflex often seen in children with cerebral palsy. When the neck is extended, the arms extend and the hips flex. When the neck is flexed, the arms flex and the hips extend

sympathetic nervous system one of two divisions of the autonomic nervous system. It is defined anatomically by preganglionic fibers that originate from the thoracic and lumbar levels of the spinal cord and by postganglionic fibers that originate in a chain of ganglia close to the vertebral column. The main neural neurotransmitter released by the postganglionic fibers is norepinephrine; effects include heart rate increase; bronchiole and pupil dilation; skin, viscera, and skeletal muscle vasodilation; peristalsis moderation; liver conversion of glycogen to glucose; and secretion of epinephrine and norephinephrine by the adrenal medulla. Sympathetic tends to prepare the body to deal with stress

symphysis cartilaginous joint uniting two bones with fibrocartilage

symptom patient's subjective experience of a disease or morbid condition

syn- prefix: with or together

synapse a connection between two neurons or between a neuron and a muscle at which signals are relayed. In chemical-type synapses, the presynaptic neuron releases a transmitter like acetylcholine into the open cleft that separates it from the postsynaptic neuron or muscle. The transmitter interacts with receptors to initiate specific responses. Another type of synapse is called electrical, in which there is direct propagation of bioelectrical potential from the presynaptic to the postsynaptic membrane

- **axoaxonic synapse** axon of one neuron actually touching axon of second neuron

- **axodendritic synapse** direct contact between axon and dendrite

- **axodendrosomatic synapse** axon of one neuron touches dendrites and cell body of second neuron

- **dendrodendritic synapse** relay between two dendrites

synaptic cleft the region between two communicating neurons into which a neurotransmitter is released

synaptic transmitter the chemical messenger released by the presynaptic terminal of a neuron on arrival of an action potential; released as a packet that moves across the synaptic cleft to link with receptors on the postsynaptic membrane. More than one type of transmitter can be released from one neuron and more than one type of postsynaptic receptor can combine with the transmitter

synaptic vesicle saccule at the end of a presynaptic membrane that contains neurotransmitter substance

synchrondrosis cartilaginous union between two bones formed by hyaline cartilage or fibrocartilage

synchronized intermittent mandatory ventilation (SIMV) mode of cycled ventilation in which the patient can breathe spontaneously between timed breaths; ventilatory mode synchronizes with spontaneous breathing efforts of the patient; only imposes a breath after a preset interval

syncope temporary loss of consciousness from transient diminished cerebral blood flow

- **swallow syncope** loss of consciousness or faint feeling during swallowing; mostly caused by an excessive vagal effect on the heart

syndrome a combination of signs and symptoms that, when associated with a single morbid process, form a recognizable pattern; from a common cause

- **Aarskog syndrome** x-linked recessive mutation of hypertelorism, hypodontia, brachydactyly, inguinal hernias, shawled scrotum, short stature, occasional cognitive impairment, with jaw and dental anomalies leading to articulation disorders; possible hypernasality and VPI from clefting

- **adult respiratory distress syndrome (ARDS)** severely impaired lung function with a number of etiologies, marked by alveolar and/or interstitial hemorrhage and edema

- **aglossia-adactylia syndrome** concurrent congenital absence of the tongue and digits

- **Alagille syndrome** may include speech-language delay secondary to mild cognitive impairment, evidenced by small stature, broad forehead, heart anomalies, vertebral anomalies, hepatic anomalies, occasional cognitive impairment, small genitals

- **Alport syndrome** dysphagia, apnea, nephritis, sensorineural hearing loss, myopia, stridor, apnea, with normal speech and language development

- **Anderson syndrome** articulation impairment secondary to malocclusion caused by abnormal jaw growth and position, evidenced by maxillary hypoplasia, mandibular prognathism, scoliosis, thin calvarium

- **ankyloglossia superior syndrome** congenital malformation, with tongue attached to the hard palate

- **Apert syndrome** speech production often delayed secondary to cognitive impairment, chronic upper airway obstruction, and severe occlusal anomalies, with compensatory articulation from possible cleft palate; language often delayed and/or impaired; condition marked by craniosynostosis, syndactyly, symphalagism, short upper arms, hydrocephalus, choanal stenosis/atresia, acne

- **Ascher syndrome** articulation impaired by redundant and loose tissue of the upper lip; marked by drooping eyelids and benign thyroid enlargement

- **Baller-Gerold syndrome** speech production onset and language may be delayed secondary to cognitive impairment and/or motor delay; marked by craniosynostosis, hypoplasia of the radius

- **Bamatter syndrome** speech production may be delayed secondary to hypotonia, with articulation hampered by lax facial skin and muscle, as well as malocclusion from prognathism; face has aged appearance

- **Beckwith-Wiedemann syndrome** hypotonia and cognitive impairment can lead to speech-language delay, with articulation disorders secondary to large tongue and malocclusion (prognathism) common; marked by large birth size, ear lobe creases, and enlarged liver, spleen, and kidneys

- **cardiofaciocutaneous (CFC) syndrome** delayed speech and language secondary to cognitive impairment and hypotonia; marked by large-appearing forehead with bitemporal depressions, sparse scalp hair, depressed nasal root, short neck, ptosis

- **Carpenter syndrome** delayed speech-language production onset secondary to cognitive impairment and articulatory impairment secondary to constricted maxilla; marked by craniosynostosis, polydactyly

- **cat eye syndrome** speech and language usually delayed secondary to cognitive impairment, with possible compensatory articulation secondary to cleft palate; marked by coloboma of iris, choroid, and retina, as well as hypertelorism and kidney anomalies

- **Cockayne syndrome** after toddler years, progressive speech and language deterioration, with dysarthric component, secondary to progressive cognitive functioning deterioration; short stature, deficient subcutaneous fat, progressive peripheral neuropathy; central hearing impairment

- **Cohen syndrome** delayed speech and language from cognitive impairment, with hypotonia influencing speech problems, along with misarticulations from open bite and maxillary constriction; also marked by obesity, short stature, delayed puberty, scoliosis, hypertensible joints, microcephaly

- **Cornelia de Lange syndrome** leads to neurogenically based articulation disorders, along with severely delayed speech production onset; cognitive impairment, microcephaly, seizures, hypertonia, cleft palate, with possible Robin sequence

- **Cowden syndrome** speech development may be impaired by lesions on lips, tongue, and gingiva, with hoarseness and breathiness secondary to laryngeal polyps

- **distal arthrogryposis syndrome** jaw limitation may lead to late speech production onset, with articulatory impairment from contractures, which usually respond positively to therapeutic management; marked by multiple contractures of limbs and digits, occasional limitation of jaw opening and cleft palate, along with possibility of Robin sequence

- **Down syndrome** upslanting eyes, strabismus, large protruding tongue, cognitive impairment, maxillary hypoplasia, occasional cleft palate/lip, airway obstruction; marked by delayed speech and language onset, uncoordinated labored articulation secondary to hypotonia and malocclusion combined with large tongue, plus dysfluency and rapid speech bursts

- **ectrodactyly-ectodermal dysplasia-clefting (EEC) syndrome** frequent compensatory articulation secondary to clefting (often bilateral complete); occasional speech and language delay secondary to cognitive impairment; misarticulations secondary to missing or malformed teeth; also marked by absence of fingers or toes, sparse hair lacking pigmentation, photophobia

- **Escobar syndrome** impaired articulation secondary to limited mouth opening and poor oral movements, with possible compensatory articulations secondary to cleft palate and/or tongue backing from micrognathia; hypernasality common, along with abnormal oral resonance

- **fetal hydantoin syndrome** speech delay secondary to cognitive impairment and compensatory articulation secondary to clefting, with language delay and impairment secondary to cognitive limitations; marked also by growth deficiency

- **FG syndrome** speech delay secondary to cognitive impairment and compensatory articulation secondary to clefting, with language delay and impairment secondary to cognitive limitations; also marked by macrocephaly, strabismus, micrognathia, hearing loss

- **Freeman-Sheldon syndrome** impaired articulation secondary to limited oral opening and compensatory articulation secondary to clefting and VPI; also marked by a whistling face and appearance of keel-shaped forehead, micrognathia, and Robin sequence

- **Golabi-Rosen syndrome** speech and language delay and impairment are common and variable depending on degree of cognitive deficiency, with articulation impairment caused by large tongue; also marked by macrostomia

- **Goldberg-Shprintzen syndrome** impaired speech secondary to cognitive impairment and cleft palate, with language delay and impairment secondary to cognitive impairment and hypernasality secondary to cleft palate; also marked by lower lip pit or mount, short stature, long curled eyelashes

- **Goldenhar syndrome** marked by misarticulation secondary to tongue motion asymmetry, malocclusion, and possible compensatory articulation secondary to clefting, with hypernasality common and hoarseness caused by unilateral vocal cord paresis; language is delayed and impaired in presence of cognitive impairment

- **Goltz syndrome** dental anomalies can lead to articulation problems and oral mucosal lesions; cognitive impairment can lead to speech delay, along with delayed and impaired language; also marked by syndactyly, small eyes, strabismus

- **Hallermann-Streiff syndrome** severe micrognathia leads to articulation impairment from problems with tongue manipulation; also marked by obstructive apnea, microphthalmia, cataracts, nystagmus

- **Hurler-Scheie syndrome** late articulatory problems from chronic mucous secretion and thickening of the tongue and lips; mucopolysaccharidosis I–H; marked by growth deficiency and congestive heart failure

- **Kabuki makeup syndrome** speech delay and compensatory articulation secondary to clefting is common, with language delay and

impairment secondary to cognitive impairment; also marked by protuberant large ears, scoliosis, heart anomalies

- **Lesch-Nyhan syndrome** later speech production hampered by by dysarthria and athetosis, with associated nasal and oral resonance abnormalities, variable breath support, and delayed language in cases with cognitive impairment; also marked by self-mutilation, mild growth deficiency, gout, high uric acid levels

- **Maffucci syndrome** articulation and oral resonance may be impaired by oral hemangiomas; also marked by bone deformity, neoplasms

- **Möbius syndrome** inanimate articulators leads to severe articulation impairment, along with muffled oral resonance and delayed expressive language development

- **Mohr syndrome** articulatory impairment secondary to lingual anomalies and possible compensatory articulation secondary to cleft palate; also marked by hyperplastic frenulae, maxillary hypoplasia

- **Nager syndrome** severe articulatory impairment, including compensatory articulation secondary to clefting and acute tongue backing secondary to prominent micrognathia; also marked by cleft or absent palate

- **Noonan syndrome** delayed or impaired speech and language in presence of cognitive impairment, with articulatory impairment secondary to malocclusion; also marked by small stature, webbed neck, vertebral anomalies, occasional cleft palate

- **oculo-dento-digital syndrome** dysarthria commonly seen, with articulation impairment secondary to dental anomalies; also marked by microphthalmia, broad lower jaw, occasional cleft palate and neuropathy

- **Opitz syndrome** delayed speech and language onset, with impaired language development and possible compensatory articulation pattern secondary to clefting; also marked by hypertelorism, cognitive impairment, cleft palate and lip

- **Pfeiffer syndrome** articulatory distortions secondary to maxillary deficiency, malocclusion and anterior skeletal open bite; also marked by craniosynostosis, hypertelorism

- **Prader-Willi syndrome** speech and language delayed, with articulatory impairment secondary to hypotonia and language impaired; marked by obesity, cognitive deficiency

- **Rapp-Hodgkin syndrome** compensatory articulation pattern secondary to clefting and hypernasality and articulatory placement problems secondary to clefting and maxillary deficiency; hoarseness secondary to hypohidrosis and dry vocal folds; marked also by ectodermal dysplasia

- **Refsum syndrome** probable late speech deterioration with ataxia onset in adult years, which can lead to dysphonia; also marked by retinitis pigmentosa, peripheral sensory and motor neuropathy

- **Schwartz-Jampel syndrome** tonic contractions of facial muscles, with progressive myotonia, skeletal dysplasia, and limited joint mobility; marked by later difficulty with articulation related to limited mouth movement and opening, accompanied by high-pitched voice and nasal resonance disorder secondary to progressive muscle contractions

- **short syndrome** small stature, deficient subcutaneous fat, delayed dental eruption; speech onset can be delayed, with abnormal dental eruption pattern leading to articulation distortion and an expressive language delay

- **Shprintzen-Goldberg syndrome** craniosynostosis, micrognathia, contractures, cognitive impairment, hypertrophy of palate, airway obstruction; cognitive impairment can lead to severely delayed speech delay, with misarticulations secondary to malocclusion and hypertrophic soft tissue of the hard palate; cognitive impairment can also lead to severe expressive language delay and impairment

- **Shprintzen syndrome** cleft palate, heart anomalies, learning disabilities, and ADHD; usually accompanied by delayed speech production onset, with global glottal stop substitutions in conjunction with clefts or VPI

- **Simpson-Golabi-Behmel syndrome** cleft palate, cognitive deficiency, macrencephaly; delayed speech production onset secondary to cognitive impairment and misarticulation from poor oral motor coordination, along with possible compensatory articulation secondary to cleft palate; language can be delayed and impaired from cognitive deficiency

- **Sjögren-Larsson syndrome** severe skin dryness and scaling, cognitive deficiency, spasticity; marked by delayed speech and language onset, along with dysarthria

- **Sotos syndrome** large stature, cognitive impairment, hypotonia, behavioral disturbances; marked by delayed speech onset secondary to hypotonia and developmental delay and articulation distortion from abnormal dental spacing

- **Steinert syndrome** has both early onset and late onset (adult) forms, with delayed speech and language in early onset type, along with severe articulatory impairment secondary to neuromuscular disease; late onset form leads to articulatory impairment secondary to malocclusion and progressing myotonia

- **Stickler syndrome** micrognathia, maxillary deficiency, cleft palate, Robin sequence; marked by articulatory distortion secondary to malocclusion, with possible compensatory articulation secondary to clefting and VPI

- **Sturge-Weber syndrome** cognitive impairment, seizures, intracranial calcification, malocclusion; speech delayed and language delayed and impaired secondary to cognitive impairment, with articulation impairment secondary to malocclusion caused by unilateral maxillary hyperplasia

- **Treacher Collins syndrome** micrognathia, absent or hypoplastic cheek bones, cleft palate, Robin sequence, airway obstruction, hearing loss; marked by misarticulations secondary to malocclusion and anterior skeletal open bite and severe tongue backing secondary to micrognathia

- **Usher syndrome** hearing loss, retinitis pigmentosa, and night blindness followed by adult deterioration and blindness in about half of the cases, along with occasional ataxia; marked by hearing loss speech and language impairment

- **velo-cardio-facial syndrome** cleft palate, heart anomalies, learning disabilities, and ADHD; usually accompanied by delayed speech production onset, with global glottal stop substitutions in conjunction with clefts or VPI

- **von Recklinghausen type neurofibromatosis (NF I)** occasional mild dysarthria or dyspraxia; if cognitive impairment is present speech and language can be delayed; marked by café au lait skin spots, cutaneous neurofibromas, macrencephaly

- **Weaver syndrome** skeletal anomalies, hypotonia, delayed development, macrocephaly; marked by delayed speech and language onset, with sluggish articulation secondary to hypotonia

- **Williams syndrome** cognitive impairment, hypercalcemia, microcephaly, large mouth, thick lips, microdontia, hyperopia; marked by echolalia, overtalkativeness, with a sophisticated but abnormal language ability known for cliché overuse and friendly cocktail party manner and conversational style

synergist a body part, medium, or substance that augments the activity or result of another body part, medium, or substance

synonym two or more words or phrases in the same language with the same or very similar meanings

synovial fluid clear, viscous fluid secreted by the membranes in an articular capsule that lubricates joints, bursae, and tendons

syntagmatic-paradigmatic shift a transition in which word associations shift from a syntactic to semantic basis

syntax the rules governing the arrangement, grammar, and ordering of language units

- **cause-effect pattern** language development syntactic devices in text grammar that signal a cause-effect relationship is being proposed

- **collection patterns** language development syntactic devices associated with text grammar that indicate a listing of items

- **comparison patterns** language development syntactic devices associated with text grammar signaling that similarities or differences are being noted

- **descriptive patterns** syntactic devices found in text grammar that signal a topic is being described

- **linear syntactic relationships** in language development, an aspect of children's early grammar describing the additive meaning of words combined in utterances

synthesis combining often disparate entities into a coherent whole; systematic use of inflected forms as a characteristic of language

- **articulatory synthesis** a type of speech synthesis (machine-generated speech) in which the organs of the vocal tract are simulated and controlled to produce speechlike patterns

- **copy synthesis** a type of speech synthesis (machine-generated speech) in which stored copies of speech segments are retrieved and assembled to form an utterance

- **formant synthesis** a type of speech synthesis (machine-generated speech) in which resonators are controlled to produce formantlike patterns

- **phonemic synthesis** blending of discrete phonemes into the correctly sequenced, coarticulated sound patterns

- **speech synthesis** the production of speech by artificial means; especially the generation of speech by computers, computer-controlled, or digital devices

synthesize to combine separate elements into a whole; to produce speech by artificial means

system complex whole consisting of correlated and loosely related parts; collection of anatomical structures that are functionally related

systematic regularities exhibited by speakers of a language that make occurrences in the language predictable

systemic condition relating to whole bodily system or group of organs

systems theory study of systems as an entity rather than a conglomeration of parts; provides a conceptual framework for understanding the organization, interaction, and dynamics of elements composing systems

T

Trachea

the windpipe that conducts air from the nose and mouth
through the larynx to the bronchi; made up of rings of hyaline
cartilage connected by an annular ligament (membrane)

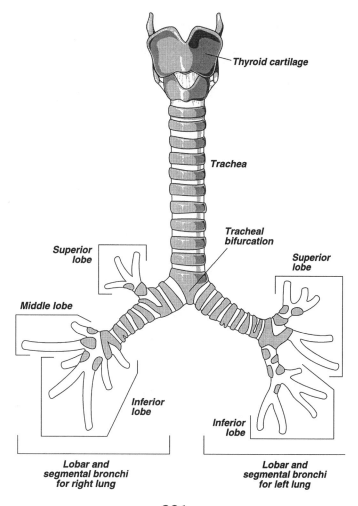

Thyroid cartilage

Trachea

Tracheal
bifurcation

Superior
lobe

Superior
lobe

Middle lobe

Inferior
lobe

Inferior
lobe

Lobar and
segmental bronchi
for right lung

Lobar and
segmental bronchi
for left lung

231

tachy- prefix: swift; fast

tachycardia rapid heart rate; more than 100 beats per minute for adults; can be caused by physiological or pathological factors

tachypnea abnormally rapid respiration

tact primary verbal operant that occurs in response to an object, event, or relationship and the form of the response exhibits a conventional correspondence to others' responses; the behavioral equivalent of naming, describing, or labeling

- **extended tact** a primary verbal operant in which responses to stimuli other than the original stimuli occur because of stimulus generalization; the behavioral equivalent of figurative language

tactile about the sense of touch

tactile aid vibrotactile hearing aid; aid that transduces sound to mechanical vibration and delivers it to the skin to provide sound awareness and gross sound identification

tactile symbols symbols with discernible differences in tactile qualities (as in various textures), used with individuals with visual impairments or dual sensory impairments

tag small polyp or outgrowth; a language structure added to the end of a statement

tag question question added to the end of a statement

talker variability different talkers producing the same phonetic unit (such as /a/) or other speech pattern with considerable variance in physical characteristics; especially true for male/female talkers or when comparing adult to child talkers. Nonetheless, the sounds are heard as belonging to the same phonetic category

talking tracheostomy tube a tracheostomy tube adapted to permit phonation in conjunction with an inflated cuff. Talking, or speaking, tracheostomy tubes have an external air port that connects to a separate air source and allows air to enter the airway above the level of the tracheostomy tube cuff

tardive dyskinesia an extrapyramidal disorder characterized by involuntary movements resulting from long-term exposure to neuroleptics such as phenothiazine or long-term use of levodopa

- **orofacial tardive dyskinesia** a dyskinesia involving the oral and perioral muscles

targeting augmentative or assistive communication ability of an individual to access a desired symbol using direct selection or scanning. Targeting accuracy is affected by the layout of symbols, symbol size, and spacing on a communication display

-tarsal combining form: ankle

taste receptor gustatory cell of a taste bud, peripheral taste organs situated on the surface of the tongue and mouth roof; basic tastes registered chemically are bitter, sour, sweet, and salty

taxonomic organization scientific classification, especially ordering of plants and animals according to believed associations

team group associated in work or activity

- **cochlear implant team** group of professionals who are part of the cochlear implant process; usually includes an otolaryngologist, audiologist, and clinical coordinator and may include an educator, aural rehabilitation specialist, speech-language pathologist, psychologist, and/or social worker

- **collaborative team model** an approach that views communication within the user's natural environments, considers the individual and family as central to the process, and integrates natural supports, including friends and community members

- **interdisciplinary team model** team members perform only those tasks specific to their respective disciplines, but share information with each other and attempt to unify their findings for optimal assessment and treatment

- **multidisciplinary team model** team members from multiple disciplines provide services in isolation from each other and perform only those tasks specific to their respective disciplines. Team members then meet to discuss results and develop recommendations

- **transdisciplinary team model** team members from different disciplines engage in a high degree of collaboration, focusing on holistic goals for an individual, rather than just discipline-specific goals

technetium-99m radionuclide commonly used for evaluation of the gastrointestinal tract in nuclear medicine scans; may be linked to food or other radioisotopes for injection into the body to be taken up by various organs; emitted energy appropriate for typical imaging techniques, with a short half-life

technetium-99m sulfur colloid radiopharmaceutical consisting of technetium bound to sulfur colloid particles that may be used to evaluate the gastrointestinal transit or uptake of the tracer by the reticuloendothelial system as part of nuclear scanning

tectorial membrane gel-like layer within the ear's cochlear partition, with cilia of outer hair cells embedded in the membrane; displacement of hair cells results in shearing movement between upper surface of hair cell and tectorial membrane

tectum rooflike structure

tegmen a roof or cover

tele- prefix: pertaining to distant or the end

telecoil (T-coil) special hearing aid input channel permitting the aid to pick up electromagnetic signals directly by induction rather than via a microphone. Useful for direct input devices such as telephone receivers

telecoil switch (T-switch) switch on a hearing aid that activates the telecoil, which is a series of interconnected wire loops in hearing aid that respond electrically to a magnetic signal to enhance telephone intelligibility

telecommunication device for the deaf (TDD; TT: text telephone; TTY) telephone device for persons with deafness or significant hearing loss in which messages are typed on a keyboard, transmitted over telephone wires, and displayed on a small monitor screen

telegraphic speech a traditional concept of children's grammar that viewed their utterances as reduced forms of adult grammar; also, spoken language patterns that are characterized by the omission of function words and, sometimes, incorrect word order

telencephalon embryonic structure from which cerebral hemispheres and rhinencephalon develop

telephone amplifier assistive listening device designed to increase the intensity of a signal from a telephone receiver

telephony any device that permits sound communication over long distances with or without wires

telereceptive about response to stimuli originating outside of the body, such as hearing, sight, and smell

Television Decoder Circuitry Act of 1990, Public Law (P.L.) 101-431 requires all televisions manufactured in the USA with a 13-inch diagonal or larger screen to contain circuitry necessary for closed captioning

telo- prefix: far from, toward the extreme

telodendria terminal arborization of an axon

template pattern or mold

temporal bone pair of large bones forming portion of lower cranium; each half includes mastoid, squamous, petrous, and tympanic parts

temporal gap transition the transition from a continuous sound to a series of pulses in the perception of vocal registers

temporal processing (auditory) auditory mechanisms and processes responsible for temporal patterning (e.g., phase locking, synchronization) of neural discharges and the following behavioral phenomena: temporal resolution (i.e., detection of changes in durations of auditory stimuli and time intervals between auditory stimuli over time), temporal ordering (i.e., detection of sequence of sounds over time), temporal integration (i.e., summation of power over durations less than 200 milliseconds), and temporal masking (i.e., obscuring of probe by pre- or poststimulatory presentation of masker)

temporal words words that relate events in time

temporary threshold shift (TTS) transient hearing loss following exposure to excessive noise

temporomandibular joint (TMJ) the jaw joint; a synovial joint between the mandibular condyle and skull anterior to the ear canal

tendon fibrous tissue attaching muscle to bone or cartilage

tenor highest of the male voices, except countertenors. Must be able to sing to C5; singer's formant is around 2800 Hz

- **countertenor** male singing voice that is primarily falsetto, in the contralto range. Most countertenors are also able to sing in the baritone or tenor range. Countertenors are also known as contraltino or contratenor

- **dramatic tenor** tenor with heavy voice, often with a suggestion of baritone quality. Suitable for dramatic roles that are heavily orchestrated. Also referred to as *tenora robusto*, and helden tenor. The term helden tenor (literally "heroic" tenor) is used typically for tenors who sing Wagnerian operatic roles

- **lyric tenor** tenor with a light, high flexible voice

- **tenore serio** dramatic tenor

tense in phonetics, a speech sound produced with relatively high muscular tension, increased duration or both; for vowels, synonymous with fortis; in linguistics, an affix that indicates time

tensile strength the most stress a material can stand without being torn apart

tensor a muscle that tenses

tensor tympani middle ear muscle just above the bony aspect of the eustachian tube that adjusts the tympanic membrane tension

teratogen an agent that causes abnormal embryonic development; literally "monster producing"

terminal contour the final pitch direction at the end of an utterance

tertiary contraction simultaneous, nonpropulsive contraction that occurs at any level of the esophagus

test an examination

- **acid-perfusion test** acid is dripped into the distal esophagus through a nasogastric tube and the patient's symptoms are recorded. Used to help determine whether a patient has gastroesophageal reflux (GER); also known as Bernstein test

- **controlled oral word association test (COWAT)** a measure of word fluency or production in which the subject is asked to produce as many words as possible beginning with a given letter in a limited period of time; the Boston Naming Test is one example of a COWAT

- **criterion-referenced test** nonstandardized probe for study of a language construct in more depth than typically associated with standardized tools

- **dichotic test** test in which the listener must identify one or both of two different acoustic signals presented separately and simultaneously, one to each ear

- **performance versus intensity (PI) function** curve illustrating percentage correct score to speech intensity. Useful for all types of speech test materials. Ordinarily, performance increases monotonically with increasing intensity

- **pulmonary function tests** a variety of assessment techniques that can provide both diagnostic and therapeutic information. These involve tests of lung volumes and capacities and expired airflow

- **sound field testing** determination of hearing sensitivity or speech recognition ability with the stimuli presented through loudspeakers; often used in pediatric testing or hearing-aid evaluations

- **test-retest reliability** measure of test consistency from one presentation to the next

testosterone the hormone responsible for development of male sexual characteristics, including laryngeal growth

tetra- prefix: four

tetrodotoxin neurotoxin mainly found in a Japanese puffer fish and California newt eggs that blocks sodium channels in the neuronal membrane

text grammar characteristic styles associated with language found in textbooks

textual primary verbal operant that occurs in response to written, printed, or graphic stimuli; the behavioral equivalent of reading

thematic organization associating words based on their relationship to a theme or context

theory explanation of information and phenomena in a particular discipline; theories not only account for the experimental data in a field, but also speculate about how and why particular phenomena exist; theories are educated guesses containing predictions that have to be tested experimentally; scientific theories are considered more certain than hypotheses, but less certain than laws

therapy restorative treatment

- **contextual therapy** occurs within a person's natural environment and attends to interactions between the individual and others, also employing the resources of others who have influence on the person being treated

- **family therapy** simultaneous treatment of more than one member of a family; may be supportive, directive, or interpretive

- **occupational therapy (OT)** a rehab specialty that employs therapeutic work, self-care, and play activities to enhance independent function; can include adaptation of tasks or environment for achievement of maximum independence and to improve performance of activities of daily life (ADLs)

- **physical therapy (PT)** a rehabilitation specialty that targets the restoration of optimal functioning following trauma; daily functions of standing, transferring, and walking are common goals

- **recreational therapy (RT)** a rehabilitation specialty that targets the use of leisure or recreational activities as part of the therapeutic process

thermoreceptor sensor responsive to temperature

thoracic pertaining to the chest

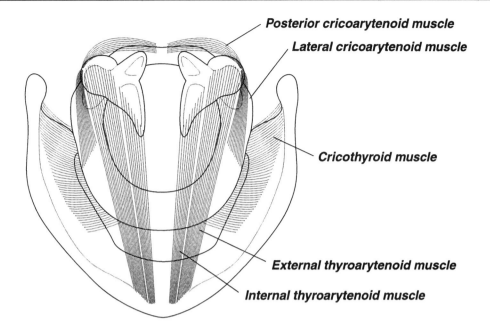

Posterior cricoarytenoid muscle

Lateral cricoarytenoid muscle

Cricothyroid muscle

External thyroarytenoid muscle

Internal thyroarytenoid muscle

Intrinsic Laryngeal Muscles

thyroarytenoid muscle (also called **vocalis**) muscle that relaxes (decreases tension) of the vocal folds and lowers the pitch of the voice tone; runs from the inner surface of the thyroid cartilage to the muscular process and outer surface of the arytenoid

---

thorax the part of the body between the diaphragm and the 7th cervical vertebra; cage of bone and cartilage housing the main organs of respiration and circulation

three-dB rule time-intensity tradeoff that states for every 50% decrease in noise-exposure, a 3-dB-A increase in noise level is permitted without increasing the risk of noise-induced hearing loss

threshold point of joining or starting; when a physiological or psychological effect begins to be produced

- **neuronal threshold** point of cell membrane stimulus depolarization at which ionic channels open to sodium and an action potential is recorded

- **threshold, aided** hearing threshold obtained from a patient using hearing aids, indicated by an "A" on the audiogram

- **threshold level** a level of language competence a person must reach to gain benefits from owning two languages

- **threshold sensitivity** faintest sound that patient can just detect. The intensity level below which the patient almost never hears the

sound, but above which he or she usually does hear the sound. Defined statistically as the level yielding a correct response on 50% of repeated trials

- **threshold shift** change in hearing sensitivity expressed in dB

- **threshold shift, temporary (TTS)** transient hearing loss following exposure to excessive noise

thrombosis formation of a blood clot in the vascular system

thrombus the debris at the site of a thrombosis

thrush mouth candidiasis marked by white exudate patches on tongue and buccal mucosa

thymus primary lymphatic system gland, located in the mediastinum

thyroarytenoid muscle (also called **vocalis**) muscle that relaxes (decreases tension) of the vocal folds and lowers the pitch of the voice tone; runs from the inner surface of the thyroid cartilage to the muscular process and outer surface of the arytenoid

thyroid cartilage the largest laryngeal cartilage. It is open posteriorly and is made up of

T

two plates (thyroid laminae) joined anteriorly at the midline. In males, there is a prominence superiorly known as the "Adam's apple"

thyroid gland ductless gland lying in the front and to the sides of the upper trachea that secretes thyroid hormone (several metabolically active substances)

- **hyperthyroidism** hyperactivity of the thyroid gland, which is usually enlarged; marked by weight loss, tremor, fatigue, heat intolerance

- **hypothyroidism** underactivity of the thyroid gland; marked by weight gain, lethargy, arthritis

- **parathyroid glands** small paired endocrine glands usually embedded on posterior surface of the thyroid gland that secrete a hormone regulating calcium and phosphorus metabolism

tic habitual, mainly involuntary muscle contraction most evident when a person is stressed, ranging from throat clearing, sniffing, lip pursing, excessive blinking, to a number of muscle twitches/spasms

tidal volume the volume inspired and expired during normal, quiet respiration. Also, the amount of air that moves in and out of the lungs during respiration. Vital capacity is inspiratory reserve volume and expiratory reserve volume combined with tidal volume. For mechanically ventilated patients, this value is set on the ventilator to ensure that a patient is adequately ventilated

- **exhaled tidal volume** the amount of volume that a patient receiving mechanical ventilation exhales or returns to the ventilator. The exhaled tidal volume display on the ventilator is monitored to assess if the patient is receiving adequate amounts of air. If a leak develops in this system, the exhaled tidal volume return alarm will sound. A leak deliberately created in the system (e.g., by cuff deflation) can be compensated for with increased volume from the ventilator

- **quiet tidal volume** the volume of air exchanged during one cycle of quiet respiration

- **resting lung volume** the volume of air remaining within the lungs after quiet tidal expiration; also called expiratory reserve volume

timbre the quality of a sound; associated with complexity, or the number, nature, and interaction of overtones

time-activity curves a graph of the amount of radioactivity recorded in an organ or in the blood over a specified time; quantifies physiologic events with radionuclide use

time-compressed speech speech that has been accelerated by means of removing segments from the waveform and compressing the remaining segments together, without changing its frequency composition

time-domain operation a study performed in a time period that is relevant to what is being measured

time-talk a language-stimulation technique of an adult purposely incorporating time-related language into conversation

time-weighted average (TWA) index of daily noise exposure that is the product of durations of exposure relative to the allowable durations of exposure for a particular sound level

tinnitus noise in the ears such as ringing, whistling, buzzing

tinnitus masker electronic hearing aid that generates and outputs noise at low levels to mask an individual's tinnitus

tissue a population of cells with a similar structure and function

titubation unsteady gait plus head and trunk swaying motion, often related to cerebellar damage

tomography sectional imaging

-tomy suffix: surgical incision

tone musical or vocal sound of a specific quality; especially musical specifics of timbre and manner of expression; also sound of a certain vibration and pitch

- **complex tone** tone composed of a series of simultaneously sounding partials (partial = sinusoid that is part of a complex tone; in voiced sounds, the partials are harmonic implying that the frequency of the nth partial equals n times the fundamental frequency)

- **overtone** partial above the fundamental in a spectrum

- **pure tone** sinusoid, the simplest tone; produced electronically; in nature, even pure-sounding tones are complex

tongue main organ of taste that also helps in mastication and swallowing of food, as well as articulation

tongue advancement articulatory description of the relative position of the tongue in the

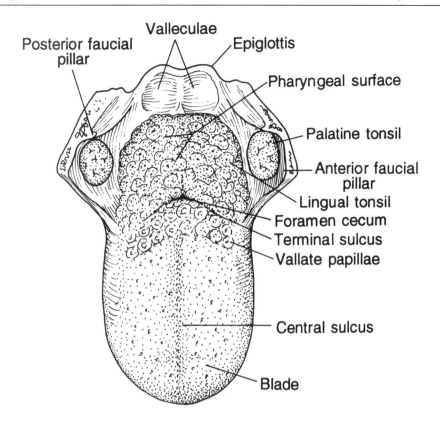

tongue   main organ of taste that also helps in mastication and swallowing of food, as well as articulation

---

anterior-posterior (front-back) dimension of the vocal tract. As applied to vowels, tongue advancement relates primarily to the relative frequency of F_2, or to the frequency difference between F_1 and F_2. Front vowels tend to have relatively high F_2 values and a relatively large value of the F_2–F_1 difference

tongue height an articulatory description referring to the relative position of the tongue in the inferior-superior (low-high) dimension of the vocal tract. As applied to vowels, tongue height relates primarily to the relative frequency of F_1; the higher the vowel, the lower F_1 tends to be. Tongue height also varies with jaw position, such that high vowels tend to have a closed jaw position

tongue pumping repeated rockinglike motion of the tongue preceding swallowing

tongue thrust immature form of swallow in which the tongue is pushed forward against the central incisors

tonic pertaining to muscular contraction

- **asymmetrical tonic neck reflex (ATNR)** a

postural reflex often seen in children with cerebral palsy. When the head is rotated, the ATNR causes an extension in the arm and leg on the side to which the face is turned, while the opposite site increases in flexion; can be elicited by turning an infant's head laterally in a supine position. Visible evidence includes extension of the extremities on the chin side or flexion on the occiput side. The ATNR is commonly persistent in children with severe motor deficits

- **symmetrical tonic neck reflex (STNR)** a postural reflex often seen in children with cerebral palsy. When the neck is extended, the arms extend and the hips flex. When the neck is flexed, the arms flex and the hips extend

- **tonic bite** form of hyperreflexia in which the bite reflex is exaggerated and leads to a tight closure of the jaws in response to slight oral stimulation

tonotopic arrangement spatial arrangement of auditory nerve fibers such that fibers innervating the apex process low-frequency information, while fibers in the basal region process

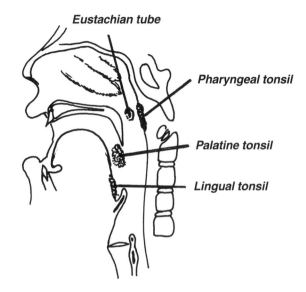

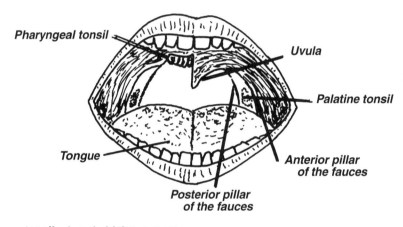

tonsil   lymphoid tissue mass

---

high-frequency information

tonsil lymphoid tissue mass

- **lingual tonsil** lymphoid tissue in the posterior (pharyngeal) regions of the tongue

- **palatine tonsils** lymphoid tissue between the fauces in the oropharynx lateral wall; generally known as tonsils

- **pharyngeal tonsil** the mass of lymphatic tissue within the nasopharynx; also called adenoids (especially when enlarged)

tonsillectomy surgical removal of the palatine tonsils; if the adenoids are removed in the same surgical procedure, it is called a tonsillectomy and adenoidectomy (T&A)

tonsillitis inflammation of tonsil, particularly the palatine tonsils

tonus continuous state of slight muscle contraction typical of normal body state

tooth hard calcified structure set in the alveolar processes of the jaws for biting and mastication of food

top-down analysis analysis of an incoming message that is processed through use of sources of information stored in the brain to form hypotheses about the message

top-down model the model that proposes reading progresses from confirming ideas about overall content as additional written material is decoded; any model that proposes an important role of higher level knowledge in the processing

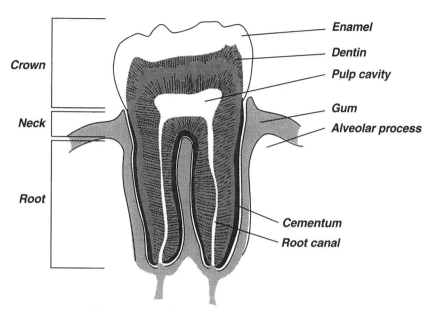

Diagrammatic Cross-Section of a Tooth

UPPER ARCH

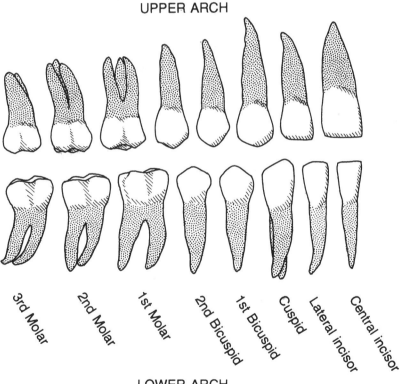

3rd Molar 2nd Molar 1st Molar 2nd Bicuspid 1st Bicuspid Cuspid Lateral incisor Central incisor

LOWER ARCH

tooth hard calcified structure set in the alveolar processes of the jaws for biting and mastication of food

and interpretation of sensory information

top-down processing information processing that is knowledge, or concept, driven, with higher level constraints guiding data processing, leading to data interpretation consistent with the constraints

topical anesthetic anesthetics applied to a local region through injection or direct application by touch or spray

topic initiation introducing a topic in discourse

topic maintenance continuation of a topic in discourse through successive utterances about the topic

topic shading subtle shifts in a conversational topic made by addressing an isolated aspect of a previous utterance

TORCH+S complex group of perinatal medical problems often linked to hearing loss. *T* = toxoplasmosis; O = other (e.g., associated ophthalmologic disease); R = rubella; C = cytomegalovirus; H = herpes; S = syphilis

torso the trunk of the body

total acceptance point moment in the real-time word recognition process when a listener recognizes the target word with a high level of confidence

total communication (TC) the simultaneous use of multiple modes of expression to enhance communication

total parenteral nutrition (TPN) nutritional needs provided exclusively through intravenous access and not the gastrointestinal tract; typically long-term, with nutrition administered through a catheter in the superior vena cava

touch pad a small touch-activated surface that operates as a substitute for a mouse to control computer cursor movement. The user moves a finger along the touch area in the direction that the cursor needs to move

touch screen a monitor or a screen placed over a monitor that consists of two electrically conductive flat surfaces separated by nonconductive spacers. Touching the screen lightly presses the two surfaces together, which sends an electronic signal to the AAC (augmentative and assistive communication) system

toxin poisonous substance produced from the metabolic activity of plants or animals

trachea the windpipe that conducts air from the nose and mouth through the larynx to the bronchi; made up of rings of hyaline cartilage connected by an annular ligament (membrane)

tracheal button a closure plug used to close the stoma of a tracheostomized patient; often utilized during the decannulation process

tracheal intubation placement of a tube into the trachea, either translaryngeally or by tracheostomy

tracheal stenosis congenital or acquired narrowing of the trachea

tracheoesophageal fistula (TEF) abnormal tubelike passage between the trachea and the esophagus; occurring during the 4th week of development because of incomplete division of the cranial part of the foregut into respiratory and digestive portions. Incidence is 1 in 2,500 births, with majority in males. TEF is the most common malformation of the respiratory tract in infancy; often affiliated with esophageal atresia

tracheoesophageal separation a type of subglottic closure where the subglottic trachea is brought to the skin as a tracheotomy, but the supraglottic portion of the trachea is attached to the esophagus so that all ingesta entering the larynx can exit into the esophagus

tracheoesophageal shunt surgery promoting laryngectomee speech by constructing a passageway between the esophagus and trachea

tracheoesophageal speech facilitated by voice prostheses, which are devices employed following laryngectomy and vocal fold excision to enable speech production; most commonly a surgical passage, tracheoesophageal puncture (TEP), is created inside the stoma from the back wall of the trachea into the esophagus, with a valved tube enabling tracheoesophageal speech

tracheomalacia pathologic softening of the tracheal cartilages, often the result of tracheal ischemia during endotracheal intubation

tracheostomy an artificial airway; surgical opening through the neck for insertion of an indwelling tube (see illustration, p. 242)

tracheostomy tube a tube placed in the trachea to keep the airway to the lungs open following tracheostomy surgery

- **one-way speaking valve** valve placed on the hub of a tracheostomy tube to allow air to enter on inspiration. On expiration, the valve closes and air cannot escape the tracheostomy tube. Rather, the trapped air is redirected through the vocal folds and into the upper airway to use for speaking and swallowing

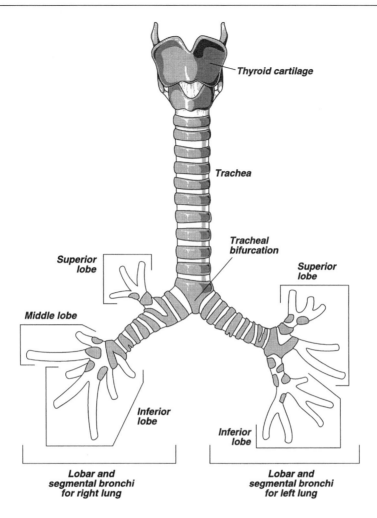

Thyroid cartilage

Trachea

Tracheal bifurcation

Superior lobe

Superior lobe

Middle lobe

Inferior lobe

Inferior lobe

Lobar and segmental bronchi for right lung

Lobar and segmental bronchi for left lung

trachea   the windpipe that conducts air from the nose and mouth through the larynx to the bronchi; made up of rings of hyaline cartilage connected by an annular ligament (membrane)

- **partial leak** intentional leak maintained in a tracheostomy tube cuff to allow a patient access to airflow through the upper airway for speaking, swallowing, and airway clearance

- **talking tracheostomy tube** a tracheostomy tube adapted to permit phonation in conjunction with an inflated cuff. Talking, or speaking, tracheostomy tubes have an external air port that connects to a separate air source and allows air to enter the airway above the level of the tracheostomy tube cuff

tracheotomy making an incision into the trachea through the neck below the larynx; allows access to the airway below a blockage by a tumor, foreign body, or glottic edema; may be done as either an emergency or planned procedure

trackball a ball set within the surface of a keyboard or a free-standing box that operates as a substitute for a mouse to control computer cursor movement

tracking gathering in homogenous groups (also called setting, streaming, banding, ability grouping); also, the use of observation and/or questioning to develop an understanding of sequences of events that occur between people. In education, grouping students based on standardized test results

tracts in the central nervous system, a bundle of nerve fibers with a shared origin, termination, and function

trademark brand name or proprietary name of an item; in pharmacology, the formulation a drug that has a name specifically assigned as its identi-

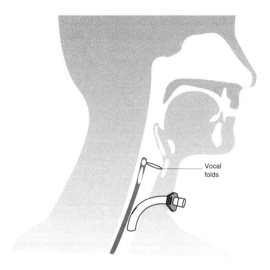
Vocal folds

tracheostomy an artificial airway; surgical opening through the neck for insertion of an indwelling tube

ty by its manufacturer, whether registered or not

traditional approach a treatment approach developed by Charles Van Riper (1905–1994) for remediating articulation errors. It is based on discriminating and practicing new speech sounds in syllables, words, and sentences to establish new production patterns for specific sounds

tragus flap-like landmark of the ear's auricle approximating the concha

trajectory in chaos theory, the representation of the behavior of a system in state space over a finite, brief period of time

trans- prefix: beyond or on the other side

transcript a written record of utterances spoken; often is a record of speech therapy sessions

transcription, narrow phonetic transcription in which sound modifications are marked, in addition to transcribing the phonemes in an utterance; usually involves the use of special symbols called diacritics or diacritic marks

transdisciplinary team model team members from different disciplines engage in a high degree of collaboration focusing on holistic goals for the individual, rather than on just discipline-specific goals

transduce to change from one form of energy to another, as in sense organs converting physical energy into a nervous signal

transducer mechanism for converting energy

from one form to another

transformational generative grammar linguistic theory proposing that universal rules generate underlying structures that may be transformed by rules to derive the specific sentence forms of each language

transformational rules the linguistic rules applied in each language to transform underlying sentence structure into the varying surface structures produced in each language

transglottal flow air that is forced through the glottis by transglottal pressure

transient ischemic attack (TIA) a small or ministroke; a brief, usually reversible episode of brain attack symptoms that may last for a period of minutes or hours; often an indicator of a person being at risk for subsequent stroke

transitional bilingual education (TBE) required courses are taught in English, with a portion in the native language; designed to prepare students for all-English instruction without falling behind in subject areas

transitional utterances in language development, any of several utterance types that appear to represent a progression from single word utterances to multiword utterances reflecting syntactic order

transition services services required by federal law that promote passage from school to postschool activities

transitive verb lexical verbs capable of carrying a grammatical object affected by the action of the verb

transit time, oropharyngeal the time elapsed between the beginning of swallowing and bolus passage out of the oropharynx

translucency property of signs or symbols that become readily guessable once the relationships between the signs or symbols or their referents are shown or taught

transmitter a device that emits electromagnetic rays that transmit radio and television signals; a component of an FM assistive listening system that modulates the frequency of a radio signal in an audio frequency signal and transmits the waves through air to an amplifier/receiver

transparency property of symbols and signs that are highly suggestive and therefore readily guessable by an untrained observer with no additional cues required; having no deception or artifice; easily understood

transverse anatomic plane that crosses the

long axis of the body, perpendicular to a given structure or phenomenon, such as a muscle fiber or airflow

trapezoid body transverse fiber knot in the lower brainstem's ventral portion

- **medial nucleus of the trapezoid body** nucleus in which some second-order neurons synapse with third-order neurons of the ascending auditory pathways; important region for mediating crossed acoustic reflex

trauma physical or mental injury

traumatic brain injury (TBI) damage to the brain caused by external mechanical forces applied to the head. Injury may involve the cranium or the brain or both. TBI results in impairment of cognitive abilities and/or physical, emotional, and behavioral functioning

traveling wave in the ear, the wave-like action of the basilar membrane arising from stimulation of the perilymph of the vestibule

traveling wave theory frequency analysis in the cochlea that ascribes the ability of the ear to analyze sounds strictly to the mechanical gradient of stiffness along the organ of Corti; Georg von Békésy's (1899–1972) Nobel Prize-winning work led to this theory

Treacher Collins syndrome micrognathia, absent or hypoplastic cheek bones, cleft palate, Robin sequence, airway obstruction, hearing loss; marked by misarticulations secondary to malocclusion and anterior skeletal open bite and severe tongue backing secondary to micrognathia

treatment broad range of planned and continuing inpatient, outpatient, and residential services including, but not limited to, diagnostic evaluation, counseling; medical, psychiatric, psychological, and social service care; and occupational services

- **auditory discrimination training** designed to teach clients to distinguish between correct and incorrect productions of speech sounds

- **breath chewing** technique involving the production of exaggerated chewing motions while vocalizing

- **breathing exercises** process that focuses on promoting adequate respiratory support for speech

- **buzzing** technique of choral reading aloud of rhyming sentences

- **chanting** repetitive tone vocalization process

- **chant-talk** technique that resembles chant-ing; consists of soft glottal attacks, raised pitch, prolonged syllables, even stress, and smooth blending of words; considered appropriate for hyperfunctional voice problems; helps reduce excessive muscular effort and tension associated with voice production

- **choral/unison reading** technique involving two (unison) or more (choral) speakers simultaneously reading selected passages aloud

- **coaching** client is reminded to continue using previously practiced behaviors

- **compensatory strategies** patterns previously atypical for a particular client are taught in seeking to promote mastery of a target behavior

- **contrastive sets/minimal pairs** person is exposed to two (minimal pairs) or more (contrastive sets) sets of stimuli that differ in only one dimension. Usually, the individual is expected to discriminate between the sets of stimuli

- **contrastive stress drills** used to promote both articulatory proficiency and natural prosody, especially the stress and rhythm aspects of spoken language. Used in treating apraxia of speech (AOS) in adults; varying phrases and sentences are used to teach placing stress on different words; stressed words or terms may be used to promote articulatory proficiency or simply to vary prosodic features of speech

- **easy onsets** technique that involves producing speech by directing breath through relaxed vocal folds, initiating vocalization, and then initiating articulatory movements

- **exaggeration** overemphasis of a selected prosodic or articulatory behavior

- **fading** cues, prompts, and/or coaching are gradually withdrawn

- **family therapy** simultaneous treatment of more than one member of a family; may be supportive, directive, or interpretive

- **gentle phonatory onset** stuttering treatment target; initiating voice in a gentle, soft, easy, relaxed manner; also a treatment target in treating hard glottal attack

- **humming** technique employing the production of a single continuing speech sound such as /m/ or /n/

- **imagery** visualization used to facilitate the production of a target behavior

- **intersystemic reorganization** strategy that pairs speaking with a rhythmic activity such

T

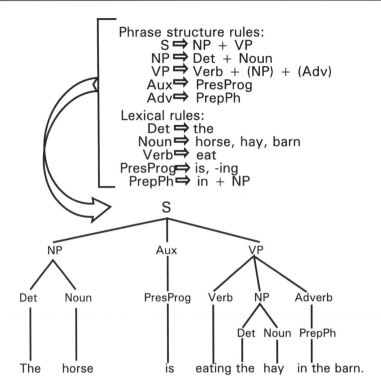

tree diagram   a graphic representation of syntactic constituent structure that uses nodes and links in a hierarchical structure

---

as pushing a button or squeezing a ball

- **intoning** technique of vocalizing or verbalizing while maintaining a simple intonation contour

- **narration** production of monologues having a story plot

- **pacing** use of an external source to cue the rate of speaking

- **pantomiming** employing facial and body gestures to express meaning

- **prompting** technique in which a client is provided hints or cues

- **pushing** speaker presses against an immovable object while vocalizing

- **rehearsal, covert** practicing targeted behaviors when alone

tree diagram a graphic representation of syntactic constituent structure that uses nodes and links in a hierarchical structure

tremolo in music, esthetically displeasing, excessively wide vibrato; also instrumental musical ornament employed by composers and performers

tremor repetitive and rhythmic contraction of opposing muscles, often involuntary, most often the hands, feet, jaw, tongue, or head

- **essential tremor** rhythmic movements of body parts, often during routine motor acts; an inherited (autosomal dominant) trait

- **frequency tremor** a periodic (regular) pitch modulation of the voice (an element of vibrato)

- **intention tremor** a tremor of a body part that occurs with intended movement; contrasts with resting tremor, which is evident for resting states

- **pill rolling tremor** rhythmic motions of finger on thumb as though a pill is being rolled between them; seen especially in individuals with Parkinson disease

- **vocal tremor** a periodic variation in vocal frequency and/or amplitude observed especially during sustained phonation

tri- prefix: three

triage medical patient screening to provide treatment order priorities

trifurcate to divide into three parts

trigeminal nerve cranial nerve V (CN V), primary facial sensory nerve and the motor nerve of the masticatory muscles; has three major sensory divisions and one motor division; innervates the head and oral cavity

- **motor trigeminal nucleus** a cranial motor nucleus with motor neurons that innervate several muscles of the mandible such as the jaw-closing muscles (i.e., masseter) and a jaw-opening muscle (i.e., anterior digastric) as well as muscles of the floor of the mouth

- **trigeminal sensory nuclei** a collection of three sensory nuclei in the brainstem, with the mesencephalic, main sensory, and spinal trigeminal the three components. Most of the sensory input from the head and neck synapses within these nuclei

trill speech sound formed by rapid oscillations of one or more structures; in early music (Renaissance) it referred to an ornament of same-note repetition, now known as a trillo

trillo originally a trill, but in recent pedagogy a rapid repetition of the same note, which usually includes repeated voice onset and offset

trochleariform process bony outcropping of the middle ear from which the tendon for the tensor tympani arises

-trophic suffix: related to nourishment or resulting from disruption of the nerve supply

trophoblast cell layer covering the embryonic blastocyst; attaches the embryo to the uterine wall and serves as the nutrient pathway

-trophy suffix: condition of growth or nutrition

-tropy suffix: having affinity for specified thing

trunk the body, excluding head and limbs

T-switch tetecoil switch on hearing aid

tubal feeding supplying liquid nutrition to the enteral tract via tubes, which may be placed through the mouth or nose or percutaneously

tubercle anatomical nodule that is a solid rounded elevation on the skin, mucous membrane, or organ surface or rounded portion of bone for muscle or ligament attachment

tumor new tissue growth noted by incremental uncontrolled cell proliferation (can be either benign or malignant); swelling or enlargement

tune-up mapping; establishing a map for a cochlear implant speech processor

tuning curve a graph depicting the response of a neuron, plotted as a function of stimulus intensity and frequency. The lowest sound level to which the neuron response is represented by the tip of the tuning curve (i.e., characteristic frequency)

tunnel of Corti region of the organ of Corti produced by articulation of the rods of Corti

turbulence a condition of airflow in which eddies (rotating volume elements of air) are associated with noise energy (turbulence noise); contrasts with **laminar flow**; also, a flow condition in which rotating elements of varying pressure and velocity are formed; condition under which noise is generated by an airstream

turbulence noise source sound produced with a continuous spectrum; results from the random variation of air pressure created when air particles pass through a narrow constriction at high velocity

turnabouts in language development, comments and replies used by caregivers to maintain momentum in a conversation and shift a turn to the child

turn taking the alternation of speaking and listening behaviors in a conversation

- **interturn pause** gap in vocalizing that occurs at the end of a speaking turn when the speaker stops talking

- **mean length speaking turn (MLT)** used in the assessment of conversational interactions, computed by determining the average number of words a person speaks during a set number of conversational turns

two-way bilingual/immersion program two languages are used for approximately equal time in a curriculum

tympanic membrane thin, taut membranous separation between the outer and middle ears, responsible for initiating the mechanical impedance-matching process of the middle ear

tympanogram graphic representation of how the immittance of the middle-ear system changes as air pressure is varied in the external ear canal. A dynamic measure of middle-ear function (see illustration, p. 246)

- **type A** normal tympanogram; sharply defined peak at or near zero air pressure

- **type Ad** normal shape, but amplified peak amplitude; usually associated with discontinuity of ossicular chain

- **type As** normal shape, but attenuated peak amplitude; usually associated with increased stiffness of ossicular chain, as in otosclerosis

T

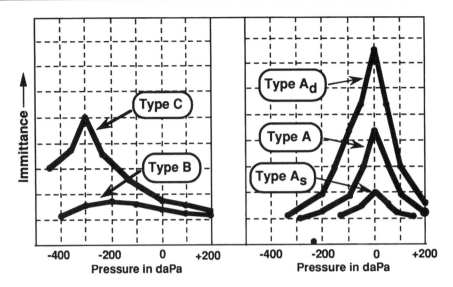

tympanogram   graphic representation of how the immittance of the middle-ear system changes as air pressure is varied in the external ear canal. A dynamic measure of middle-ear function

- **type B** relatively flattened tympanogram without sharp peak; usually associated with fluid in the middle-ear space

- **type C** peak has shifted significantly in the direction of negative air pressure in the external ear canal; usually associated with re-

U

Uvula

the small appendage suspended from the soft palate

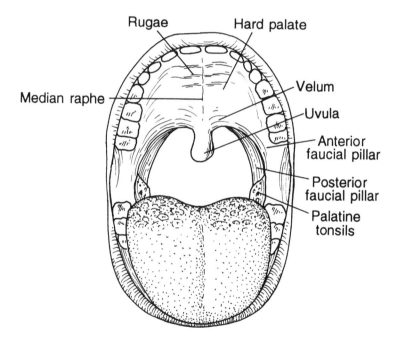

Rugae

Hard palate

Median raphe

Velum

Uvula

Anterior
faucial pillar

Posterior
faucial pillar

Palatine
tonsils

ulcer open sore or lesion of mucous membrane or skin caused by necrosis from an infectious, inflammatory, or cancerous process

- **glottal contact ulcer** benign lesion on the posterior third of the glottal margin; possibly due to trauma, reflux, or vocally abusive behaviors; voice symptoms include low pitch, effortful phonation, and vocal fatigue

ultra excess

ultrafast computed tomography (CT) synonymous with fast CT scanning. A technique of CT scanning in which the X ray rapidly scans the patient in several planes; fast enough to freeze rapid motions such as occur in the oropharynx during swallowing

ultrafast magnetic resonance imaging (uMRI) scanning technique allowing rapid magnetic resonance imaging scans to be performed, allowing enhanced swallowing studies

ultrasound imaging high-frequency sound wave used for soft tissue visualization, with tissue contrast provided by the differences in each tissue's ability to reflect sound

- **real-time ultrasound** sonographic procedure providing rapid, multiple images of an anatomical structure in the form of motion

umbo any projection of a rounded object in the body

- **umbo of tympanic membrane** the most distal point of attachment of the inner tympanic membrane to the malleus

un- prefix: not

unaided communication communication aspects that use only the communicator's body, with vocalizations, gestures, facial expressions, manual sign language, and head nods being examples

uncertainty behavior (or verbal fragmentation) excessive interjections and filler sometimes heard in utterances of aging individuals

uncomfortable level (UL) level at which sound is judged to be so loud as to be uncomfortable to a listener

uncrossed acoustic reflex stapedius muscle contraction recorded with sound stimulus and immittance recording probe in the same ear

underextension a word that is used for less than its full range of appropriate referents; a word that occurs only in response to a specific stimulus or context

understanding the process of decoding meaning from an encoded message, as in comprehending the significance of words and sentences

uni- prefix: one

unilateral pertaining to one side

unilateral upper motor neuron dysarthria motor speech disorder caused by damage to the upper motor neurons that supply cranial and spinal nerves involved in speech production; the dominant speech problem is imprecise production of consonants, but slow diadochokinesis and voice disorder also commonly occur

unilateral vocal fold paralysis immobility of one vocal fold from neurological dysfunction

unisensory older educational philosophy of presenting stimulation primarily through audition

unmarked semantic aspect of words about a dimension (e.g., length); in phonology, the less natural value of a feature

unstressed syllable any syllable in a word or utterance that is not the most prominent syllable

upper esophageal sphincter (UES) formed by the cricopharyngeus muscle, which by its tonic contraction closes the lumen between the pharynx and the esophagus. The cricopharyngeus relaxes briefly during swallowing. Opening of the UES segment is enhanced by the pull from the hyoid ascent and the pressure exerted by the luminal bolus

Usher syndrome hearing loss, retinitis pigmentosa and night blindness followed by adult deterioration and blindness in about half of the cases, along with occasional ataxia; marked by hearing loss, speech and language impairment

utero pertaining to the uterus

utricle regions of the ear's vestibule housing the otolithic organs of the vestibular system; a small sac

uvula the small appendage suspended from the soft palate (see illustration, p. 247)

V

Vocal Folds

muscles and connective tissue located within the larynx used to produce voice (through vocal fold vibration). The two vocal folds are attached anteriorly to the thyroid cartilage and posteriorly to the arytenoid cartilages

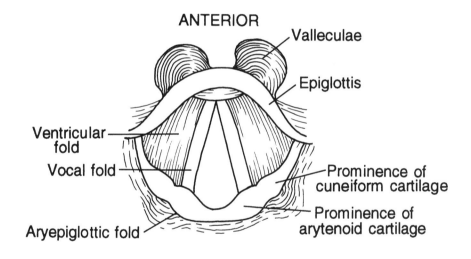

ANTERIOR

Valleculae

Epiglottis

Ventricular fold

Vocal fold

Prominence of cuneiform cartilage

Prominence of arytenoid cartilage

Aryepiglottic fold

SUPERIOR VIEW

vagotomy surgical cutting of at least one vagus nerve section

vagus nerve the tenth cranial nerve (CNX), which arises from the side of the medulla oblongata and innervates a wide variety of visceral organs, including the tongue (sensory), pharynx (sensory and motor), larynx (sensory and motor), lungs and heart (parasympathetic and visceral afferent)

validity degree of a measure's appropriateness for the matter being studied and/or its ability to measure what it is purported to measure

- **concurrent validity** criterion-related validity index employed to predict real-life performance

- **construct validity** statistical term meaning the extent to which a test measurement corresponds to theoretical concepts (as when a measure expected to vary over time does so)

- **content validity** statistical term meaning the extent to which a test adequately samples the domain studied (measurement for delirium would evaluate cognition)

- **criterion-related validity** test effectiveness of an individual's behavior or abilities in specific situations

- **external validity** (generalizability) means results can lead to unbiased inferences about the target population and not just the study subjects

- **face validity** how well test items represent what they claim to test

- **internal validity** variability between the control and comparison groups; may, other than sampling error, be from the effect being studied

vallecula a small depression or crevice

- **epiglottic vallecula** hollow immediately beyond the tongue root and before the epiglottis; residue in the vallecula after a swallow indicates a problem in tongue base movement

Valsalva maneuver the closure of the true and false vocal folds to assist in fixing the thorax for effortful activities (i.e., coughing and lifting); from Antonio Valsalva (1666–1723)

valve, one-way speaking valve placed on the hub of a tracheostomy tube to allow air to enter on inspiration. On expiration, the valve closes and air cannot escape the tracheostomy tube. Rather, the trapped air is redirected through the vocal folds and into the upper airway to use for speaking and swallowing

variability the amount of change or ability to change

- **talker variability** different talkers producing the same phonetic unit (such as /a/) or speech pattern with considerable variance in physical characteristics; especially true for male/female talkers or when comparing adult to child talkers. Nonetheless, the sounds are heard as belonging to the same phonetic category

variable, supplementary stimulus, such as an audience, that has a secondary influence on the likelihood of verbal behaviors

variance the mean squared difference from the average value in a data set

varicosity marked by being very swollen or dilated

varix vein that is grossly enlarged; varices at the gastroesophageal junction are common in chronic liver disease

varus bent inward or toward the midline

vasculature distribution of blood vessels in the body, including their connection and purposes

vasculitis inflammation of the small blood vessels

vasoconstrictor an agent that produces constriction of blood vessels; often used to treat hypotension

vasodilation dilation of blood vessels

vasospasm a brief abnormal constriction of a blood vessel

vasovagal reflex vagus nerve stimulation causing laryngeal or tracheal irritation; leads to pulse rate slowing

vector quantity with size and direction commonly shown by a directed line segment whose length represents the size and whose orientation in space represents the direction; organism (as an insect) that transmits a pathogen; sequence of genetic material employed for introducing certain genes into an organism's genome

vegetative sounds infant oral sounds (e.g., clicks, burps) associated with feeding and digestion

- **quasiresonant nuclei (QRN)** early infant oral sighlike sounds that lack resonance of mature vowel sounds

vein a vessel that returns blood to the heart from the capillaries

velar relating to the velum, or palate

velar assimilation substitution of a velar consonant for a nonvelar (e.g., /g/ for /d/)

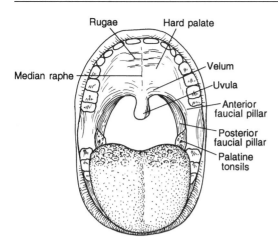

Rugae   Hard palate
Median raphe
Velum
Uvula
Anterior faucial pillar
Posterior faucial pillar
Palatine tonsils

velum generally means veil, or covering; in the vocal tract, is the soft palate and adjacent nasopharynx that closes during normal swallowing and phonation of certain sounds

---

velo-cardio-facial syndrome cleft palate, heart anomalies, learning disabilities, and ADHD; usually accompanied by delayed speech production onset, with global glottal stop substitutions in conjunction with clefts or VPI

velocity the rate of change of displacement of a body with respect to time (measured in meters per second, with the appropriate direction)

velopharyngeal insufficiency (also velopharyngeal incompetence) (VPI) functional or congenital deficiency in the superior constrictor muscle or soft palate leading to escape of air, liquid, or food from the oropharynx into the nasopharynx or nose when the nasopharynx should be closed by approximation of the soft palate and pharyngeal tissues

velopharyngeal opening the opening between the posterior portion of the oral cavity (actually oropharynx) and the nasal cavity

velopharyngeal port the passage that connects the oral and nasal cavities

velum generally means veil, or covering; in the vocal tract, is the soft palate and adjacent nasopharynx that closes during normal swallowing and phonation of certain sounds

venipuncture collection of blood from a vein or introduction of solution by puncturing the vein

vent bore drilled into a hearing aid earmold that permits the passage of sound and air; used for aeration of the external auditory canal or for acoustic modification of amplified sound

ventilation air inhaled per unit time; process of moving air into and out of lungs

- **assist-control mode (A/C)** a mode of mechanical ventilatory support. The ventilator will respond to the patient's spontaneous breathing efforts by delivering volume and provide a preset number of breaths if a patient fails to inspire within a set period

- **bilevel ventilation (BiPAP)** a method of noninvasive mechanical ventilation that provides an inspiratory pressure as well as a lower expiratory pressure. It is a variation of CPAP

- **continuous positive airway pressure (CPAP)** a mode of mechanical ventilatory support that is noncycled; the ventilatory provides a continuous flow of air to maintain a fairly constant pressure in the airway and at the alveolar level

- **controlled mode ventilation (CMV)** a mode of ventilation that cycles to provide inspiratory breaths independent of the breathing efforts of the patient

- **dead space ventilation** the volume of inhaled gas that does not come in contact with alveoli and hence does not contribute to gas exchange

- **hyperventilation** ventilation that exceeds the needs of the body. Reflected in abnormally low levels of CO_2 in the arterial blood

- **hypoventilation** ventilation that is inadequate to meet the needs of the body. Reflected by increased levels of CO_2 in the arterial blood

- **intermittent mandatory ventilation (IMV)** a mode of cycled ventilation where the patient may breathe spontaneously between timed mandatory breaths

- **manual bagging** the process of supplying breaths by a manual resuscitation bag, often used to oxygenate a patient before attempting intubation or when a patient is temporarily disconnected from mechanical ventilation

- **mechanical ventilation** mechanical assistance in the breathing process; it may be used to augment the efforts of a patient who has spontaneous, but weak, breaths or for individuals who do not breathe on their own

- **minute ventilation (V_E)** expired volume per unit time per kilogram of body weight. Oral feeding results in an impairment of ventilation during continuous sucking. The subsequent recovery during intermittent sucking

V

depends on postconceptional age. The recovery or increase may be a complex phenomenon that begins with respiratory inhibition caused by frequent sucking and swallowing, followed by an increase in V_E as arterial CO_2 rises and the frequency of sucking and swallowing decreases

- **negative pressure ventilation** noninvasive ventilatory support mode that employs negative pressure around the thorax to decrease intrathoracic pressure in relation to atmospheric pressure, causing inspiration. Expiration is passive. As a noninvasive mode, negative pressure ventilation does not require an endotracheal tube or tracheostomy, but can be physically restricting to a patient

- **peak inspiratory pressure** the highest measured airway pressure during the inspiratory phase of mechanical ventilatory support; pressures significantly exceeding this level causes the high pressure alarm on the ventilator to sound

- **positive end expiratory pressure (PEEP)** the application of a small amount (typically 5–20 cm H_2O) of positive airway pressure during mechanical ventilation to minimize alveolar collapse; the maintenance of airway pressures above atmospheric throughout the expiratory phase of a ventilatory cycle; designed to improve oxygenation. PEEP can be set at differing levels according to patient need

- **positive pressure ventilation** a means of mechanical ventilation that can be administered via invasive or noninvasive means by creating pressure higher than atmospheric and pushing air into the lungs

- **restrictive ventilatory defect** classification of respiratory pathology in which the patient's ability to fully inflate the lungs is diminished. May be a result of neuromuscular diseases (causing respiratory muscle weakness), to defects in the thoracic spine, ribs, or pleura (causing a mechanical obstruction to lung inflation), or to fibrosis or surgical removal of the lungs

- **synchronized intermittent mandatory ventilation (SIMV)** a mode of cycled ventilation in which the patient may breathe spontaneously between timed breaths. Unlike IMV, this mode of ventilation synchronizes with the spontaneous breathing efforts of a patient and waits, within a preset time, to allow the patient to inspire, without necessarily imposing a preset breath

ventilatory circuitry the tubing and connectors that connect a patient with a mechanical ventilator

ventral pertaining to the belly

ventral horns the anterior areas of the spinal cord containing nuclei for relaying outgoing motor impulses to the body

ventricle of Morgagni also known as laryngeal ventricle, laryngeal sinus, and ventriculus laryngis. The ventricle is a fusiform pouch bounded by the margin of the vocal folds, the edge of the free margin of the false vocal fold (ventricular fold), and the mucous membrane between them that forms the pouch. Anteriorly, a narrowing opening leads from the ventricle to the appendix of the ventricle of Morgagni

ventricular dysphonia disorder caused by use of the ventricular (false) vocal folds; sometimes associated with enlarged ventricular folds; condition is characterized by low pitch, monotone, decreased loudness, harshness, and arrhythmic voicing; diagnosis depends on endoscopy, X ray, or stroboscopy, as condition is very difficult to diagnose from voice sound, alone

ventricular folds so-called false vocal folds, situated above the true vocal folds

ventricular ligament narrow band of fibrous tissue that extends from the angle of the thyroid cartilage below the epiglottis to the arytenoid cartilage just above the vocal process. It is contained within the false vocal fold. The caudal border of the ventricular ligament forms a free crescentic margin, which constitutes the upper border of the ventricle of Morgagni

ventricular septal defect congenital abnormality in which the two lower chambers of the heart are connected

ventro-, ventri- combining form: pertaining to the belly, or anterior part of the body

venule tiny vein

verb class of words that usually express action

- **action verb** word that refers to activity that is observable

- **auxiliary verb** grammatical verb serving as helper by conveying number and tense

- **copula** grammatical verb that links its subject to a noun phrase, adjective, or prepositional phrase

- **grammatical verb** verb that plays a grammatical role without conveying specific action

- **intransitive verb** lexical verb that is incapable of carrying or containing a direct object

- **lexical verb** verb that expresses a specific activity

- **modal auxiliary verb** auxiliary verb that expresses the speaker's attitude or mood regarding the main verb

- **process verb** referring to unobservable activity or gradual change

- **state verbs** words that links a subject to a stable or unchanging condition or attribute

- **transitive verb** lexical verb that carries or contains a direct object affected by the action of the verb

verbal auditory closure the ability to use spoken contextual information to facilitate speech recognition

verbal behavior paradigm, interlocking B. F. Skinner's model illustrating the interactive nature of verbal exchanges between speaking partners

verbal communication the use of symbols (i.e., words), whether spoken, written, or gestured by a speaker to express ideas

verbal fragmentation (or uncertainty behavior) excessive interjections and filler sometimes heard in utterances of aging individuals

verbal operant conditioning language acquisition concept from B. F. Skinner that learning a language is a process in which correct grammar is shaped by positive reinforcement, which leads to reuse, and poor grammar is negatively reinforced and not repeated

vermillion zone the red part of the lip where the lip mucosa borders the skin

vernacular language (often informal) or dialect intrinsic to an area or nation, as opposed to a literary or cultured language; sometimes considered nonstandard

vertical phase difference asynchrony between the lower and upper surfaces of the vibratory margin of the vocal fold during phonation

vertigo sensation of rotary motion. A form of dizziness

vesicle a small fluid-filled sac

vestibule a cavity that serves as an entrance to a canal; specifically the ovoid central cavity of the ear's osseous labyrinth

- **gastroesophageal vestibule** bulging esophageal portion just above the cardiac orifice

- **oral vestibule** mouth portion bounded by the lips and cheeks and teeth and/or gums; also known as buccal cavity

- **rima vestibuli** space between the false (ventricular) vocal folds

- **scala vestibuli** peripheral cavity of the cochlea that communicates with the middle ear via the vestibule and the oval window

- **vestibule of larynx** upper portion of the laryngeal cavity, ranging from the superior aperture to the vestibular (false vocal) folds, marked anteriorly by epiglottis and laterally by the quadrangular membrane mucosa and posteriorly by the arytenoid cartilage mucosa and arytenoideus muscle

vestibulocochlear nerve acoustic nerve, eighth cranial nerve (CN VIII), which emerges from the brain behind the facial nerve between the pons and medulla oblongata

vibration periodic particle motion in an elastic body or medium alternating in opposite directions from equilibrium when the position of equilibrium has been disturbed—as when particles of air transmit sounds to the ear or a stretched string makes a musical sound

- **cycle of vibration** one full return to the point at which a function begins to repeat itself

vibrato in classical singing, vibrato is a periodic modulation of the frequency of phonation. Its regularity increases with training. The rate of vibrato (number of modulations per second) is usually in the range of 5–6 per second. Vibrato rates over 7–8 per second are esthetically displeasing to most people; extent of vibrato (amount of variation above and below the center frequency) is usually one or two semitones. Vibratos extending less then ±0.5 semitone are rarely seen in singers although they are encountered in wind instrument playing. Vibrato rates greater than two semitones are usually esthetically unacceptable

- **frequency tremor** a periodic (regular) pitch modulation of the voice (an element of vibrato)

vibratory instability irregular vocal fold vibration

vibrotactile pertaining to the detection of vibrations through the sense of touch

vibrotactile hearing aid an assistive listening device that converts acoustic energy into vibratory patterns that are delivered to the skin

videofluoroscopic examination (VFE) dynamic (moving) X-ray examination of oral and pharyngeal swallowing function; also called dysphagia diagnostic study (DSS), functional assessment of swallowing (FAS), videofluoroscopic swallow study (VSS), cookie swallow test, and modified barium swallow (MBS). The primary purpose of this examination is to determine the cause(s) of dysfunction of the oral and/or pharyngeal stages of swallowing

videotaped scenarios videotaped examples of communication interactions that may include use of communications strategies and language-stimulation techniques

vigilance (sustained attention) ability to inhibit interference; requires sustained focus while waiting for a target stimulus to happen

villus, (pl., **villi)** slender process on a mucous membrane

virus tiny microorganism that can only replicate within a plant or animal cell; can cause disease in humans, animals, and plants; typically has a genetic RNA or DNA center surrounded by a protein coating

viscera internal organs within a cavity

visceral pertaining to internal organs

visceral pleura outer surface of the lung

viscerocranium facial bones of facial skeleton; skull portion derived by embryonic pharyngeal arches; distinct from braincase

viscoelastic material substance that exhibits characteristics of both elastic solids and viscous liquids. The vocal fold is an example

viscosity property of a liquid associated with its resistance to deformation; associated with the "thickness" of a liquid

viseme groups of speech sounds that appear identical on the lips (e.g., /p, m, b/)

visual alerting systems assistive devices that include alarm clocks, doorbells, and smoke detectors in which the alerting mechanism is a flashing light

visual association area the cortical area surrounding the primary visual cortex and responsible for interpretation of the significance of visual stimuli

visual reinforcement audiometry (VRA) audiometric technique used with young children in which a correct response to a stimulus presentation is reinforced by a visual reward, such as the activation of a lighted toy

vital capacity maximum possible breathing capacity: total volume of air that can be expired at

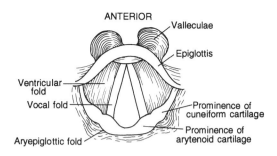

ANTERIOR
Valleculae
Epiglottis
Ventricular fold
Vocal fold
Prominence of cuneiform cartilage
Prominence of arytenoid cartilage
Aryepiglottic fold

SUPERIOR VIEW

vocal folds muscles and connective tissue located within the larynx used to produce voice (through vocal fold vibration). The two vocal folds are attached anteriorly to the thyroid cartilage and posteriorly to the arytenoid cartilages

a typical rate following a maximum inspiration; inspiratory reserve volume added to the tidal volume plus the expiratory reserve volume

vital signs (VS) prime indicators of life; measures of pulse rate, body temperature, and respiration rate, with blood pressure often included; used for monitoring patients

vocabulary all words used by a language, group, individual, or in area of knowledge

- **core vocabulary** highly functional, high-frequency words and phrases, typically related to basic needs

- **fringe vocabulary** words and expression that are typically content-rich, topic-related, and specific to particular individuals, activities, or environments

vocabulary development formation of a stock of words accessible for everyday use

- **horizontal vocabulary development** the process of adding associated features that expand the meaning of a word

- **vertical vocabulary development** the process of associating additional meanings and contexts for a word

vocabulary spurt sharp increase in new words from one month to the next after a child has acquired a small number of words in the second year

vocal cord old term for vocal fold

vocal folds muscles and connective tissue located within the larynx used to produce voice (through vocal fold vibration). The two vocal folds are attached anteriorly to the thyroid cartilage and posteriorly to the arytenoid cartilages

- **false vocal folds** folds of tissue located slightly higher than and parallel to the actual vocal folds

- **hyperadduction of the vocal folds** overly strong adduction of muscles that causes the vocal folds to be pressed at midline

- **hypoadduction of the vocal folds** reduced vocal fold adduction resulting in disordered voice (flaccid or hypokinetic); usually of neurological origin

- **longitudinal tension** stretching of the vocal folds

- **medial compression** the degree of force that may be applied by the vocal folds at their point of contact

- **surface wave** a wave that moves along a surface; the vertical-phase difference observed on the vocal fold during vibration

- **vertical phase difference** asynchrony between the lower and upper surfaces of the vibratory margin of the vocal fold during phonation

- **vocal fold abduction** the vocal folds are positioned near the side of the airway in the trachea; the vocal folds are open

- **vocal fold adduction** the vocal folds are positioned near midline in the trachea; the vocal folds are closed

- **vocal fold augmentation** the injection of an absorbable or nonabsorbable substance to achieve vocal fold closure and prevent aspiration related to vocal fold paralysis

- **vocal fold body** vocalis muscle

- **vocal fold paralysis, bilateral** loss of the ability to move both vocal folds caused by neurologic dysfunction

- **vocal fold paralysis, unilateral** immobility of one vocal fold, due to neurological dysfunction

- **vocal fold stiffness** the ratio of the effective restoring force (in the medial-lateral direction) to the displacement (in the same direction)

- **vocal fold stripping** a surgical technique, no longer considered acceptable practice under most circumstances, in which the vocal fold is grasped with a forceps, and the surface layers are ripped off

vocal fry a "rumble-crackling" of sound resulting from abnormal vibration of the vocal folds, or a low-frequency vibration of the false vocal folds; also known as pulse register and strohbass

vocal hyperfunction vocally abusive behaviors that cause nodules, polyps, and associated voice disorders; specifically, speaking with excessive muscular effort and force

vocal intensity sound pressure level associated of a given speech production

vocalis muscle (also called thyroarytenoid) relaxes (decreases tension) of the vocal folds and lowers the pitch of the voice tone; runs from the inner surface of the thyroid cartilage to the muscular process and outer surface of the arytenoid; originates at the concavity of the thyroid cartilage laminae and inserts at vocal process of arytenoid

vocal jitter cycle-by-cycle variation in fundamental frequency of vibration

vocal ligament intermediate and deep layers of the lamina propria. Also forms the superior end of the conus elasticus

vocal nodules small benign growths (that resemble calluses) that form on the vocal folds at the point of maximum vocal fold adduction; usually paired and fairly symmetric; generally caused by chronic, forceful vocal fold contact (voice abuse)

vocal play infant sound productions exhibiting long strings of varied syllables

vocal polyp small bulge of tissue on vocal fold mucosal surface; usually unilateral and benign

vocal tract the cavities and structures above the vocal folds capable of modifying the vocal tone and airflow into distinctive speech sounds. The vocal tract can include the nasal airway during the production of nasal sounds (see illustration, p. 256)

vocal tract model a model that illustrates the shaping of the vocal tract for the production of speech sounds

vocal tremor rhythmic shaking of the voice that is observed in some neurological disorders; the frequency of tremor varies with the neurologic disorder

vocative a word representing the individual to which a message is addressed (e.g., the name "Crystal" in "Crystal, don't eat the chocolates.")

voce coperta in singing, covered registration

voce di petto in music, chest voice

voce di testa in music, head voice

voce mista in singing, mixed voice

voce piena in music, full voice

voce sgangherata in music, white voice; means immoderate or unattractive; lacks strength in the lower partials

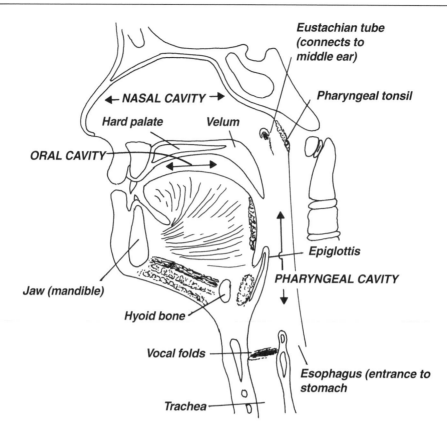

Eustachian tube (connects to middle ear)

NASAL CAVITY

Pharyngeal tonsil

Hard palate   Velum

ORAL CAVITY

Epiglottis

PHARYNGEAL CAVITY

Jaw (mandible)

Hyoid bone

Vocal folds

Esophagus (entrance to stomach

Trachea

vocal tract   the cavities and structures above the vocal folds capable of modifying the vocal tone and airflow into distinctive speech sounds. The vocal tract can include the nasal airway during the production of nasal sounds

---

voice the tone produced by vibration of the vocal folds and modified by the resonating cavities of the vocal tract

- **chest voice** heavy registration with excessive resonance in the lower formants

- **creaky voice** the perceptual result of subharmonic or chaotic patterns in the glottal waveform. According to I. R. Titze, if a subharmonic is below about 70 Hz, creaky voice may be perceived as pulse register (vocal fry)

- **normal voice** sound produced with normal vibration of the vocal folds

- **voice abuse** use of the voice in specific activities that are deleterious to vocal health, such as screaming

- **voice bar** a band of energy, typically reflecting the first harmonic of the voice source, that appears on a spectrogram; it is indicative of voicing

- **voice onset time (VOT)** a measure of the time between a supraglottal event and the onset of voicing; for stops, VOT is the interval between release of the stop (usually determined acoustically as the stop burst) and the appearance of periodic modulation (voicing) for a following sound

- **voice quality** perceptual characteristics of the vocal tone (normal, breathy, harsh, hoarse)

- **voice recognition** the determination that a particular speaker produced a given speech signal; also called speaker recognition

- **voice rest, absolute** total silence (nonuse) of the phonatory system

- **voice rest, relative** restricted, cautious voice use

voice box nontechnical term for larynx

voice coach in singing, a professional who works with singers, teaching repertoire, language pronunciation, and other artistic components of performance (as opposed to a singing teacher, who teaches technique); voice coach is also used as term for acting-voice teachers who specialize in vocal, body, and interpretive techniques to enhance dramatic performance

voiced speech produced using the vibrating vocal folds

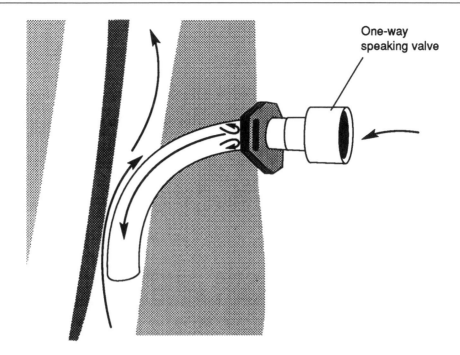

One-way speaking valve

voice prosthesis following laryngectomy and vocal fold excision, device used to facilitate speech production. Most commonly a surgical passage, tracheoesophageal puncture (TEP), is created inside the stoma from the backwall of the trachea into the esophagus, with a valved tube enabling tracheosophageal speech; a small silicone device that has a valve at the back end and an opening at the front end is inserted into a tracheoesophageal puncture that allows air into the esophagus, which vibrates to create sound that can be shaped into speech

voice disorder abnormal voice quality resulting from anatomic, physiologic, or psychogenic causes

voiced-voiceless a phonetic feature of speech distinguished by voice onset time, an acoustic feature that describes the timing between two events in speech, the onset of laryngeal voicing and the onset of other acoustic events that mark the release of the sound; voiced sounds are produced when these two events occur nearly simultaneously, voiceless sounds when the release of the sound precedes voicing by more than 40 ms

voiceless phoneme produced without the vibration of vocal folds

voice misuse habitual phonation using phonatory techniques that are not optimal and lead to vocal strain. For example, speaking with inadequate support, excessive neck muscle tension, and suboptimal resonance

voice prosthesis following laryngectomy and vocal fold excision, device used to facilitate speech production. Most commonly a surgical passage, tracheoesophageal puncture (TEP), is created inside the stoma from the backwall of the trachea into the esophagus, with a valved tube enabling tracheosophageal speech; a small silicone device that has a valve at the back end and an opening at the front end is inserted into a tracheoesophageal puncture that allows air into the esophagus, which vibrates to create sound that can be shaped into speech

voice source sound generated by the pulsating transglottal airflow; the sound is generated when the vocal fold vibrations chip the airstream into a pulsating airflow

voice turbulence index a measure of the relative energy level of high-frequency noise

volume amount of sound; best measured in terms of acoustic power or intensity; amount of material in a container

volume conduction passive conduction of a current from a potential source through tissue or body fluid, not limited to a plane such as a membrane surface

volume control manual or automatic control used to adjust the output of a listening device

volume velocity measure of airflow that takes account of both amount and speed of air

von Recklinghausen type neurofibromatosis (NF I) occasional mild dysarthria or dyspraxia; if cognitive impairment is present speech and language can be delayed; marked by café au lait skin spots, cutaneous neurofibromas, macrencephaly

vortex theory holds that eddies, or areas of organized turbulence, are produced as air flows through the larynx and vocal tract

vowel speech sound class member that when articulated does not block the oral portion of the breath channel, preventing constriction and audible friction; most noticeable sound in a syllable

- **cardinal vowel system** set of vowel reference points introduced by the linguist Daniel Jones. It uses 8 primary vowels in a front-back arrangement, with variations in vertical tongue position for both front and back vowels

- **central vowel** the major articulator for a central vowel is the tongue blade, with the American English central vowel [ə]

- **corner vowels** /a/, /i/, and /u/; vowels at the corners of a vowel triangle; they necessitate extreme placements of the tongue. Also, the vowels /a/, /æ/, /i/, and /u/ that define the points of the vowel quadrilateral

- **long vowels** vowels that have an inherently long duration:, e.g., /i/, /e/, /a/, /ɔ/, /u/

- **point vowels** the three vowels (/i/, /a/, and /u/) that are at the articulatory and acoustic extremes in vowel space

- **short vowels** vowels with an inherently short duration; [ɪ], [ə], [ʊ]; also known as lax vowels

Vygotsky approach cognitive psychological approach that bases cognition and personality development on social interaction, dealing with macro- and microsocial influences during development; from Lev Semyonovich Vygotsky (1896–1934), variant contemporary spelling of the original Russian is Vygotskii

W

Wernicke's Area

cortical area in the posterior temporal lobe
primarily responsible for interpreting oral language

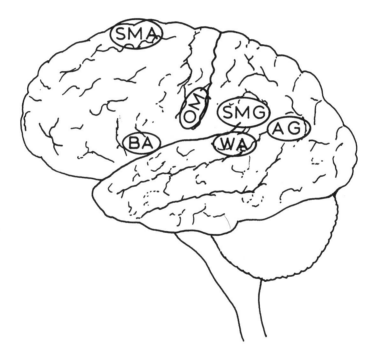

Lateral aspect of the left cerebral hemisphere, with major speech-
language areas labeled. BA = Broca's area, WA = Wernicke's area,
AG = angular gyrus, SMG = supramarginal gyrus, SMA = supplementary motor area, and OM = orofacial motor cortex.

Waldeyer's ring a ring of lymphatic (tonsillar) tissue at the oral-pharyngeal-nasal junction

warm spot receptive field of sensory nerve fibers that discharges when a stimulus that produces a temperature across a specific range is placed within its receptive field

warping of acoustic space a change in the perceived distance between various phonetic stimuli that is brought about by exposure to a specific language

wave a propagation of a disturbance through a medium

- **mucosal wave** undulation along the vocal fold surface traveling in the direction of the airflow

- **sound wave** the acoustical manifestation of physical disturbance in a medium

- **surface wave** a wave that moves along a surface; the vertical phase difference observed on the vocal fold during vibration

- **traveling wave** in the ear, the wave-like action of the basilar membrane arising from stimulation of the perilymph of the vestibule

waveform usually a graphic representation of a wave shape that illuminates its characteristics, as in showing the amplitude versus time function for a continuous signal such as the acoustic signal of speech, which is also known as the time series

- **complex periodic waveform** a waveform constructed of two or more sinusoids whose frequencies are multiples of the frequency of the waveform

wavefront initial disturbance in a propagating wave

wavelength the distance that a periodic sound travels in one complete cycle. Wavelength = speed of sound/frequency

weaning process of removing a patient from mechanical ventilatory support. May be a gradual reduction of support or a more abrupt process; also describes the process of gradually decannulating a patient from a tracheostomy

Weaver syndrome skeletal anomalies, hypotonia, delayed development, macrocephaly; marked by delayed speech and language onset, with sluggish articulation secondary to hypotonia

weighting scale sound level meter filtering network, in which the measurement of one band of frequencies is emphasized over another (e.g., dBA scale)

Wernicke's aphasia a type of aphasia named after the Polish neurologist who first described its features (Karl Wernicke, 1848–1905); characterized by fluent flow of jargon, but with little or no comprehension of the spoken word; a severe fluent (sometimes nonsensical) aphasia

Wernicke's area cortical area in the posterior temporal lobe primarily responsible for interpreting oral language

wheelchair mounting systems custom-made or commercial adaptations for wheelchairs designed to support an AAC device at the correct height and viewing angle

whisper sound created by turbulent glottal airflow in the absence of vocal fold vibration

whistle register the highest of all registers (in pitch). It is observed only in females, extending the pitch range beyond F_6

white noise noise having equal energy at all frequencies audible to the human ear; random-like signal with a flat frequency spectrum, in which each frequency has the same magnitude; analogous to white light, which contains every possible color. Typically described as a relative power density in volts squared per hertz; power varies directly with bandwidth, so white noise would have twice as much power in the next higher octave as in the current one

whole language educational theory incorporating teaching strategies and experiences to promote learning of reading, writing, speaking, and listening in natural language situations. Instruction with a whole language approach is informal and transactional, following a psychosociolinguistic approach. Also, an amorphous cluster of ideas about language development in the classroom; generally supports a holistic and integrated teaching of reading, writing, spelling, and oracy (function matters rather than the form of language)

wholistic associations extension of a word to items sharing a number of features with the original referent for that word

wh-question interrogative sentence beginning with a wh-word, such as who, what, where, when, how, and why

wide-band analysis analysis in which a relatively large analyzing bandwidth is used (such as 300 Hz in speech analysis). A wide-band analysis is preferred when the primary concern is to reveal formant pattern or to increase time resolution

wide-band noise white noise

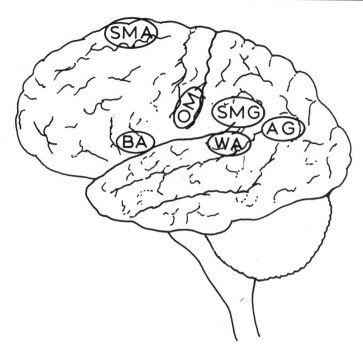

Lateral aspect of the left cerebral hemisphere, with major speech-language areas labeled. BA = Broca's area, WA = Wernicke's area, AG = angular gyrus, SMG = supramarginal gyrus, SMA = supplementary motor area, and OM = orofacial motor cortex.

Wernicke's area   cortical area in the posterior temporal lobe primarily responsible for interpreting oral language

Williams syndrome cognitive impairment, hypercalcemia, microcephaly, large mouth, thick lips, microdontia, hyperopia; marked by echolalia, overtalkativeness, with a sophisticated but abnormal language ability known for cliché overuse and friendly cocktail party manner and conversational style

window a weighting function applied to a waveform so that its amplitude gradually increases and decreases; the window acts like an acoustic "lens" to focus analysis on a representative part of a signal

wireless system an assistive listening device in which wires are not necessary to connect the sound source to the listener; includes FM and infrared systems

withdrawal syndrome a cluster of characteristic symptoms and reactions of varying intensity, sometimes fatally severe, that follow on abrupt cessation or reduction in amount of alcohol and/or other drug for which the body has developed a physical dependence

wobble in singing, slow, irregular vibrato; esthetically unsatisfactory; sometimes referred to as a tremolo; may have a rate of less than 4 oscillations per second and an extent of greater than ±2 semitones

word, action relational word acquired early that relates actions with an object of interest

word awareness conscious awareness that words are objects with phonetic structure and can have multiple meanings

word formation rule a process by which a word or stem is combined with an affix to form a new word with a somewhat altered meaning

word predictability amount of fill-in-the-blank meaningfulness in a preceding spoken context. In predictability-high (PH) sentences, preceding semantic-contextual information is presented in the form of clue words; no such clue words are available in predictability-low (PL) sentences

word prediction memory-resident utility word processing ancillary software that provides keyboard assistance. As the user inputs each keystroke, the software presents a list of possible words or phrases that it predicts the user may intend. The user then selects the appropriate word from the prediction list. Statistical weighting and grammatical knowledge are often incorporated into the software to improve prediction tasks

word processing the entry and manipulation of written words using a computer or other device to electronically record words. Word processing features include methods for entering, deleting, editing, merging, and saving written material

word recognition a spoken language processing event marking the conclusion of a word selection phase; also is a listener's ability to perceive and correctly identify a set of words usually presented at suprathreshold hearing level

word recognition score percentage of words correct

world knowledge individual's understanding of the world based on his or her accumulated experiences and memory

X-linked

a 50% chance of males inheriting an abnormal trait because of the presence of a mutant gene on one of the mother's X chromosomes

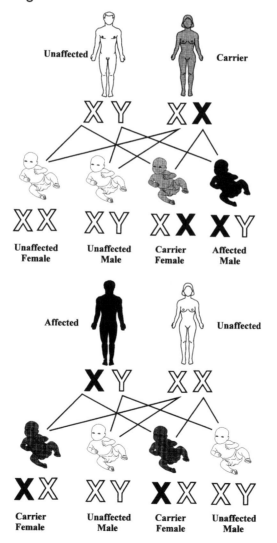

xerostomia a condition of excessively dry mouth caused by abnormal saliva production; can occur as a result of medication, disease, or radiation therapy

X-linked a 50% chance of males inheriting an abnormal trait because of the presence of a mutant gene on one of the mother's X chromosomes (see illustration, p. 2)

xyphoid sword-shaped; the bony inferior extension of the sternum

Y in the manual alphabet

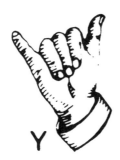

Young's modulus the ratio between magnitudes of stress and strain (Thomas Young, 1860–1905)

Z

zygomatic bone

bone pairs forming the cheek prominence (zygoma), eye orbit lower portion, and parts of the temporal processes

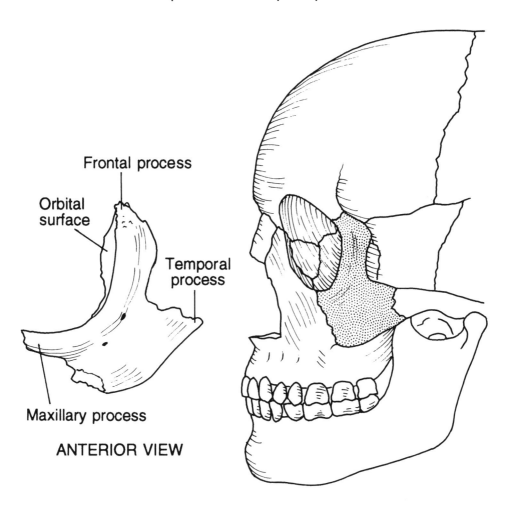

Frontal process

Orbital surface

Temporal process

Maxillary process

ANTERIOR VIEW

Zenker's diverticulum herniation of the pharyngeal mucosa at the level of the upper esophageal sphincter. The diverticulum usually protrudes between the fibers of the cricopharyngeus and inferior constrictor muscles. These herniations most commonly occur on the left side, less commonly on the posterior wall and the midline, and only rarely on the right side (after German pathologist Friedrich Zenker, 1825–1898)

zygomatic arch prominent portion of the zygomatic bone that is attached to the lateral surface of the squamous portion of the temporal bone

zygomatic bone bone pairs forming the cheek prominence (zygoma), eye orbit lower portion, and parts of the temporal processes; see illustration, p. 267

zygote the single cell formed at conception containing the genetic codes of both a father and mother

Abbreviations, Acronyms, and Initialisms

AAA American Academy of Audiology, 9

AAC augmentative (assistive) and alternative communication; see also **scanning**, 23

AACPDM American Academy for Cerebral Palsy and Developmental Medicine

AAMFT American Association of Marital and Family Therapy

AAMR American Association on Mental Retardation

AAO-HNS American Academy of Otolaryngology—Head and Neck Surgery

AAC augmentative (assistive) and alternative communication, 23

AAP American Academy of Pediatrics

AARP American Association of Retired Persons

AAUAP American Association of University Affiliated Programs for Persons with Developmental Disabilities

ABG arterial blood gas, 16

ABR auditory brainstem response, 22

A/C assist-control mode, 19

ACh acetylcholine, 3

ACSW Academy of Certified Social Workers

ADA Academy of Dispensing Audiologists

ADA Americans with Disabilities Act, 9

ADD attention deficit disorder, 21

ADHD attention deficit hyperactivity disorder, 21

ADL activity of daily living, 4

AEP auditory evoked potential, 22

Ag antigen, 13

AGC automatic gain control, 24

AIDS acquired immunodeficiency syndrome, 4

AIR American Institutes for Research

ALD assistive listening device, 19

ALS amyotrophic lateral sclerosis, 10

AM amplitude modulation

AMA American Medical Association

ANSI American National Standards Institute, 9

AP action potential, 4

APA American Psychiatric Association; American Psychological Association

APQ amplitude perturbation quotient, 10

APTA American Physical Therapy Association

APUD amine precursor uptake and decarboxylation (cells), 15

aq. water (Latin: *aqua*)

ARDS adult respiratory distress syndrome, 5

ASD atrial septal defect, 20

ASHA American Speech-Language-Hearing Association, 9

ASL American Sign Language, 9

ATNR asymmetrical tonic neck reflex, 19

Ba barium chemical symbol

BAER brainstem auditory evoked response

BBB blood-brain barrier, 33

BICS basic interpersonal communication skills, 29

b.i.d. 2 times a day (Latin: *bis in die*)

BiPAP bilevel ventilation, 32

BEA Bilingual Education Act

BP blood pressure, 34

BTE behind-the-ear hearing aid, 31

BW body weight

BX biopsy, 32

CAD central auditory disorder, 42

CALP cognitive academic language proficiency, 48

CANS central auditory nervous system, 42

CAPD central auditory processing disorder; continuous ambulatory peritoneal dialysis, 42

CAT outdated term for CT scan, 59

CBA cost–benefit analysis, 56

CBF cerebral blood flow, 43

CDS child-directed speech, 44

CEA cost-effectiveness analysis, 56

CFC cardiofaciocutaneous syndrome, 40

CEC Council for Exceptional Children

CGRP calcitonin gene-related peptide, 40

CHI closed-head injury, 46

cib food (Latin: *cibus*)

CIC completely-in-the-canal hearing aid

cm centimeter

CMRR common mode rejection ratio, 50

CMV controlled mode ventilation; cytomegalovirus, 54

CN cranial nerve, 57

CN VIII eighth cranial nerve, 57

CNS central nervous system, 42

CNT could not test

COPD chronic obstructive pulmonary disease, 45

COWAT controlled oral word association test, 54

CPU central processing unit, 43

CPR cardiopulmonary resuscitation

CREST Raynaud phenomenon/esophageal dysfunction/sclerodactyly/telangiectasis, 57

CSF cerebrospinal fluid, 43

CT computed tomography, 52

CUP common underlying proficiency (in two languages), 50

CV consonant-vowel, 53

CVA cerebrovascular accident, 43

CVC consonant-vowel-consonant, 53

DAF delayed auditory feedback, 63

DAI direct audio input

DAT diet as tolerated

dB decibel, 62

DBE dual bilingual education

DC direct current

DDK diadochokinesis, 66

DDS dysphagia diagnostic study

DFT discrete Fourier transform

DHHS Department of Health and Human Services, 64

DL difference limen; dual language

DPOAE distortion-product evoked otoacoustic emissions, 68

DMA direct memory access (computer)

DMFT decayed, missing, and filled teeth

DNA deoxyribonucleic acid, 64

DSP digital signal processing, 66

Dx diagnosis, 66

EBV Epstein-Barr virus, 76

EC European Community

ECG electrocardiography, 73

ECoG, EcochG, ECOG electrocochleography, 73

E. coli escherichia coli

ECU environmental control unit, 75

EEC ectrodactyly-ectodermal dysplasia-clefting, 73

EEG electroencephalography, 74

EFL English as a foreign language, 75

EGG electroglottography, 73

EKG electrocardiography, 73

EMG electromyography, 74

ENG electronystagmography, 74

ENT ear, nose, and throat

e.o.d. every other day

EPROM erasable programmable read-only memory, 76

ESEA Elementary and Secondary Education Act

ESOL English for speakers of other languages, 75

ESR erythrocyte sedimentation rate, 77

EUS endoscopic ultrasound, 75

FAPE free and appropriate education

FAS fetal alcohol syndrome/functional assessment of swallowing, 83

FB foreign body

FDA Food and Drug Administration, 85

FFT fast Fourier transform

FGG flow glottogram

FIM functional independence measure, 90

FM frequency modulated, 89

fMRI functional magnetic resonance imaging, 90

F₀, f₀, F0 fundamental frequency, 90

FRC functional residual capacity, 90

GABA gamma-aminobutyric acid, γ-aminobutryic acid, 94

GER gastroesophageal reflux, 94

GERD gastroesophageal reflux disorder, 94

GRBAS hoarse voice scale; G = overall grade, R = rough, B = breathy, A = asthenic, S = strained, 99

GSR galvanic skin response

HAE hearing aid evaluation, 104

HAO hearing aid orientation, 104

HAS high-amplitude sucking, 106

HDL high-density lipoproteins

HL hearing level, 104

HME heat moisture exchange filter, 105

HMM hidden Markov model, 106

HMO health maintenance organization

HPV human papilloma virus, 107

Hx history

ICIDH International Classification of Impairments, Disabilities, and Handicaps

IDEA Individuals with Disabilities Education Act, 113

IEC International Electrotechnical Commission

IEP individualized educational plan, 113

IFSP individualized family service plan, 113

IMV intermittent mandatory ventilation, 116

INF intravenous nutritional fluid

I/O input/output, 115

IPA International Phonetic Alphabet, 116

ISO International Organization for Standardization

ITC in the canal (hearing aid)

ITE in-the-ear (hearing aid), 117

IV intravenous

JND just noticeable difference, 122

Kb, Kbyte kilobyte; one thousand bytes, 124

LAD language acquisition device, 128

LCD liquid crystal display, 134

LDL loudness discomfort level, 135

LDL low-density lipoproteins

LED light-emitting diode, 131

LEP limited-English proficiency

LES lower esophageal sphincter, 135

LMS language-minority students

L1/L2 first language, second language, 126

LPC linear predictive coding, 133

LPR laryngopharyngeal reflux, 129

LRE least restrictive environment, 131

LTAS long-term average spectrum, 135

MAO monoamine oxidase, 147

M & R measure and record

MBS modified barium swallow, 147

MCL most comfortable loudness

MHC major histocompatibility complex, 140

MI myocardial infarction, 151

MIT melodic intonation therapy, 143

ml milliliter, 146

MLR middle-latency response, 146

MLT mean length speaking turn

MLU mean length of utterance, 143

mm millimeter, 146

MPO maximum power output

MRI magnetic resonance imaging, 140

MS multiple sclerosis, 150

N newton

NAD National Association of the Deaf, 154

NATS National Association of Teachers of Singing

N & V nausea and vomiting

NECCI Network of Educators of Children with Cochlear Implants, 156

NG nasogastric (tube), 154

NHR noise-to-harmonic ratio, 160

NIHL noise-induced hearing loss, 160

NIPTS noise-induced permanent threshold shift, 160

NITTS noise-induced temporary threshold shift, 160

NLM native language magnet (theory), 155

NPO nothing by mouth (Latin: *non per os*)

NPO p MN nothing by mouth after midnight

NR no response

NX nourishment

O$_2$ oxygen, 168

OAE otoacoustic emission, 167

OCR Office of Civil Rights

OHCP occupational hearing conservation program

OT occupational therapy, 164

OSHA Occupational Safety and Health Administration, 164

Pa pascal, 172

Pad Passavant's ridge, 172

PaCO$_2$ partial pressure of carbon dioxide in arterial blood, 172

PB phonetically balanced, 176

p.c. after meals (Latin: *post cibum*)

PCS picture communication symbols, 178

PDA pitch determination algorithm, 179

PE pressure equalization

P-E pharyngeal-esophageal, 175

PECS picture exchange communication system, 178

PEEP positive end expiratory pressure, 180

PEG percutaneous endoscopic gastrostomy, 173

PET positron emission tomography, 181

pH potential hydrogen

PH predictability high, 182

PKU phenylketonuria, 176

PL predictability low, 182

PI performance versus intensity, 173

PMH past medical history

PNS peripheral nervous system, 173

p.o. by mouth (Latin: *per os*)

poc plan of care

pp after meals (Latin: *postprandial*)

PSS progressive systemic sclerosis, 184

PT physical therapy, 178

PTA posttraumatic amnesia; pure-tone average; Parent-Teacher Association, 181, 186

q.a.m. every morning (Latin: *qaque ante meridiem*)

q.d. every day (Latin: *qaque die*)

q.h. every hour (Latin: *qaque hora*)

q.i.d. 4 times a day (*quarter in die*)

QRN quasiresonant nuclei

QWERTY standard keyboard arrangement, from the six leftmost letters in the second row from the top of keyboards, 188

R Reynold's number, 199

rad radiation absorbed dose, 190

RAM random access memory

RAST radioallergosorbent test, 190

REM rapid eye movement, 190

RF rheumatoid factor, 199

RHI right hemisphere impairment, 199

RLN recurrent laryngeal nerve, 193

RO renew order

R/O rule out

ROM range of motion; read-only memory, 190

RP received pronunciation, 191

RT recreational therapy; reverberation time, 193

RTC return to clinic

Rx recipe; prescription

SAIP special alternative instructional program

SD standard deviation, 219

Sd discriminative stimulus, 220

SDT speech detection threshold

SEE seeing essential English, 205

SEE2 signing exact English, 208

SEP somatosensory evoked potential, 212

SGA small for gestational age, 210

SHHH Self Help for Hard of Hearing People, 279

SIMV synchronized intermittent mandatory ventilation, 226

SL sensation level, 206

SLI specific language impairment, 279

SLN superior laryngeal nerve, 223

SLP speech-language pathologist, 216

S/N signal-to-noise, 208

SNHL sensorineural hearing loss, 206

SOAE spontaneous otoacoustic emission

s.p. status post, 219

SPECT single-photon emission computed tomography, 209

SPI soft phonation index

SPL sound pressure level, 212

sPPQ smoothed pitch perturbation quotient

SRT speech reception threshold, 217

SSPL saturation sound pressure level, 202

ST spondee threshold, 218

STNR symmetrical tonic neck reflex, 225

T&A tonsillectomy and adenoidectomy, 238

TBE transitional bilingual education, 242

TBI traumatic brain injury, 243

TDD telecommunication device for the deaf, 233

TEF tracheoesophageal fistula, 240

TEFL teaching English as a foreign language

TEP tracheoesophageal puncture

TESOL teachers of English to speakers of other languages

TIA transient ischemic attack, 242

TLESR transient LES relaxation

TMH trainable mentally handicapped

TMJ temporomandibular joint, 233

TORCH+S toxoplasmosis/associated ophthalmologic disease/rubella/cytomegalovirus/herpes/syphilis, 240

TPN total parenteral nutrition, 240

TPOAE transient-evoked, distortion-product otoacoustic emissions

TPR total physical response

TT/TTY text telephone

TTS temporary threshold shift, 233

TWA time-weighted average, 236

Tx therapy or treatment, 234

UCL uncomfortable loudness level

UES upper esophageal sphincter, 248

ULL uncomfortable loudness level, 248

UNESCO United Nations Educational, Scientific, and Cultural Organization

V$_E$ minute ventilation, 251

VFE videofluoroscopic examination, 254

VIP vasoactive intestinal peptide

VOT voice onset time, 256

VPI velopharyngeal incompetence/velopharyngeal insufficiency, 251

VRA visual reinforcement audiometry, 254

VS vital signs, 254

VSS videofluoroscopic swallow study

VTI voice turbulence index, 257

WHO World Health Organization

WNL within normal limits

W/U work up

APPENDIX

The International Phonetics Alphabet

THE INTERNATIONAL PHONETIC ALPHABET (revised to 1993, updated 1996)

CONSONANTS (PULMONIC)

	Bilabial	Labiodental	Dental	Alveolar	Postalveolar	Retroflex	Palatal	Velar	Uvular	Pharyngeal	Glottal
Plosive	p b			t d		ʈ ɖ	c ɟ	k g	q ɢ		ʔ
Nasal	m	ɱ		n		ɳ	ɲ	ŋ	N		
Trill	B			r					R		
Tap or Flap				ɾ		ɽ					
Fricative	ɸ β	f v	θ ð	s z	ʃ ʒ	ʂ ʐ	ç ʝ	x ɣ	χ ʁ	ħ ʕ	h ɦ
Lateral fricative				ɬ ɮ							
Approximant		ʋ		ɹ		ɻ	j	ɰ			
Lateral approximant				l		ɭ	ʎ	L			

Where symbols appear in pairs, the one to the right represents a voiced consonant. Shaded areas denote articulations judged impossible.

OTHER SYMBOLS

ʍ	Voiceless labial-velar fricative
w	Voiced labial-velar approximant
ɥ	Voiced labial-palatal approximant
H	Voiceless epiglottal fricative
ʕ	Voiced epiglottal fricative
ʡ	Epiglottal plosive

ɕ ʑ	Alveolo-palatal fricatives
ɺ	Alveolar lateral flap
ɧ	Simultaneous ʃ and X

Affricates and double articulations can be represented by two symbols joined by a tie bar if necessary.

k͡p t͡s

TONES AND WORD ACCENTS

LEVEL			CONTOUR		
e̋ or	˥	Extra high	ě or	˩˥	Rising
é	˦	High	ê	˥˩	Falling
ē	˧	Mid	e᷄	˧˥	High rising
è	˨	Low	e᷅	˩˧	Low rising
ȅ	˩	Extra low	e᷈	˧˩˧	Rising-falling
↓		Downstep	↗		Global rise
↑		Upstep	↘		Global fall

Reprinted courtesy of the International Phonetic Association.

275

CONSONANTS (NON-PULMONIC)

	Clicks		Voiced implosives		Ejectives
⊙	Bilabial	ɓ	Bilabial	ʼ	Examples:
|	Dental	ɗ	Dental/alveolar	pʼ	Bilabial
!	(Post)alveolar	ʄ	Palatal	tʼ	Dental/alveolar
ǂ	Palatoalveolar	ɠ	Velar	kʼ	Velar
‖	Alveolar lateral	ʛ	Uvular	sʼ	Alveolar fricative

VOWELS

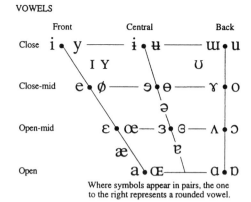

Where symbols appear in pairs, the one to the right represents a rounded vowel.

DIACRITICS   Diacritics may be placed above a symbol with a descender, e.g. ŋ̊

̥	Voiceless	n̥ d̥	̤	Breathy voiced	b̤ a̤	̪	Dental	t̪ d̪
̌	Voiced	s̬ t̬	̰	Creaky voiced	b̰ a̰	̺	Apical	t̺ d̺
ʰ	Aspirated	tʰ dʰ	̼	Linguolabial	t̼ d̼	̻	Laminal	t̻ d̻
̹	More rounded	ɔ̹	ʷ	Labialized	tʷ dʷ	̃	Nasalized	ẽ
̜	Less rounded	ɔ̜	ʲ	Palatalized	tʲ dʲ	ⁿ	Nasal release	dⁿ
̟	Advanced	u̟	ˠ	Velarized	tˠ dˠ	ˡ	Lateral release	dˡ
̠	Retracted	e̠	ˤ	Pharyngealized	tˤ dˤ	̚	No audible release	d̚
̈	Centralized	ë	̴	Velarized or pharyngealized	ɫ			
̽	Mid-centralized	e̽	̝	Raised	e̝	(ɹ̩ = voiced alveolar fricative)		
̩	Syllabic	n̩	̞	Lowered	e̞	(β̞ = voiced bilabial approximant)		
̯	Non-syllabic	e̯	̘	Advanced Tongue Root	e̘			
˞	Rhoticity	ɚ a˞	̙	Retracted Tongue Root	e̙			

SUPRASEGMENTALS

ˈ	Primary stress	
ˌ	Secondary stress	
		ˌfoʊnəˈtɪʃən
ː	Long	eː
ˑ	Half-long	eˑ
̆	Extra-short	ĕ
|	Minor (foot) group	
‖	Major (intonation) group	
.	Syllable break	ɹi.ækt
‿	Linking (absence of a break)	

APPENDIX

List of Illustrations

alveolus, alveoli, p. 8 (From *Anatomy and Physiology for Speech, Language and Hearing*, by J.A. Seikel, D.W. King, and D.G. Drumright, 1997, p. 72. Reprinted with permission.)

Angle's classification of malocclusion, p. 12 (From *The Speech Sciences*, by R.D. Kent, 1997, p. 165. Reprinted with permission.)

articulators, p. 17 (From *Introduction to Communication Sciences and Disorders*, by F.D. Minifie (Ed.), 1994, p. 401. Reprinted with permission.)

ASL (American Sign Language), p. 9 (From *Introduction to Language Development*, by S. McLaughlin, 1998, p. 9. Reprinted with permission.)

audiogram, p. 21 (From *Introduction to Communication Sciences and Disorders*, by F.D. Minifie (Ed.), 1994, p. 616. Reprinted with permission.)

Basal ganglia (basal nuclei), p. 30 (From *The Speech Sciences*, by R.D. Kent, 1997, p. 252. Reprinted with permission.)

Blissymbols, p. 34 (From *Handbook of Augmentative and Alternative Communication*, by S.L. Glennen and D.C. DeCoste, 1997, p. 120. Reprinted with permission.)

Brodmann's areas, p. 36 (From *The Speech Sciences*, by R.D. Kent, 1997, p. 247. Reprinted with permission.)

bronchioles, p. 27 (From *Anatomy and Physiology for Speech, Language and Hearing*, by J.A. Seikel, D.W. King, and D.G. Drumright, 1997, p. 68. Reprinted with permission.)

cleft (cleft palate, cleft lip), p. 46 (From *The Speech Sciences*, by R.D. Kent, 1997, p. 431. Reprinted with permission.)

cochlear implant, p. 47 (From *Foundations of Aural Rehabilitation*, by N. Tye- Murray, 1998, p. 145. Reprinted with permission.)

cranial nerves, p. 58 (From *The Speech Sciences*, by R.D. Kent, 1997, p. 258. Reprinted with permission.)

dental arch, deciduous, p. 64 (From *The Speech Sciences*, by R.D. Kent, 1997, p. 161. Reprinted with permission.)

dermatome, p. 65 (From *Anatomy and Physiology for Speech, Language and Hearing*, by J.A. Seikel, D.W. King, and D.G. Drumright, 1997, p. 397. Reprinted with permission.)

ear, p. 72 (From *The Speech Sciences*, by R.D. Kent, 1997, p. 211. Reprinted with permission.)

endoscope, p. 76 (From *Communication and Swallowing Management*, by K.J. Dikeman and M.S. Kazandjian, 1995, p. 152. Reprinted with permission.)

A Poor Man's Tour of Physical Quantities and Units[1]

Michael R. Chial, Ph.D.
Professor, Department of Communicative Disorders
Professor, Department of Professional Development and Applied Studies
University of Wisconsin-Madison

INTRODUCTION

Physical quantities are objective events that can assume numerical values. *Basic quantities* are limited to mass, time, displacement (or length) and electric charge. *Derived quantities* are generated through algebraic combination of basic quantities and other derived quantities. These include velocity, acceleration, pressure, force, work, power, and temperature, as well as the quantities of electricity and electronics (except for electric charge). *Units of measurement*, on the other hand, are standardized amounts of quantities. In most cases, units are named in honor of the individuals whose scientific efforts clarified our understanding of the respective phenomenon. Finally, *values* are specific amounts of units.

In the expression, "she was 5 feet, 4 inches tall," feet and inches are units, the numbers 5 and 4 are values, and "tall" denotes the quantity of vertical length.

QUANTITIES AND UNITS

Quantities differ from units. For example, the basic quantity length is defined as the distance between two points. Any particular length can be expressed by a host of units, including inches, centimeters, feet, meters, rods, furlongs, miles, kilometers, etc. Similarly, the derived quantity force (F) is defined by Newton's second law of motion as mass (M) times acceleration (a), whereas, the metric unit for force is defined as the newton (N).

---

[1]Reprinted courtesy of M. R. Chial

Force (quantity):　F = M * a
Force (MKS unit):　1 N = 1 kg * 1 m / sec²

Although physical quantities are well-standardized, the symbols and abbreviations used to represent them are not. Indeed, they differ considerably among authors, scholarly journals, and scientific or professional disciplines. Symbols for units are formally defined by international standards bodies and are even the subject of treaties among nations. Generally, honorific units (those named in honor of individuals) are written without capitalization (to distinguish the unit from the person); when abbreviated, honorific units are capitalized.

MEASUREMENT SYSTEMS

Physical measurement always requires specification of both a value (i.e., a number representing "how much") and a unit (i.e., "of what"). *Systems of measurement* are formal strategies for indexing amounts of specified physical quantities. Such systems include (1) definitions of quantities, (2) units of measurement—the names we give quantities when we want to be specific, (3) standards of measurement—formally defined reference values for units, and (4) procedures (rules) of measurement for applying standards to specific things or events.

Units of measurement and the physical standards underpinning them become progressively more precise as science and technology develop. In other words, newer standards are capable of accommodating smaller *differences* in the amounts of the quantities measured. Standard units (e.g., the standard second and the standard meter) also are periodically redefined in pursuit of greater objectivity and repeatability. The second originally was standardized as the duration between heartbeats (problem: whose heart and after what activity?). Today, the standard second is defined in terms of atomic events, allowing resolution of time to 10^{-12} seconds (one trillionth of a second, or 1 picosecond).

The most common systems of units are the English system (foot-pound-second or FPS), the early metric system (centimeter-gram-second or CGS), and the *Systeme International d'Unites* (meter-kilogram-second or MKS). All three systems use the same units for the basic quantities of time (the second) and electric charge (the coloumb). Different units are employed for mass. The CGS system uses the gram, the MKS system uses the kilogram, and the FPS system uses the *slug* or *poundal*. The more familiar *pound* is a unit of weight (a force), not a unit of mass. Both metric systems employ a powers-of-ten

(decimal) number scheme, whereas the English system is based on doublings, triplings, or other multiples (e.g., 2 cups = 1 pint, 2 pints = 1 quart; 3 feet = 1 yard). Confusions related to the inconsistencies of the English FPS system are among the reasons it is seldom used in science and engineering.

The *Systeme International d'Unites* (abbreviated SI) is the contemporary version of the metric system originally developed by the French Academy of Science in 1791. The SI also is referred to as the *rationalized MKS system*, so-called because both basic and derived units are defined as having unity (1) values, even though derived units may be given new names. *Basic units* and *basic quantities* are not the same (see above). Basic units (see Table 1) are required in the SI to accomplish the goal of unity value for derived units. Note that two of the basic units of the SI are honorific. Those for displacement, mass, time, light intensity and molecular substance are not.

The quantities in Table 1 define the MKS system and also underpin the FPS and CGS systems. Many everyday quantities are missing from Table 1, for example, area, volume, velocity (or speed), and power. These and other *derived quantities* are defined as combinations of the quantities listed in Table 1. The methods by which basic quantities are combined to form derived quantities (and, for that matter, by which derived quantities may be combined to define still other derived quantities) are inherently algebraic. These mathematical methods are based upon known lawful relations of the physical universe and generally are quite simple. Thus, formal systems of measurement constitute a worldview about how the universe and everything in it works. Table 2 lists commonly used derived SI units.

METRIC PREFIXES

A distinct advantage of the SI system is a set of prefixes that can be applied to units to indicate scale of measurement, i.e., to overall size or magnitude of a measured quantity. The most commonly used prefixes are noted in Table 3. Note that prefixes employ a base-10 exponential progression such that prefixes close to the <unit> (i.e., from milli to kilo) are based upon small differences in exponents, while extremely large and extremely small magnitudes are based upon numerically greater differences in exponents. Table 4 gives instructions for converting values expressed with one common prefix to identical values expressed with another common prefix.

Table 1. Base units of measurement in the *Systeme International d'Unites* (also called the "rationalized MKS system"). Asterisks in the left-hand column designate basic quantities. All other quantities are derived.

Quantity	Unit	Symbol	Physical Definition
*Displacement (Length)	meter	m	distance traveled by light in a vacuum in 1 / 299 792 458 of a second
*Mass	kilogram	kg	mass equal to that of a prototype platinum-iridium cylinder kept in Paris, France
*Time	second	s	duration of 9 192 631 770 periods of radiation of the cesium 133 atom in transition between two states
Electric current	ampere	A	coulomb / s
Temperature	kelvin	K	1 / 273.2 of the triple point of water
Light intensity	candela	cd	directional radiant intensity of 1 / 683 watt per steradian at a monochrome frequency of 540×1012 hertz
Molecular substance	mole	mol	amount of substance equal to that of 0.012 kg of carbon-12

Table 2. Some derived units of measurement in the *Systeme International d'Unites*. Many additional derived units are in common use. Basic and derived units of measurement (including those honoring individuals) always are given in lower-case letters when written out in full. Thus, people can be distinguished from the physical units named after them. When abbreviated, units named to honor people are capitalized. Asterisks in the right-hand column designate multiplication.

Quantity	Unit	Symbol	Other Definition	
Area	m^2	m^2	displacement squared	
Volume	m^3	m^3	displacement cubed	
Density	kg / m^3	kg / m^3	mass / unit volume	
Velocity	m / s	m / s	Δ displacement / unit time	
Acceleration	m / s^2	m / s^2	Δ velocity / unit time	
Plane angle	radian	rad	2π rad = 360°	
Angular velocity	rad / s	ω	2π rad / s = 360° / s	
Solid angle	steradian	sr	(complex)	
Energy	joule	J	$kg * m^2 / s^2$	= N * m
Force	newton	N	$kg * m / s^2$	= J / m
Pressure or stress	pascal	Pa	$(kg * m / s^2) / m^2$	= N / m^2
Power	watt	W	$kg * m^2 / s^3$	= J / s
Electric charge	coulomb	C	A * s	
Electric potential (emf)	volt	V	$kg * m^2 / s^3 * A = J / A * s$	= W / A
Electric resistance	ohm	Ω	$kg * m^2 / s^3 * A^2$	= V / A
Electric capacitance	farad	F	$A^2 *s^4 / kg * m^2$	= A * s / V
Electric inductance	henry	H	$kg * m^2 / s^2 * A^2$	= V * s / A
Frequency	hertz	Hz	cycle / s	= s^{-1}
Magnetic flux	weber	Wb	$kg * m^2 / s^2 * A$	= V * s
Magnetic flux density	telsa	T	$kg / s^2 * A$	= Wb / m^2
Luminous flux	lumen	lm	cd * sr	
Customary temperature	degree Celsius	°C	K − 273.15	

STANDARDS ORGANIZATIONS

The SI is but one part of a larger process by which scientific, technical, and professional communities strive to standardize measurements. In the United States, the National Technical Institute (NTI—formerly called the National Bureau of Standards) is responsible for defining and in-

Table 3. Metric prefixes. Note the use of capital letters to distinguish among abbreviations for prefixes.

Prefix	Symbol	Power of 10	Numerical Value
exa	E	10^{18}	1 000 000 000 000 000 000
peta	P	10^{15}	1 000 000 000 000 000
tera	T	10^{12}	1 000 000 000 000
giga	G	10^{9}	1 000 000 000
mega	M	10^{6}	1 000 000
kilo	k	10^{3}	1 000
hecto	h	10^{2}	100
deka	da	10^{1}	10
—<unit>—	(none)	10^{0}	1
deci	d	10^{-1}	0.1
centi	c	10^{-2}	0.01
milli	m	10^{-3}	0.001
micro	μ	10^{-6}	0.000 001
nano	n	10^{-9}	0.000 000 001
pico	p	10^{-12}	0.000 000 000 001
femto	f	10^{-15}	0.000 000 000 000 001
atto	a	10^{-18}	0.000 000 000 000 000 001

Table 4. Metric conversions. To convert a unit of measurement expressed with an original value prefix to the same unit expressed with a different value prefix, start by finding the correct cell in the table below. Then move the decimal point of the original value the number of places indicated by the digit in the direction indicated by the arrow. For example, 5 kilometers equals 500,000 centimeters (5⇒ move the decimal 5 spaces to the right); 12.5 milliseconds equals 0.0125 seconds (⇐3 move the decimal 3 spaces to the left).

Original Prefix ⇓	giga	mega	kilo	—(unit)—	centi	milli	micro	nano	pico
giga	⇐0⇒	3⇒	6⇒	8⇒	11⇒	12⇒	15⇒	18⇒	21⇒
mega	⇐3	⇐0⇒	3⇒	6⇒	8⇒	11⇒	12⇒	15⇒	18⇒
kilo	⇐6	⇐3	⇐0⇒	3⇒	6⇒	8⇒	11⇒	12⇒	15⇒
—(unit)—	⇐9	⇐6	⇐3	⇐0⇒	3⇒	6⇒	8⇒	11⇒	12⇒
centi	⇐10	⇐9	⇐6	⇐3	⇐0⇒	3⇒	6⇒	8⇒	11⇒
milli	⇐12	⇐10	⇐9	⇐6	⇐3	⇐0⇒	3⇒	6⇒	8⇒
micro	⇐15	⇐12	⇐10	⇐9	⇐6	⇐3	⇐0⇒	3⇒	6⇒
nano	⇐18	⇐15	⇐12	⇐10	⇐9	⇐6	⇐3	⇐0⇒	3⇒
pico	⇐21	⇐18	⇐15	⇐12	⇐10	⇐9	⇐6	⇐3	⇐0⇒

Desired Prefix ⇓

creasing the precision of the physical standards that underpin scientific and commercial measurement. A branch of the US Department of Commerce, the NTI was originally formed to insure that materials and equipment purchased by the federal government (including the military) conformed to consistent standards of measurement.

Other national groups, such as the American National Standards Institute (ANSI) and international groups, such as the International Standards Organization (ISO) and the International

Electrotechnical Commission (IEC), are voluntary organizations that exist for the purpose of documenting generally accepted practices for making and reporting measurements. A major goal of these groups is to facilitate communication among scientists, technical workers, and various professionals so as to insure that differences in measurement practices do not cause differences in the meaning of reported data.

Standards published by standards organizations fall into four distinct categories.

(1) **Definition standards** which formally define physical quantities, units, and related concepts,

(2) **Data standards** which precisely define reference quantities for units, for technical instruments, or for technical procedures,

(3) **Instrument standards** which specify the tolerances of devices used to make measurements for different purposes, and

(4) **Procedure standards** which detail the steps to be taken in making measurements of interest to the public or particular scientific, technical, or professional groups.

Five groups currently active within ANSI are highly relevant to scientists and clinicians who work with persons who have disorders of speech, language, or hearing. These are designated as ANSI Committee S1-Acoustics (dealing with the physical measurement of sound), ANSI Committee S2-Vibration (dealing with physical measurement of mechanical events), ANSI Committee S3-Bioacoustics (dealing with the measurement of hearing), ANSI Committee S12-Noise (dealing with the physical measurement of generally unwanted acoustical signals, as well as ways to assess and prevent unwanted effects of such sounds), and ANSI Committee S14-Electroacoustics (dealing with sound recording and reproduction).

Hundreds of other industry, government, and professional groups exist to standardize everything from the size of photographic film, to computer languages, to audiogram symbols, to envelope sizes, to screw threads and wire gauges, to the dimensions of the cardboard cores found in toilet paper, to the speed of audio tapes, to the capacity of CD-audio disks. Some of these eventually become standards endorsed by ANSI, ISO, or both. Others do not. In France, for example, a government agency requires that common baked goods such as croissants be prepared using specified recipes. Non-standardized industries include shoe and clothing manufacturing. If such products were more rigorously standardized, we would have little use for phrases such as "if the shoe fits. . . ."

REFERENCES

Adams, H. (1974). *SI metric units: An introduction* (rev. ed.) Toronto, ON: McGraw-Hill Ryerson, Limited.

Anderson, H. (Ed.). (1989). *A physicist's desk reference: The physics vade mecum* (2nd ed.). New York, NY: American Institute of Physics.

Klein, H. (1974). *The science of measurement: A historical survey.* New York, NY: Simon & Schuster, Inc. Republished (1988) by Dover Publications, Inc.

SELECTED CONVERSION FACTORS

The following material is not intended to encourage you to translate metric measures into the arguably more familiar foot-pound-second (FPS) measures in common use in the United States, but instead to illustrate the complexity of the FPS system and the simplicity of the *Systeme International d'Unites*, even for routine measurement. The superiority of the SI system is particularly evident for dry and liquid volume measurements. The English FPS system employs two entirely different sets of units for such measurements, while the SI uses only one. It is noteworthy that the English FPS system is no longer used in England, or in any of the nations of the former British Commonwealth.

Linear Measure

1 inch = 2.54 centimeters
1 foot = 12 inches = 30.48 centimeters
1 yard = 3 feet = 36 inches = 0.914 4 meters
1 rod = 5.25 yards = 5.029 meters
1 furlong = 40 rods = 201.17 meters
1 statute mile = 5280 feet = 1760 yards = 8 furlongs = 1 609.344 meters
1 league = 3 miles = 4.83 kilometers

1 meter = 39.370 08 inches = 3.280 840 feet = 1.093 613 yards

1 meter = 100 centimeters = 1 000 millimeters = 0.001 kilometers

Square Measure

1 square inch = 6.452 square centimeters
1 square foot = 144 square inches = 929 square centimeters
1 square yard = 9 square feet = 0.836 1 square meters
1 square rod = 30.25 square yards = 25.29 square meters

1 acre = 4 840 square yards = 0.404 7 hectacres

1 square mile = 640 acres = 2.59 square kilometers

1 square meter = 10.763 91 square feet = 1.195 990 square yards

1 square meter = 10 000 square centimeters = 0.000 1 hectacre

Cubic Measure

1 cubic inch = 16.387 cubic centimeters

1 cubic foot = 1 728 cubic inches = 0.028 3 cubic meters

1 cubic yard = 27 cubic feet = 0.764 6 cubic meters

1 cord = 128 cubic feet = 3.625 cubic meters

1 cubic meter = 1 000 liters

Volume or Capacity (Dry Measure)

1 bushel = 4 pecks = 32 dry quarts = 64 dry pints = 2 150.42 cubic inches
= 35.239 07 liters = 0.035 239 07 cubic meters

1 liter = 1.816 166 dry pints

1 liter = 1 000 milliliters = 0.001 cubic meters

Volume or Capacity (Liquid Measure)

1 gallon = 4 liquid quarts = 8 liquid pints = 32 gills = 128 liquid ounces = 728 teaspoons
= 61 440 minims = 3.785 411 784 liters
= 0.003 785 411 784 cubic meters

1 liter = 202.884 136 211 teaspoons = 2.113 376 liquid pints = 0.264 172 05 gallons

1 liter = 1 000 milliliters = 0.001 cubic meters

Nautical Measure

1 fathom = 6 feet = 2 yards = 1.829 meters

1 nautical mile = 1.508 statute miles

60 nautical miles = 1 degree of a great circle of the earth

1 knot = 1 nautical mile per hour (a measure of speed)

1 kilometer = 1 000 meters

Weight

1 avoirdupois pound = 16 avoirdupois ounces
= 12 troy ounces = 0.000 5 short tons
= 0.000 446 428 6 long tons = 256 avoirdupois drams = 7 000 grains
= 0.453 592 37 kilograms

1 kilogram = 15, 432.36 grains = 35.273 96 avoirdupois ounces = 32.150 75 troy ounces
= 0.001 102 31 short tons = 0.000 984 2 long tons = 2.204 623 avoirdupois pounds
= 2.679 229 troy pounds

1 kilogram = 1 000 grams = 0.001 metric tons

REFERENCES

Anderson, K. N., Anderson, L. E., & Glanze, W. D. (Eds.). (1998). *Mosby's medical, nursing, & allied health dictionary* (5th ed.). St. Louis: Mosby-BYear Book, Inc.

Bleile, K. M. (1994). *Manual of articulation and phonological disorders*. San Diego: Singular Publishing Group, Inc.

Chermak, G. D., & Musiek, F. E. (1997). *Central auditory processing disorders*. San Diego: Singular Publishing Group, Inc.

DeCoste, D. C., & Glennen, S. L. (1997). *Handbook of augmentative and alternative communication*. San Diego: Singular Publishing Group, Inc.

Dikeman, K. J., & Kazandjian, M. S. *Communication and swallowing management of tracheostomized and ventilator-dependent adults*. San Diego: Singular Publishing Group, Inc.

Drumright, D. G., King, D. W., & Seikel, J. A. (1997). *Anatomy and physiology for speech, language and hearing* (exp. ed.). San Diego: Singular Publishing Group, Inc.

Gilbert, P. (1995). *The a–z reference book of childhood conditions*. San Diego: Singular Publishing Group, Inc./Chapman Hall.

Gilbert, P. (1996). *The a–z reference book of syndromes and inherited disorders*. San Diego: Singular Publishing Group, Inc.

Guilmette, T. J. (1997). *PocketGuide to brain injury, cognitive, and neurobehavioral rehabilitation*. San Diego: Singular Publishing Group, Inc.

Hargrove, P. M., & McGarr, N. S. (1994). *Prosody management of communication disorders*. San Diego: Singular Publishing Group, Inc.

Hegde, M. N. (1996). *PocketGuide to treatment in speech-language pathology*. San Diego: Singular Publishing Group, Inc.

Kayser, H. (1998). *Assessment and intervention resource for Hispanic children*. San Diego: Singular Publishing Group, Inc.

Kent, R. D. (1997). *The speech sciences*. San Diego: Singular Publishing Group, Inc.

Kent, R. D., & Read, C. (1992). *The acoustic analysis of speech*. San Diego: Singular Publishing Group, Inc.

Lyon, J. G. (1998). *Coping with aphasia*. San Diego: Singular Publishing Group, Inc.

McLaughlin, S. (1998). *Introduction to language development*. San Diego: Singular Publishing Group, Inc.

Miller, A. (1998). *The neuroscience of swallowing and dysphagia*. San Diego: Singular Publishing Group, Inc.

Minifie, F. D. (1994). *Introduction to communication sciences and disorders*. San Diego: Singular Publishing Group, Inc.

Perlman, A. L., & Schulze-Delrieu, K. (1997). *Deglutition and its disorders: Anatomy, physiology, clinical diagnosis, and management*. San Diego: Singular Publishing Group, Inc.

Sataloff, R. T. (1997). *Professional voice: The science and art of clinical care*. San Diego: Singular Publishing Group, Inc.

Shprintzen, R. J. (1997). *Genetics, syndromes, and communication disorders*. San Diego: Singular Publishing Group, Inc.

Speaks, C. E. (1999). *Introduction to sound* (3rd ed.). San Diego: Singular Publishing Group, Inc.

Stedman, T. L. (1995). *Stedman's medical dictionary* (26th ed.) Baltimore: Williams & Wilkins.

Sorti, S. A. (1997). *Alcohol, disabilities, and rehabilitation*. San Diego: Singular Publishing Group, Inc.

Tye-Murray, N. (1998). *Foundations of aural rehabilitation: Children, adults, and their family members. San Diego*: Singular Publishing Group, Inc.